Instructor's Resource Manual
to accompany

Psychiatric Mental Health Nursing

Second Edition

Katherine M. Fortinash, MSN, RNCS, CNS
Certified Clinical Specialist,
Adult Psychiatric Mental Health Nursing;
Clinical Nurse Specialist/Senior Systems Specialist
Sharp Mesa Vista Hospital
Sharp Behavioral Health Services
San Diego, California;
Consultant
San Diego, California

Patricia A. Holoday-Worret, MSN, RNCS, CNS
Certified Clinical Specialist,
Adult Psychiatric Mental Health Nursing;
Professor, Psychiatric Mental Health Nursing
Palomar College
San Marcos, California;
Consultant
San Diego, California

Contributors

Marjorie F. Bendik, RN, DNSc
Professor, Nursing Education
Consultant
San Diego, California

Joanne Lavin, RN, EdD, CNS
Associate Professor of Nursing
Kingsborough Community College
Brooklyn, New York

Mildred Gooch Parker, MS, RN, CS
Certified Clinical Specialist,
Adult Mental Health Nursing
Assistant Professor,
Department of Nursing
Norfolk State University
Norfolk, Virginia

Deenie Porter-Mahoney, RN, MS, CS
Associate Professor,
Department of Nursing
Endicott College
Beverly, Massachusetts
Consultant in Private Practice

Mosby

St. Louis Baltimore Boston Carlsbad
Chicago Minneapolis New York Philadelphia Portland
London Milan Sydney Tokyo Toronto

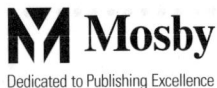
Dedicated to Publishing Excellence

Editor-in-Chief: Sally Schrefer
Developmental Editor: Jeff Downing
Project Manager: Gayle May Morris
Designer: Kathi Gosche

SECOND EDITION

Copyright © 2000 by Mosby, Inc.

All rights reserved. No part of this publication may be reproduced or transmitted in any form or by any means, electronic or mechanical, including photocopy, recording, or any information storage and retrieval system, without permission in writing from the publisher.

Permission to photocopy or reproduce solely for internal or personal use is permitted for libraries or other users registered with the Copyright Clearance Center, provided that the base fee of $4.00 per chapter plus $.10 per page is paid directly to the Copyright Clearance Center, 222 Rosewood Drive, Danvers, Massachusetts 01923. This consent does not extend to other kinds of copying, such as copying for general distribution, for advertising or promotional purposes, for creating new collected works, or for resale.

Mosby, Inc.
A Harcourt Health Sciences Company
11830 Westline Industrial Drive
St. Louis, Missouri 63146

Printed in the United States of America

International Standard Book Number
0-323-01112-8

Preface

This resource manual has been developed to enhance instruction from the textbook *Psychiatric Mental Health Nursing* through supplemental information and activities. It follows the format of the textbook, emphasizing the nursing process as the core of the helping relationship discussed in the chapters. The following resources are provided:

Critical Thinking Questions: Open-ended questions designed to promote independent student thinking. Answers may vary from student to student, and there may be more than one correct answer. An answer key is not provided, given the nature of these questions.

Enrichment Activities: Learning activities developed to assist students in applying theoretical concepts in the practice setting. Emphasis has been placed on developing experiences that will provide students with a reality-oriented perspective of psychiatric mental health nursing.

Multimedia Resources: An annotated listing of audiovisual, CAI, and vidiodisc materials related to the topics of each chapter.

Teaching Strategies: A discussion of issues and strategies related specifically to the teaching of psychiatric mental health nursing. The strategies focus on instruction that promotes critical thinking and problem solving through innovative methods.

Suggested Course Outlines: Outlines that suggest ways to use the textbook in 5-week, 8-week, and 16-week courses, to accommodate varying course lengths.

Student Worksheets: A variety of learning exercises, such as fill-in-the-blank, definition, matching, true/false, and critical thinking questions. An answer key is provided.

Test Bank: A 600-item test bank of multiple-choice questions. The answer key provides rationales for correct and incorrect answers and the applicable nursing process step and cognitive level of each question. The test bank is also available in a computerized version for either IBM or Macintosh.

Kathi Fortinash
Pat Holoday-Worret

Contents

1 Foundations of Psychiatric Mental Health Nursing, *1*
2 Clinical Experiences: Rewards, Challenges, and Solutions, *4*
3 Theoretic Perspectives, *6*
4 Psychobiology, *7*
5 Legal-Ethical Issues, *8*
6 Cultural Issues, *10*
7 The Nursing Process, *12*
8 Principles of Communication, *14*
9 Children and Adolescents, *16*
10 The Adult, *18*
11 The Elderly, *19*
12 Anxiety and Related Disorders, *21*
13 Mood Disorders: Depression and Mania, *22*
14 The Schizophrenias, *24*
15 Personality Disorders, *26*
16 Substance-Related Disorders, *27*
17 Delirium, Dementia, and Amnestic and Other Cognitive Disorders, *30*
18 Disorders of Childhood and Adolescence, *32*
19 Eating Disorders, *34*
20 Sexual Disorders, *35*
21 Adjustment Disorders, *36*
22 Interactive Therapies and Methods of Implementation, *37*
23 Psychopharmacology and Other Biologic Therapies, *39*
24 Alternative Therapies, *40*
25 Crisis Intervention, *42*
26 Activity Therapies, *44*
27 Survivors of Family Violence, *45*
28 Suicide, *47*
29 Grief and Loss, *49*
30 Persons With HIV/AIDS, *51*
31 Psychologic Aspects of Physiologic Illness, *54*
32 Persons With Chronic Mental Illness, *55*
33 Community Psychiatric Mental Health Nursing, *57*
34 Spirituality, *59*

Strategies for Teaching Psychiatric Mental Health Nursing, *61*
Suggested Course Outlines, *67*
Student Worksheets, *71*
Student Worksheets Answer Key, *123*
Test Bank, *147*
Test Bank Answer Key, *211*

Chapter 1

Foundations of Psychiatric Mental Health Nursing

Critical Thinking Questions

1. Following is a list of the "Myths of Mental Illness." As psychiatric-mental health nurses, students will be challenged with these myths by the general public. How will students respond?

   Myths of Mental Illness
   (1) Mental illness does not strike the average person.
   (2) The mentally ill rarely recover.
   (3) Former psychiatric clients cannot go to college.
   (4) Most people who need psychiatric care are hospitalized.
   (5) Everyone mentally ill acts crazy.
   (6) Drugs do nothing more than sedate clients.
   (7) Psychiatric attendants are all brawn and no brains.
   (8) Most therapists are Freudian.
   (9) Life in a mental hospital is totally unlike life outside.
   (10) People in mental hospitals have no civil rights.
   (11) Mental illness rarely strikes children.
   (12) People who cannot handle emotional problems have no will power.
   (13) Former psychiatric clients cannot get or hold jobs.
   (14) Research into mental illness is getting nowhere.
   (15) Most alcoholics are drunks.
   (16) Everyone gets senile as they get older; it is useless to treat elderly clients with mental problems.
   (17) In treatment, one need focus only on the individual client.
   (18) In many ways, clients in mental hospitals are like children.
   (19) Mental illness has nothing to do with the physical condition of the body, and vice-versa.
   (20) Recovered mental clients remain erratic and unpredictable, and may be dangerous.

2. Why would a nurse choose psychiatric-mental health nursing as a specialty? What qualities of the nurse are essential? What are the rewards and frustrations in this field?

3. What are the economic and social realities that are affecting psychiatric-mental health nursing today? How will the science of psychiatric-mental health nursing assist or hinder the nurse in meeting these challenges?

Enrichment Activities

At the beginning of the course, it is important to not only introduce the student to psychiatric-mental health nursing, but to emphasize how it relates to other nursing specialties. Indeed, the principles of psychiatric-mental health nursing obtain throughout all forms of nursing and all interactions with others, whether they are ill or well. The following enrichment activities are designed to show how the concepts learned in this course will assist the student throughout his or her professional and social life.

1. Each student should be assigned to select a situation where they can overhear the interaction between two persons. For example, one might enter a restaurant at a time when it is not so busy, and sit in a booth next to a couple having a discussion. (A disagreement or argument makes a good example to analyze.) Look for the use of various defense mechanisms in the statements of the participants. (Example: "Well, it was your fault that I was late—you insisted on this restaurant rather than one nearer to my work!" This is an example of projection). Make notes on these defense mechanisms, and bring them to class for discussion. Challenge the class to think of other ways to handle the situation that would be more effective in resolving conflicts.

2. A class exercise that would raise student awareness to their hidden prejudices involves the use of a brief questionnaire that students can complete on the first day of class. These are not shared or collected at this time. Each student is asked to save it. The same questionnaire is completed again at the conclusion of the course. On comparing the two questionnaires, students will probably be surprised at how their attitudes have changed. A debriefing, in the form of an open class discussion on the last day of class, should include student comments on their attitude changes and client situations that may have been instrumental in fostering change. The questionnaire follows:

SITUATION: You have heard through the grapevine that a neighbor, with whom you have a casual acquaintanceship, had been on the psychiatric unit of the hospital for a brief time. Think of how you would handle the following situations.

   a. Your neighbor is giving a Christmas buffet party and invites you and other neighbors to attend.
      I would go _____. Not go _____.
      RATIONALE:

   b. You and your spouse have been invited to an important social function for adults. The neighbor offers to babysit.
      I would accept the offer _____.
      I would not accept _____.
      RATIONALE:

   c. You learn that the neighbor is a substitute teacher in the elementary school your children attend, and is often called to teach a class.
      This is fine with me _____.
      I would protest to the school _____.
      RATIONALE:

   d. One of your relatives has been dating the neighbor. They are the same age, and the relationship seems to be serious. In fact, your relative is considering marriage to your neighbor.
      I would be happy for the couple _____.
      I would advise my relative not to marry this person _____.
      RATIONALE:

   e. You are a bank loan officer. The neighbor comes to you to request a loan to buy a new car.
      I would draw up a contract _____.
      I would refuse the loan _____.
      RATIONALE:

   f. An opportunity for a full-time teaching position opens in the elementary school, and other teachers are recommending your neighbor for this position.
      I would support my neighbor _____.
      I would object _____.
      RATIONALE:

   g. There is an elective position soon to be vacated on the town council. Your neighbor wants to run for the office, and asks your help in campaigning, as you have done this for others.
      I would offer to help _____.
      I would not assist _____.
      RATIONALE:

h. There have been some acts of vandalism and petty theft in the neighborhood. A policeman with whom you are acquainted asks you if there are any suspicious persons in your area.
I would tell the officer about my neighbor _____.
I would say that I saw no evidence of any such person _____.
RATIONALE:

i. Your neighbor wants to obtain a higher degree, and the university requires letters of recommendation along with the application. Your neighbor asks you for a character reference letter.
I would write the letter, based on our acquaintanceship _____.
I would not write a letter _____.
RATIONALE:

j. Your neighbor's niece from out of town is visiting. She is eight, the same age as your daughter, and the neighbor asks if your daughter, who likes her, can "sleep over" with her Saturday night.
I would agree, if my daughter wanted to go _____.
I would not allow my daughter to go _____.
RATIONALE:

(Would the gender of your neighbor make any difference in any of these situations?)

3. Ask students to write a one-page example from another nursing specialty in which they have encountered a "difficult" client. Have them bring this to class for an instructor-led discussion of how they could interact more effectively with the client, using some of the essential facilitative qualities of the psychiatric-mental health nurse described in Box 1-1.

Chapter 2

Clinical Experiences: Rewards, Challenges, and Solutions

Critical Thinking Questions

1. Clients may target a new nursing student to act as a confidant, because they often feel that a student is to be trusted, while the staff is not. How should a nursing student respond if the client says, "I want to tell you a secret—promise me you won't tell anyone else."

2. How does the concept of "helping" differ when viewed from the perspective of the psychiatric-mental health nurse, as opposed to the acute care nurse?

3. In the past, psychiatric-mental health nurses have complained that only partial use was made of their abilities on the units, and that they had little opportunity to establish therapeutic relationships with their clients. Do you think these problems still prevail today? Under what circumstances do you think nurses have the opportunity to do real psychiatric nursing?

Enrichment Activities

To accept the challenge of psychiatric-mental health nursing, the following activities will help the nursing student.

1. The students' worst fears are that clients will get violent, and students or other clients will be hurt. While it is true that students seldom face violence on the first day of clinical, it can happen, and role-playing helps the students to cope, since they can feel that they have faced the situation before.

   First review with students the proper procedure to follow in an altercation, should one occur while on the unit. (It is true that students ideally should not be on closed psychiatric units early in their clinical assignments, but in reality, it may not be possible, in a clinical group of 10 students, to assign them all to the open unit. Choose the more mature students for the closed unit, and allow them to participate in the following scenario.)

   Stage a vignette in which two students are assigned to start an argument that escalates to threats. Three students are to play the roles of uninvolved clients, standing by. Two other students are to play the roles of nursing students. Other students can observe the interactions.

   What should follow is that one nursing student (role) will escort the uninvolved clients (roles) away from the action, while the other nursing student (role) goes to an expert for help (you, the instructor). Take the vignette no further than this at this stage in the course. Follow the scenario by a discussion of what occurred, giving the bulk of the comments over to the observers (roles): What did you see? What were the expressions of the participants as the argument escalated? What of the bystanders? How effective was the intervention by the nursing students (roles)? Was there anything about the intervention that was problematic?

   Clients arguing: What did you feel while enacting the roles?

   Uninvolved clients: What emotions were you feeling? Did these change over time?

   Nursing student: How did you feel?

   All: What could or should be done differently next time? (Instructor, please help with this last question!)

2. The following exercise will help the students to see the price of uninvolvement with clients on a client's well-being, and on their learning experience. Have one student sit quietly in a chair, head down, saying nothing, not moving. Have another student sit on a chair a few feet away, reading a book, not facing or looking at the first student. Ask the class what the quality of this interaction is. Now ask the class to imagine that the first student is a client on a psychiatric unit, and the second student is a new nursing student. What has the nursing student done to help the client? Ask the first student how it felt to be ignored. Perhaps the client does not feel like talking. What position and attitude could the nursing student assume to indicate to the client that the nursing student cares and is there to help? What could he or she say to the client?

3. Consult the psychiatric liaison nurse in the hospital, and have students accompany him or her on a visit to a unit where there are both mentally and physically compromised clients. Look at the care plans and see how the treatment addresses both the physical and the psychological problems. Following this exposure, have a discussion concerning how physical conditions affect mental status, and vice versa.

Chapter 3

Theoretic Perspectives

Critical Thinking Questions

1. Compare the therapeutic process for any two of the following theory orientations:

Psychoanalytic	Transactional analysis
Gestalt	Client-centered
Behavioral	Rational-emotive
Cognitive	Strategic
Psychobiologic	

   How would the psychiatric nurse structure the therapeutic relationship differently in each case? Why might the nursing specialist want to use one theory orientation for one client, but another orientation for a different client?

2. If you were a psychiatric nurse, which theory orientation would you probably use most, and why? Which orientation, in your opinion, would have the least value for your practice? Why?

3. What is the relationship between behaviorism and learning? Is learning essential to change? Discuss the basic premise of behaviorism. How else do people learn? Consider learning from the point of view of the different theory orientations.

Enrichment Activities

1. To see theory and therapy in action, it is useful to have students visit, and possibly participate in a gestalt therapy session, or a psychodrama session.

2. It can be enlighting and stimulating to participate in a group exercise that follows the idea of free association. The instructor reads off a list of about 10 words, asking the class to respond immediately, aloud and together. For example, consider the words:

	The usual responses:
white—	—black
hot—	—cold
grass—	—green
tight—	—loose
dark—	—light
day—	—night
clean—	—dirty
open—	—closed
summer—	—winter
sharp—	—dull
cloudy—	—clear

   When someone responds atypically, it is very apparent to the group, and the student may want to consider the meaning of the response. Make the link to psychoanalysis, explaining that if a person answered "knife" to the word "sharp", the psychoanalyst might try for an interpretation—possibly the client suffered a forgotten trauma (but still in the subconscious mind) associated with a knife in the past. (It might even have been a surgeon's knife!)

3. Demonstrate the technique of desensitization. Have one student play the role of a client who is afraid of leaving home. Play the therapist on day 1 (having the student [client] list the smallest to the greatest fear he or she has about leaving home); on day 2 (having the student [client] move closer to the door); on day 3 (having the student [client] open and close the door); on day 4 (having the student [client] step out onto the porch), etc. Discuss with the class how the procedure could help the client to overcome agoraphobia (fear of open places). Ask if the class knows anyone who was involved in an automobile accident and then was afraid to drive again; were they helped by therapy?

Chapter 4

Psychobiology

Critical Thinking Questions

1. What is the significance to nurses in knowing and understanding the anatomy and physiology of the brain and nervous system?

2. How does brain biology relate to mental disorders?

3. What is the function of neurons, the basic subunit of the brain?

4. Of what importance are electrical and chemical responses in the central nervous system?

5. How will you describe neurotransmitters to clients who ask?

6. Brain synapses are the site of important functions during medication therapy. What are these functions?

7. What behavioral symptoms of mental disorders are manifested by clients? Describe them in their biological context, according to brain dysfunction.

8. What are some potential areas for nursing research relating to psychobiology?

Enrichment Activities

1. In groups of four or five students, discuss the term the "Decade of the Brain." Share comments with the entire class.

2. Make a list of ways that the explosion of knowledge concerning the biologic basis of mental disorders has affected (1) changes in client care and (2) the role of the nurse in a psychiatric setting.

3. Name two major neuroimaging techniques, and describe their use for the psychiatric client. Discuss how have these techniques influenced care of the client with mental disorders.

4. Form two teams to debate the pros and cons of psychopharmacology.

Multimedia Resources

Audio/Visual

Lost in the Mind
Description: Documentary of the neuroscience of Alzheimer's Disease, with physiological, emotional, and social aspects of the disease.
Running time: 58 minutes
Purchase: $150
To order: Aquarius Healthcare Videos, PO Box 1159, Shearborn MA 01770, Call: (508) 651-2963 Fax: (508) 650-4216 e-mail *aqvideos@tiac.net* web: www.aquarius-productions.com

Chapter 5

Legal-Ethical Issues

Critical Thinking Questions

1. A psychologist wished to conduct a research project with mentally ill clients. He told them that some of them would receive group therapy and others would not. What do you think of the ethical ramifications of such a research design?

2. How has the concept of the least restrictive alternative contributed to the problem of the mentally ill homeless? What steps could be taken to alleviate this situation?

3. What do you think about the civil rights of mentally ill clients? What problems might arise in matters such as money management, receiving visitors, or telephoning others? How can clients be helped to use these rights prudently?

4. Can you think of examples where advocacy has the potential to set up adversarial relationships between the client and advocate and the mental health system? For example, a client has a right to visitors, but what assurance does the staff have that the visitors are not bringing drugs into a drug treatment unit? How should this situation be addressed?

5. What is the importance of thorough documentation in psychiatric-mental health nursing? Why should documentation be descriptive verus interpretive?

Enrichment Activities

1. Many communities have Mental Health Advisory Boards that meet in the evening once a month, and are open to the general public. Controversial cases, often brought before the board by family members, are discussed and resolved. The involvement by the family is dynamic and educational for students. Empathy for families is generated through this exposure.

2. Whenever possible, students should attend Reis hearings (on whether or not a client is capable of deciding to accept or refuse medication) and commitment proceedings that often take place on the unit. Supervising nurses need to be alerted to student interest in these proceedings, so permission to attend can be obtained. Permission to attend ECT sessions may also be possible to obtain from the physician and client, for interested students. Attending or "fish-bowling" group therapy sessions on the unit or in an out-patient facility is another way to understand the concepts of mental illness and mental health.

3. Psychiatric hospital units are regularly visited by patient advocates, who are usually persons having a social work or nursing background with advanced education or degrees in civil law. Inviting a patient advocate to give a presentation to the students, either in the classroom or clinical conference room, will provide them with specific information related to the laws and practice of psychiatry and psychiatric-mental health nursing in their particular state or locale.

4. For a view of forensic psychology and how it applies to the child or adolescent offender, arrange a trip for students to the Juvenile Detention Facility. Children as young as nine years of age are detained for the commission of serious crimes, and psychiatric-mental health nurses work with these clients, as they do with the adult mentally ill in prisons. They will share enhancing experiences with students.

5. A visit to court when conservatorship hearings are held is a valuable learning experience. It teaches students what provisions are made for individuals in the community who are not dangerous, but are totally or partially incapable of handling their own affairs, such as food, clothing, or shelter.

Multimedia Resources

Audio/Visual

Decisions of the Heart
Running Time: 8 minutes
Purchase: $200
Rental: $60
To order: AJN Company, 555 West 57th St., New York, NY, 10019, Attn: Interactive Video Dept., or call 1-800-CALL-AJN, or FAX to (212) 944-9055.
DESCRIPTION: Addresses the sensitive and difficult decision whether to resuscitate a seriously ill family member. Explains in lay language what resuscitative efforts entail and defines "do not resuscitate" instructions and their reasons.

Power of Attorney for Health Care
Running time: 14 minutes
Purchase: $250
Rental: $70
To order: AJN Company, 555 West 57th St., New York, NY, 10019, Attn: Interactive Video Dept., or call 1-800-CALL-AJN, or FAX to (212) 944-9055.
DESCRIPTION: This timely program will not only help you comply with the law of Patient Self-Determination Act, but will save you time and work while helping your staff and clients understand this very important right. An attorney describes both living wills and the power of attorney and explains the reasons for such documents and how to create them.

Legal Issues Confronting Today's Nurses—Part I (How to Reduce Your Risks of Being Sued) Part II (Defending a Nursing Malpractice Lawsuit)
Running time: Part I, 26 minutes; Part II, 25 minutes
Purchase: $295 or $175 each
Rental: $70 each
To order: AJN Company, 555 West 57th St., New York, NY, 10019, Attn: Interactive Video Dept., or call 1-800-CALL-AJN, or FAX to (212) 944-9055.
DESCRIPTION: Part I covers the basics of a nursing malpractice lawsuit and provides guidelines for reducing liability. This program identifies key issues such as the nursing standard of care that may affect a nurse's risk of liability. This program identifies key issues such as the nursing standard of care that may affect a nurse's risk of liability. Realistic case studies are used to emphasize key points. Part II offers an inside perspective on a nursing malpractice lawsuit. Nurses see firsthand what to expect if they are named as a defendant or called as a witness. Advice is included to help them prepare for the rigors of legal interrogation and give composed, believable testimony.

Accountability and Liability in Nursing Practice
Running time: 28 minutes
Purchase: $285
Rental: $70
To order: AJN Company, 555 West 57th St., New York, NY, 10019, Attn: Interactive Video Dept., or call 1-800-CALL-AJN, or FAX to (212) 944-9055.
DESCRIPTION: Reenacts a real case brought against a nurse, in order to present the basic legal aspects of malpractice. Addresses key considerations involved in malpractice cases: what constitutes reasonable and prudent care and what standard of care is expected from nurses. Provides detailed discussion of how nurses can prevent malpractice charges by exercising caution in troublesome situations.

Mosby's Legal and Ethical Issues in Nursing Video Series
Six Video Series
To order: Pat Newman, Mosby, Inc. 11830 Westline Industrial Dr., St. Louis, MO, 63146-9934, or call 1-800-426-4545, or FAX to 1-800-535-9935.
DESCRIPTION: Includes ethical dilemmas and decision making, documentation, basic legal terminology, minimizing legal liability, advance directives and Do Not Resuscitate Orders, and the nurse's rights as an employee. Relevant concepts and terminology in each video are defined and discussed followed by vignettes illustrating these concepts.

Interactive Video

Ethical Dilemmas and Legal Issues in Care of the Elderly
Purchase: $995 (5 1/4" or 3 1/2" diskettes available)
To order: AJN Company, 555 West 57th St., New York, NY, 10019, Attn: Interactive Video Dept., or call 1-800-CALL-AJN, or FAX to (212) 944-9055.
DESCRIPTION: This Level III interactive videodisc case study simulation focuses on four ethical situations and their legal implications: advance directives, use of restraints, reassignment of a nurse, and Do Not Resuscitate orders. Learning progresses through a decision making guide, which provides a structure to help with the decision making process in these types of situations.

Chapter 6

Cultural Issues

Critical Thinking Questions

1. What problems can ethnic stereotyping and ethnocentrism cause for the nurse practicing in a mental health setting? How can nurses learn to recognize such tendencies in themselves?

2. What are factors that make members of certain ethnic groups reluctant to seek mental health care?

3. What are areas of similarity and differences among the four groups of the emerging majority? These groups are African-, Asian-, Hispanic-, and Native Americans.

Enrichment Activities

1. Invite a physician or nurse from another culture to a post-conference session on the clinical unit, or to a class session. Have them discuss with students:

    How mental illness is viewed by another culture.

    What treatments are used that are different by the other culture.

    How the family responds to the mental illness of a member in another culture.

    How society regards its discharged clients in another culture; what provisions are made for aftercare?

    What terms are used for professionals who deal with mentally ill clients in another culture? Are the psychiatric or nursing diagnoses different?

2. Acquaint students with the Transcultural Nursing Association. Find out if there will be a conference in your city or nearby. Often students can attend at reduced rates. Urge them to attend, giving participation points for attending and reporting back to the class on the activities there. Joining the association as a student member is often a good networking strategy for the student whose ethnic background is not the majority Caucasian American, or the student who has an interest in working with clients (physically or mentally ill) from another culture or in another part of the world.

3. Encourage students to take a foreign language course as an elective subject (which fulfills a humanities requirement). In the United States, Spanish is the most common second language spoken. There may even be a course titled "Spanish for the Health Professional". Being able to discuss symptoms and feelings in the client's native language is a valuable asset in any nursing specialty field.

4. Survey local mental health facilities to discover what cultural groups use the facility; call agencies in the community. What provisions are there for service—for example, are there interpreters? Visit an agency and notice cultural artifacts, for example, different types of toys, different foods served. How does the agency individualize care for clients of different backgrounds? How do clients perceive care? Are the caregivers of the same ethno-cultural background as their clients?

5. When on vacation to another country, or another state or section of the United States, investigate the local variances in cultural beliefs and health care practices among different groups. How do religious beliefs and economic circumstances influence views? For example, how do the Pennsylvania Dutch view mental illness? The peoples of

Appalachia? People in the ghettos of New York City? The Apache Indians? The Hawaiian Islanders? What are some of the practices in Belgium that differ from those of the United States? What are the psychiatric hospitals like in Russia? (Yes, it is possible to get permission to visit them!)

6. Attend a healing ceremony of a different religious group than your own. (For example, Christian Scientists) Observe the similarities and differences in beliefs and practices. Talk to a registered nurse of the Christian Science faith. How does he or she consolidate medical and nursing knowledge within his or her faith?

Multimedia Resources

Audio/Visual

Cultural Assessment
Running time: 28 minutes
Purchase: $285
Rental: $70
To order: AJN Company, 555 West 57th St., New York, NY, 10019, Attn: Interactive Video Dept., or call 1-800-CALL-AJN, or FAX to (212) 944-9055.
DESCRIPTION: Features nursing experts as they share their experiences with patients from various cultures, with real-life vignettes. Describes an assessment tool with several key variables, including ethnic/racial identity, language, healing beliefs and practices, and religious beliefs.

Chapter 7: The Nursing Process

Critical Thinking Questions

1. Discuss the basic differences between a nursing diagnosis and medical diagnosis. To develop a nursing care plan, is it essential to wait until a medical diagnosis has been made? Why or why not?

2. Why is it important to discuss the nursing care plan with the client, and obtain his or her input? When would you consider the agreement of the family with the plan to be important? If the outcomes of the plan are not met, what should the psychiatric mental health nurse do to facilitate this?

3. When a plan is evaluated as to its effectiveness, what parts of the plan are being scrutinized? What is the relationship between outcomes, interventions, and evaluation?

Enrichment Activities

1. The following exercise will serve as a rehearsal for actual clinical situations, and help the students to sharpen their observation and documentation skills. Have each student observe another person without the person's knowledge. Using the Mini Mental Status Exam below, the student will assess the person according to the mental status parameters.

    Mini Mental Status Exam

    (1) Appearance:

    Posture _____

    Dress _____

    Grooming _____

    Gait _____

    Behavior _____

    (2) Speech:

    Clarity _____

    Rapidity _____

    Tone _____

    Productivity _____

    Sensibility _____

    (3) Affect _____

    Mood _____

    (4) Sensorium (state of mind):

    Orientation (person, place, time, situation) _____

    Attention behavior _____

    Recent memory _____

    Remote memory _____

    General knowledge level _____

    Judgment _____

    Insight _____

    For category 4, the student may ask the friend some questions or have a brief conversation, but should not be filling out the form in the person's presence. Discuss the results in class. What might rapid speech indicate, for example? Or careless grooming? Although the person who the student assessed was designated as "mentally healthy," how might the results be different if the instrument was used to assess a mentally ill person?

2. An exercise to help students formulate nursing diagnoses follows:

    Give the class the following three situations, and ask them to formulate a nursing diagnosis for each one, using the NANDA nursing diagnosis criteria.

Have the students identify qualifying statements, etiologies, risk factors, and cite evidence for the diagnosis when possible. In what category is each diagnosis placed? How would one prioritize the most important problem(s)?
   a. Accompanied by her friend, Mrs. H. came to a psychiatric-mental health nurse, a clinical specialist in private practice. Mrs. H.'s statement, when asked her reason for coming, was that she was "feeling tired all the time."
   b. Mrs. H. is distraught over the recent death of her husband, and cannot sleep at night. She has always had a gun in the house, and keeps it in the drawer of her night table.
   c. During Mr. H.'s illness, Mrs. H. "felt depressed" and complained of constipation. This problem continues to disturb her, and she wants help with it.

   Discuss the nursing diagnoses and the prioritization criteria. How are the physical complaints related to the psychiatric diagnoses?

3. Have students attend an interdisciplinary treatment planning conference on the unit to which they are assigned. At post-conference, they will report:

   Who was present at the treatment conference? Were all disciplines represented? Were nursing assistants (who are often with the clients for long periods of time) asked for their observations? If a nursing student was assigned to the particular client, did he or she contribute observations? Was the client involved in some part of the planning process? Was the meeting egalitarian or hierarchical in structure?

Multimedia Resources

Audio/Visual

The Psychosocial Nursing Assessment: A Holistic Approach
Running time: 30 minutes
Purchase: $285
Rental: $70
To order: AJN Company, 555 West 57th St., New York, NY, 10019, Attn: Interactive Video Dept., or call 1-800-CALL-AJN, or FAX to (212) 944-9055.
DESCRIPTION: This program discusses the holistic approach to nursing and can help all nurses accurately assess the patient's psychosocial needs, providing the nurse with the opportunity to identify present stressors in the patient's life as well as past and present coping methods. Included is a study guide with a questionnaire that gives the nurse the components of the holistic assessment.

Nursing Diagnosis: Concepts and Practice
Running time: 28 minutes
Purchase: $285
Rental: $70
To order: AJN Company, 555 West 57th St., New York, NY, 10019, Attn: Interactive Video Dept., or call 1-800-CALL-AJN, or FAX to (212) 944-9055.
DESCRIPTION: Provides nurses with a common language and enables them to describe problems. Distinguishes nursing diagnosis from medical diagnosis and identifies eleven functional health patterns. Uses an actual example of a patient who complains of difficulty sleeping.

Comprehensive Health History: Key to Diagnosis
Running time: 30 minutes
Purchase: $285
Rental: $70
To order: AJN Company, 555 West 57th St., New York, NY, 10019, Attn: Interactive Video Dept., or call 1-800-CALL-AJN, or FAX to (212) 944-9055.
DESCRIPTION: Portrays three nurse practitioners using individualized approaches in gathering a health history from three different patients. Video pauses intermittently for discussion by a panel of nursing experts. The program covers all segments of the health history including interview techniques, analysis, and interpretation of subjective data.

Chapter 8

Principles of Communication

Critical Thinking Questions

1. Consider interviewing a newly admitted mentally ill client. What location would you choose? What physical posture would you assume? Think about your voice tone, word choices, your dress and grooming, your affect and body language. Give your description of the ideal setting and rationales for all of the factors you would consider.

2. Explain the differences between a social conversation and a therapeutic interaction. How do they differ in terms of purpose, focus, and the necessary skills? If a psychiatric mental health nurse was to engage in social conversation with a client, how might the client interpret the communication experience?

3. Distinguish between the terms empathy and sympathy. Which of the two responses below denotes empathy? Explain.
   Client: ". . . and then he locked me out of the house. I couldn't help it; I got angry then."
   Nurse: "What an experience! I'm so sorry that happened to you."
        or
   Nurse: "I'd be angry, too, if I was treated that way."

Enrichment Activities

1. To examine the importance of body language in communication, randomly pair off students and have each pair sit back to back. (In a large class, this may have to be done with a few pairs at a time.) Have them carry on a conversation without observing the other person. A good topic might be how the other person felt before the first clinical day in psychiatric-mental health nursing. After the exercise, ask for comments as to how the position (back to back) affected the ability to hear the other person, and to be heard.

2. Read a short, emotionally laden piece to the class. Then write several words from the piece, along with some additional, related words, on the board. Ask the students to identify which words were actually from the reading. There will be discrepancies, which will illustrate how we think we heard something when we really did not. (This is a variation on the old "telephone message" game, where the message is whispered around the circle, and the last person to receive it reports a message very different from the first person who sent it!) Discuss how people make assumptions, fill in the blanks, and jump to conclusions, even when they are trying to listen.

3. To gain experience in therapeutic communication, have students write down on paper the hardest thing a client has ever said to them—one in which they did not know how to respond. Collect these and read them aloud, encouraging students to formulate helpful responses. Discuss how important congruence between verbal and nonverbal communication would be in such interactions.

4. Take an American Sign Language course, and learn how much can be communicated without uttering a word! Deaf individuals also have mental health problems, and are sometimes thought to be autistic or mentally retarded because no one understands what they are trying to communicate. They may feel hopeless, and stop trying to communicate, even if they know sign language. Nurses who know how to "sign" have a big advantage in helping these clients.

Multimedia Resources

Audio/Visual

Connecting with Your Patient: Nonverbal Communication for the Health Care Professional
Running time: 21 minutes
Purchase: $285
Rental: $70
To order: AJN Company, 555 West 57th St., New York, NY, 10019, Attn: Interactive Video Dept., or call 1-800-CALL-AJN, or FAX to (212) 944-9055.
DESCRIPTION: Discusses the ways we communicate without words: how we listen, how we stand, the expressions of our eyes and face, the tone of our voice, our touch, and the space we occupy. Teaches students and staff awareness of and control over their nonverbal communications so that they can be used therapeutically.

Mosby's Communication in Nursing Video Series
Six Video Series
Running time: 20 to 25 minutes each
To order: Pat Newman, Mosby, Inc., 11830 Westline Industrial Dr., St. Louis, MO, 63146-9934, or call 1-800-426-4545, or FAX 1-800-535-9935.
DESCRIPTION: Series includes videos on basic principles for communicating effectively in Nursing, with clients and colleagues; clients from different cultures, difficult clients and colleagues, clients with mental disorders or emotional problems, and across the lifespan. Each video is introduced by a series host and employs realistic clinical scenarios which demonstrate therapeutic and non-therapeutic communication, special techniques for more effective communication, and interviews with practicing nurses and nurse experts in the area of communication.

Chapter 9

Children and Adolescents

Critical Thinking Questions

1. Discuss the interaction of maturation and environment in a child's development. What are some examples of these interactions? What are some theoretical perspectives that consider the interaction of maturation and environment? Explain.

2. What theory of development explains the tendency of the adolescent to argue with parents and to form his or her own opinions? Assume a troubled parent asked you about her son, who "was always so obedient, and now he finds reasons for why he shouldn't do as we say." How would you explain this phenomenon to the parent, using your knowledge of the theory?

3. Consider Kohlberg's theory of moral development. What are the problems with this theory, according to Gilligan? Do you think her stand is well-taken? Can you think of situations from your own experience that would support either theorist's point of view?

Enrichment Activities

1. A visit to a school classroom for emotionally disturbed children in special education programs is a mind-opening experience for nursing students. Many times people do not think of children as being mentally ill, or believe their illness means they do not need to attend school. But this is not the case. On the psychiatric units, special education teachers work in unit classrooms with children of all ages, from kindergarten to high school. As the children improve with treatment, they are transported to local schools, where they are "mainstreamed" gradually into the school environment, and returned to the treatment center after school. If the nursing students have the good fortune to be assigned to a children's facility, they often assist in the classroom as one-on-one tutors for the children with short attention spans, dyslexia, or poor hand-eye coordination. If the facility does not treat children, an effort should be made to visit a special classroom to assist the children.

2. For the adolescent with mental illness, there are residential treatment centers. A visit to one of these centers is rewarding. The centers were designed for the adolescent who is recovering from an acute episode of mental illness, but is not quite ready to assume his or her roles in the community. Guidance and support are received from the staff, which is composed of psychiatric mental health nurses, psychologists, and mental health assistants. The adolescents live in a structured milieu, providing order and meaning that has often been lacking in their lifestyle prior to their illness. The centers also provide family therapy, in an attempt to unite and support the family that is dealing with the stigma and trauma of mental illness.

3. On occasion, there are Roger O. hearings on the child or adolescent units. The patient advocate usually arranges these, and permission from the advocate and the client is necessary to attend a hearing. The Roger O. hearings are a protection for any child over the age of 10, against being incarcerated for an insufficient reason. Prior to this protective strategy, children and adolescents could be remanded to the psychiatric units for spurious reasons, such as truancy or behavior difficult to handle at home, even though the child was not mentally ill.

Multimedia Resources

Audio/Visual

Infancy through Adolescence—Infant/Toddler/Preschool Child/School-age Child/Adolescent (5 videos)
Running time: Infant (38 minutes)/Toddler (40 minutes)/Preschool Child (41 minutes)/School-age Child (41 minutes)/Adolescent (44 minutes)
Purchase: $750 or $300 each
Rental: $70
To order: AJN Company, 555 West 57th St., New York, NY, 10019, Attn: Interactive Video Dept., or call 1-800-CALL-AJN, or FAX to (212) 944-9055.
DESCRIPTION: Depicts the growth and development from infancy through adolescence in documentary format.

Human Development: First 2½ years (4 videos)
Purchase: $880 or $280 each
Rental: $50 for 10 days
To order: Concept Media Inc., PO Box 19542, Irvine, CA, 92713-9849, or call 1-800-233-7078, or FAX to (714) 660-0206.

Physical Growth and Motor Development
Running time: 18 minutes
DESCRIPTION: Emphasizes individual differences by depicting a wide range of normal physical growth and motor development. Discusses ways in which environmental factors such as nutrition and the mother's health habits during pregnancy affect development.

Cognitive Development
Running time: 25 minutes
DESCRIPTION: Discusses the senses, perception, and memory as important aspects of cognitive development. Includes some of the work of Piaget. Presents practical advice for improving a child's chances for optimum cognitive development.

Language Development
DESCRIPTION: Discusses parent-child communication including turn-taking and "motherese." Describes the stages and sequences of language acquisition and development. Presents practical advice for improving a child's language ability.

Emotional/Social Development
Running time: 25 minutes
DESCRIPTION: Begins with a brief discussion of Erikson's first two stages of man and traces the developmental processes by which the newborn becomes a social being. Discusses temperament, attachment, and social responses such as smiling, stranger anxiety and separation anxiety. Self-awareness, development of empathy, and development of standards are discussed at length.

Human Development: 2½ to 6 years (4 videos)
Purchase: $880 or $280 each
Rental: $50 for 10 days
To order: Concept Media Inc., PO Box 19542, Irvine, CA, 92713-9849, or call 1-800-233-7078, or FAX to (714) 660-0206.

Physical Growth and Motor Development
Running time: 21 minutes.
DESCRIPTION: Discusses the patterns of growth seen in the years between 2½ and 6 and describes how the differential growth of various organs affect the child's ability to function.

Cognitive Development
Running time: 28 minutes.
DESCRIPTION: Describes Piaget's theories regarding cognitive development including the process of assimilation and accommodation. Discusses preoperational thought including concepts such as irreversibility, static thought, egocentrism, conservation, classification, magical thought, animism, and ritualistic behavior.

Psychosocial Development
Running time: 23 minutes
DESCRIPTION: Begins by discussing the tasks which are crucial to a preschooler's emotional and social development. Describes Erikson's stages pertaining to preschool children and Rene Spitz's stages of how children deal with frustration.

Role of Play
Running time: 22 minutes
DESCRIPTION: Defines play and discusses some of the functions including gross and fine motor development, cognitive development, creativity, socialization, self-awareness, and therapeutic value. The social character of play and gender differences in play are also discussed.

Chapter 10 The Adult

Critical Thinking Questions

1. If you were an employer, would you hire someone who has been treated for mental illness? Why or why not? On what would your decision depend?

2. Discuss the social forces that stimulated the study of adult development. Why is this field a difficult one for investigators to focus on? In your opinion, what theorist explained adult development most clearly? Give some examples, from your own life or the lives of people you know, that illustrate some of the concepts from the theory.

3. Consider Levinson's theory of the interface between the self and the interpersonal world in adult development. Would the stages he proposed apply equally to men and to women? Why or why not? How does a woman's socially defined sense of time influence her adult developmental stages?

4. What are some of the violations of the hierarchy that occur when applying Maslow's theory to certain individuals? Are there times when adult development seems to proceed at an uneven rate? Explain.

Enrichment Activities

1. When adults have had an episode of mental illness, it is often difficult for them to be assimilated into the community following recovery. For many young adults, they may have had their first episode of mental illness in their adolescent years, at a time when they would be making the transition to adulthood. The skills of applying for work, going for an interview, getting and holding a job, and learning how to manage time effectively may not have been possible for them to learn. A sheltered workshop does provide the opportunity to learn these skills, and gives a boost to the self-esteem by allowing clients to earn a small amount of money for productive work. Arrange a visit to a sheltered workshop for students, and support the industries that provide opportunities for discharged clients.

2. Clients who were incarcerated, either in a prison or a psychiatric hospital for the criminally insane, for a crime committed while in an episode of mental illness, will be released to the community when they are mentally stable. While they are in the institution, however, their families may be attending meetings of Prison Families Anonymous (PFA), to support them in handling stigma and community, social, or school problems. One can volunteer to help these families in their adjustment, which is especially difficult once their previously mentally ill member returns to the family and the community. Unfortunately, state psychiatric hospitals and prisons are often located a distance away from the client's home, and it may have been years since the client has seen his or her children. Students desiring to serve with PFA should contact their local clergy, or the Fortune Society.

3. Former mentally ill clients who are not functional enough for employment are often assigned to a day care program. They are transported to the center, usually three times a week. At the center they learn skills of living, such as cooking, shopping, money management and other routine tasks. They also participate in supportive group sessions, arts and crafts groups, and occasionally go on outings in the community, such as a visit to the zoo, or a picnic at the beach.

Students can ask to be assigned to the day treatment center associated with their psychiatric facility for a one day experience in this client stimulating environment.

Chapter 11: The Elderly

Critical Thinking Questions

1. Compare and contrast the disengagement theory of aging with the activity theory. From your experience, do you know of any examples of persons who seem to violate the premises of the disengagement theory? What is the meaning of the description of the theory as one of "presumed universality"? Would there be gender differences in the application of the theory?

2. Theorists today discount the old stereotypes of the elderly as not being interested in sexual pleasures and intimacy. How do you think these stereotypes came to be? Have you observed older couples who seem to be enjoying the company of each other? In some nursing homes or assisted living residences for the elderly, the genders are separated, even when both partners have been married for years! Explain what effects this policy might have on the elders' psychosocial health.

3. In many theories on aging, one detects a theme of discouragement and depression that leads to ageism. Do you know any elderly individuals who seem to belie this generalization of aging development? What factors in their life seem to influence their psychological outlook? Given any unforeseen accident, what do you think of their chances to live to a happy and productive old age? Explain.

Enrichment Activities

1. An experience that will add insight to problems suffered by certain elders is an outing with members of the Senior Team or similar organizations in the community. This organization, with teams of registered nurses and social workers, follows up on the most vulnerable members of our society—the mentally ill, and often physically ill, elders. A call by anyone to the Senior Team prompts an investigation.

2. Day care centers for seniors in the community range from organizations to promote socialization and prevent loneliness among the elder citizens, to centers that help Alzheimer's disease victims with activities of daily living. The latter provide much needed respite care for the caregivers of the clients. Students are welcome to volunteer their time to this worthy cause by attending support and current events groups at the Alzheimer's centers. Students can socialize with the elders, help to serve meals, and learn about Alzheimer's disease.

3. Activities of the Retired Senior Volunteer Program (RSVP) in the community are many and noteworthy. Seniors volunteer their time and talents in many ways, teaching children to read, acting as a foster grandparent, visiting shut-ins, and maintaining a telephone line to keep in contact with other elders engrossed in caregiving activities for a spouse or other relative. RSVP sponsors fundraising events for worthy causes, such as obtaining money for persons needing bone-marrow transplants, or to combat other serious illnesses. Senior Committee of Retired Executives (SCORE) is a group that helps young people start their own businesses in the community. Students are encouraged to discover the wisdom and productivity of groups such as these, to combat the stereotype of the elderly as senile and worthless.

Multimedia Resources

Audio/Visual

Common Problems: Knowledge Deficit
Running time: 15 minutes
Purchase: $150
Rental: $60
To order: AJN Company, 555 West 57th St., New York, NY, 10019, Attn: Interactive Video Dept., or call 1-800-CALL-AJN, or FAX to (212) 944-9055.
DESCRIPTION: Explores the case history of a 70-year-old woman with a diagnosis of lymphoma. The patient's defining characteristics reveal deficiencies of knowledge, inaccurate information, faulty procedures, and a need for help in self-administering medication. The scenario is an excellent example of how the nursing process works to help patients attain realistic short/long-term goals.

Natural Process of Aging
Running time: 30 minutes
Purchase: $199
Rental: $70
To order: AJN Company, 555 West 57th St., New York, NY, 10019, Attn: Interactive Video Dept., or call 1-800-CALL-AJN, or FAX to (212) 944-9055.
DESCRIPTION: It is necessary for the nurse to understand how the aging process affects major body systems and functions. Each system is covered. Dramatic scenes and graphic art are used to illustrate these changes. Also covered are some disease conditions common among the elderly and, when applicable, suggested interventions.

Polypharmacy in the Elderly
Running time: 30 minutes
Purchase: $285
Rental: $70
To order: AJN Company, 555 West 57th St., New York, NY, 10019, Attn: Interactive Video Dept., or call 1-800-CALL-AJN, or FAX to (212) 944-9055.
DESCRIPTION: This program examines age-related changes and risk factors that affect medications and influence medication-taking behaviors of older adults. Also discussed are risk factors such as lack of information, functional impairments, disease-related factors affecting vision and memory, and interactions with other drugs.

Medication Use by the Elderly: Implications for Nurses
Running time: 30 minutes
Purchase: $285
Rental: $70
To order: AJN Company, 555 West 57th St., New York, NY, 10019, Attn: Interactive Video Dept., or call 1-800-CALL-AJN, or FAX to (212) 944-9055.
DESCRIPTION: Showing a variety of elderly clients in various community settings, a nurse practitioner elicits drug histories. The program shows proper procedures in taking the history, how physiological aging affects drug absorption, distribution, metabolism, and excretion, and covers principles of prescribing for the elderly.

Medicating the Elderly
Running time: 28 minutes
Purchase: $285
Rental: $70
To order: AJN Company, 555 West 57th St., New York, NY, 10019, Attn: Interactive Video Dept., or call 1-800-CALL-AJN, or FAX to (212) 944-9055.
DESCRIPTION: Stresses the need for careful drug history, for using the fewest drugs and smallest doses possible, for awareness that confusion may be drug-induced, and for patient education on safety and drug purposes. Discusses balancing a drug's therapeutic effects with the various risks it poses.

Functional Assessment of the Elderly: Part I—Cognitive and Special Senses
Running time: 28 minutes
Purchase: $285
Rental: $70
To order: AJN Company, 555 West 57th St., New York, NY, 10019, Attn: Interactive Video Dept., or call 1-800-CALL-AJN, or FAX to (212) 944-9055.
DESCRIPTION: Helps recognize age-related physiological changes and changes in cognitive and emotional capabilities. Defines skills and relates them to the corresponding activities of daily life.

The Disruptive Geriatric Patient
Running time: 17 minutes
Purchase: $175
Rental: $50 for 10 days
To order: Concept Media Inc., PO Box 19542, Irvine, CA, 92713-9849, or call 1-800-233-7078, or FAX to (714) 660-0206.
DESCRIPTION: Presents practical guidance for the care giver in dealing with the disruptive geriatric patient. Describes types of behavior, possible causes, symptoms of impending hostility, and appropriate interventions. Techniques of therapeutic communication as well as non-therapeutic communication are identified and examined.

Chapter 12

Anxiety and Related Disorders

Critical Thinking Questions

1. What issues does a psychiatric mental health nurse need to consider when determining whether a person's level of anxiety is adaptive or maladaptive?

2. What behaviors are commonly seen as the anxiety level rises in an individual? Use yourself as your reference point. What physiological responses occur? What changes may be experienced in affect and behavior? What effect does rising anxiety have upon cognitive functioning?

3. Discuss the comorbidity aspect of anxiety disorders. Offer an explanation of how anxiety may produce a variety of disorders. For example, if palpitations are experienced in a panic attack, is it likely that somatization or hypochondria will occur? Make links between anxiety and other diagnoses, considering the responses of the autonomic nervous system.

Enrichment Activities

1. Students are often afflicted with state anxiety in a test-taking situation. Ask students in the class how they feel, what symptoms and sensations they experience just before taking the test. Then put them through a short session of relaxation therapy, using a tape with soothing sounds, and/or a voice tone that is low and smooth. Have them relax each muscle group in turn, and envision (visual imagery) a quiet place they love to be—beside a woodland stream, on a quiet and sunny beach cove, alone or with someone dear, etc. After about 5 minutes you can tell them to come back any time they wish. They will return to the present relaxed and more alert. Tell them they can do this whenever they feel stressed, for even a minute or two in the middle of a test! Students sometimes can bring their test score up a whole grade through this strategy.

    The discussion that follows this exercise should include the role of the autonomic nervous system, the difference between beta and alpha brain waves, and the symptoms of anxiety (tunnel vision) that make it difficult to think laterally, as they need to do. Show them an overhead on the curvilinear relationship between anxiety and performance (Ax's study).

2. Link some of the aspects of anxiety to literature:

    Why did Pontius Pilate wash his hands after sentencing Jesus?

    What was Lady MacBeth's hand-washing all about?

    Ask students to give examples of the effects of anxiety from their own experiences or observations. What perceptual cues were missed due to anxiety (something obvious that was not seen, for example).

3. With the help of two students in the class, who are to play the role of monkeys, demonstrate the methodology that was used to link anxiety as a cause of gastric ulcers, from the executive monkey study. Ask the student who plays the executive monkey what the experience was like.

Chapter 13

Mood Disorders: Depression and Mania

Critical Thinking Questions

1. Differentiate between exogenous and endogenous depression. What are the etiological factors involved, and how does the treatment differ for each type? What is the relationship between loss and anger in exogenous depression?

2. Define hopelessness in the context of mood disturbances, and explain how it contributes to feelings of apathy and helplessness in all situations. How is hope conveyed to the depressed client?

3. What clinical nursing alerts must a psychiatric mental health nurse be aware of in caring for a client with acute mania? What sort of social, perceptual, and behavioral manifestations does the client exhibit? Can acute mania be a life-threatening condition? Explain.

Enrichment Activities

1. On the notion that depression is anger turned inward, have the students do an exercise at home or in class (if space permits), and discuss the results afterward. Each student is to think of a frustrating experience which made him or her really frustrated and angry—not being able to get a class they wanted, being the victim of a bureaucratic error, etc. Then the student is to take some modeling clay, of the type used in ceramics class, and pound the air out of it, as one is instructed to do in a ceramics class. After a few minutes, the clay will be well-pounded, and the student will be relieved of pent-up anger. Have the students report out their results with this experiment at the next class meeting.

2. One way to prevent depressed feelings is to focus on the positive aspects of life. The following highlight activity recalls to awareness some of the best times of life:

    Tell the students to draw three triangles on a sheet of paper; the triangles should be about 3 inches on each side. Then they are to imagine the three happiest times of their lives, and let them fill each triangle with a name for these happy times. They can pair with another student, and share these times in a 5 minute discussion. This will relax the whole class, and everyone will benefit from the "smile break."

3. Hand out to members of the class a case study, as follows:

    Pat is thinking of dropping out of school. Pat had an accident in which an ankle was broken, and there was a week's loss of class, affecting the grades. Then Pat's grandmother died. Next semester will probably be worse, because there is a mandatory math course which must be taken. Pat has become anxious and depressed, and does not feel well physically. So, Pat is ready to give it up, at least for now.

    If you were in Pat's situation, what would you do? Why?

    Give students time to read the case study, then have a discussion based on their responses to the question. What would be the advantages/disadvantages of the proposed action? What pattern of coping would likely be established in either action?

Multimedia Resources

Audio/Visual

The Depressed Patient: Nursing in the Acute Care Setting
Running time: 28 minutes
Purchase: $285
Rental: $70
To order: AJN Company, 555 West 57th St., New York, NY, 10019, Attn: Interactive Video Dept., or call 1-800-CALL-AJN, or FAX to (212) 944-9055.
DESCRIPTION: Helps nurses meet the needs of depressed patients, a common problem in acute care settings. Describes six depressive syndromes, ranging from total withdrawal to chronic low-level depression. Vignettes illustrate each state and show what nurses can do to speed recovery.

Chapter 14: The Schizophrenias

Critical Thinking Questions

1. What evidence is available for the support of the biochemical theory of schizophrenia? Contrast the biochemical theory with the psychosocial theories of the development of schizophrenia. Which approach has the best potential for decreasing the stigma that clients and their families face on a daily basis? Give reasons for your answer.

2. What are some of the common reasons for recidivism in the client with schizophrenia who is discharged to the community? How can the mental health system be revised to lessen the rate of readmissions? How do you think the client might feel about having to return to the institution?

3. What is the difference between positive and negative symptoms in schizophrenia? How does the presence of either type correlate with prognosis for the client? Which type of symptom responds best to pharmacological therapy?

Enrichment Activities

1. Clients with schizophrenia are frequently in need of supervised aftercare on discharge from the hospital. Often they are visited regularly by the psychiatric mental health community nurse. It is possible to make arrangements for students to accompany the nurse, one at a time, as rounds are made in the community. This is an enlightening experience for students, as they see the former clients living, working, or going to school in the community, and learn how the psychiatric-mental health nurse carefully assesses treatment compliance, reality orientation, functioning ability, and general well being.

2. Two organizations that support formerly hospitalized clients with schizophrenia are the Alliance for the Mentally Ill and Schizophrenics Anonymous. Leaders from these organizations are eager to diminish the stigma of schizophrenia and to promote community understanding. They can be invited to speak at a class session.

3. Support groups in the aftercare facilities can be attended by nursing students. Encouraging students to seek an opportunity to attend group sessions can be supportive for the clients and educational for the students.

4. While students are on the clinical units, they should learn how a "take down" procedure is done. This is a very organized and orderly procedure, designed to avoid injury to client or staff, and to calm a client who was unresponsive to verbal, biologic, or medication interventions. Students can practice the procedure among themselves, with the instructor providing direction and supervision. The role play procedure is as follows:
   a. A team leader can be any staff member. It may be the first staff member on the scene, or the one who has been working with the client and has established rapport. The duties of the leader are to assess the situation, plan the intervention, and be the spokesperson or delegate this role to another staff member. The leader, being perceived by the client as the one responsible for placing him or her in restraints, should be the one to remove them when the client is calm.
   b. The charge nurse (instructor's role) is the manager and should be notified in time to start directing the intervention.
   c. Other clients are escorted safely away from the area by students playing the role of staff members.

d. The leader assigns a staff member (A,B,C,D) to manage each of the client's extremeties, including the head. The client is approached by A and B from the front sides, to avoid staff being kicked. All staff approach at the same time. Two staff (A and B) face client and take hold of client's arms above the joint area and firmly at the sides, while two other staff (C and D) stand behind them to the side, to avoid being bitten or spat upon. The client is pulled forward by C and D, with their legs in front of the client's legs. The duties of the team are to follow the directions of the leader. The spokesperson is to talk reassuringly to the client during the procedure (no one else should be talking). Each team member communicates to the leader if they need help.
e. Once a client is safely and gently lowered to the floor, he or she is restrained at this time, lifted to the stretcher, and transported to the seclusion room, where constant staff supervision is required.
f. It is important to maintain the client's dignity, with regard to clothing, which may be in disarray. Explain that the restraints are being applied for protection of the client and others, and give reassurance that they will be removed when the client is in control of his/her behavior.
g. Evaluation of the procedure is done immediately after the incident, with emphasis on what worked and what could have been done better. Allow student role players to express feelings about the procedure.

In an actual take down procedure on the unit, full documentation of the whole episode, from the escalation of behavior to the removal of the restraints and aftercare of the client in the post crisis phase, is mandatory. In most instances, the student is not involved in the physical take down procedure; he or she generally accompanies other clients out of the area, remaining with them until the incident is over.

Chapter 15

Personality Disorders

Critical Thinking Questions

1. Describe some of the characteristics of the borderline personality disorder that present a challenge to the psychiatric mental health nurse who is caring for the client. How do the behaviors of splitting and manipulation affect the relationship? What other characteristics are especially problematic?

2. What are the similarities and differences between cluster A personality disorders and schizophrenia? What is the comorbidity potential of clients diagnosed with a cluster A personality disorder?

3. What is the relationship between the diagnosis of conduct disorder in childhood and the occurrence of antisocial behavior in adolescents and adults? In your opinion, how much of the antisocial behavior is related to child-rearing situations and socioeconomic conditions? Give reasons for your answers.

4. Clients with obsessive-compulsive personality disorder are not likely to seek help. What are some of the reasons for not seeking help? What effect does this personality disorder have on interpersonal relationships, especially those with significant others such as marriage partners? In our society, is the behavior of the obsessive-compulsive client rewarded? In what ways?

Enrichment Activities

1. Clients with antisocial personality disorders often use manipulation to gain power. This can be demonstrated by a role-playing exercise. Divide the class into partners or groups of three. Have one student in each group play the therapist, using limit-setting techniques, and have the other one or two students play manipulative clients. Share the results of the exercise with the class. How difficult was it to set limits? Did feelings of empathy for the client get in the way? Were some of the clients (roles) able to manipulate the therapist (role)? What tactics did the clients use? (The usual one is turning on the charm.)

2. Assign half the class a personality disorder to role-play.

    They are to study this disorder, and at the next class each role-play participant is to be paired with a student who was not given a role to play. Chairs are arranged in a circle, and each pair goes to the center of the circle, one by one. They engage in an interaction with the role-playing student enacting the personality disorder. As soon as the other student realizes what personality disorder the partner is enacting, that non-role-playing student identifies it: "Oh! You're enacting an obsessive compulsive personality!" Follow this exercise with a general class discussion. How did the student identify the enacted personality disorder? What clues were seen?

3. As students read the chapter, they will realize that they know persons with personality disorders or traits who live in the community. Without identifying the individuals, have students discuss the symptoms manifested by these people, and cite events where the personality disorder or trait has interfered with functioning and made it difficult for the individual to relate to others in an effective way. For example, would other people tend to avoid the person with a dependent personality? Why?

Chapter 16

Substance-Related Disorders

Critical Thinking Questions

1. What drugs are being abused in the area in which you live? What population group abuses drugs—adolescents, adults, elders?

   What type of drug does each segment of the population abuse? Do you think drug abuse is more or less prevalent in your area than it is in other parts of the country? What resources does your community have for drug abusers? Explain your answers.

2. How do nurses sometimes act as enablers for their addicted colleagues? How can nurses help addicted nurses? What are the likely consequences of acting as an enabler, or ignoring the problem? Who will be affected by these consequences?

3. Describe the cultural ambivalence that exists concerning the use of alcohol, tobacco, and marijuana. Should any or all of these substances be controlled? Should the use of certain "recreational" drugs be decriminalized? Which ones? What are the pros and cons of such a decision? Give reasons for your answers.

4. Which drugs are most frequently abused by the elderly population? How do the majority of these individuals become addicted? Do they, or does society, consider them drug addicts?

5. Discuss the needle exchange program for IV drug users. If an individual is identified as an IV drug user, what are the actions your community would take? What if that IV drug user is a woman, and she is pregnant? Or, suppose the user is a man, and he has a family and a well-paying job?

Enrichment Activities

1. Have students visit an Alcoholics Anonymous meeting, an Alanon, or Alateen meeting, and later share the dynamics of the meeting with the class. They should discuss whether or not their view of alcoholism has changed through the experience, and if so, in what way? What characteristics were apparent in the persons participating in the meeting? What evidence was there of support by the group? These groups are successful—what are some reasons that you can see for their success?

2. Each student or pair of students could visit a local high school in their area and discuss the drug abuse situation that exists, with a teacher or a principal. (This is action research, and an introductory letter from the professor of this course may be necessary.) Find out what percent of the students may be using drugs, problems the school has had with keeping dealers away, and how student performance has been affected in students who may be using drugs. If the class is scattered over several residential areas, the ensuing class discussion will be more interesting, as different school district areas can be compared. Does drug abuse seem to be related to the economics of the area?

   What other factors may account for a difference in estimated rate of drug abuse in a given area?

3. Have an officer from the local police department visit the class and demonstrate the different drugs of abuse, giving the street term as well as the generic term for the drug. Officers who work with drug abuse squadrons have excellent kits that they use when addressing adolescents and children in the schools. Some of the students may never have seen marijuana ("Mary Jane" or "weed" or "pot") as it grows. Even if they have seen some of the drugs, the demonstration and discussion of drug use and abuse by the officer will help them see the whole picture and specific relationships between drugs (cocaine and crack, for example).

4. Have students visit a detoxification unit, and discuss the experience with the class.

5. Ask the hospital pharmacologist to talk to the class about designer drugs—What are they? How are they made, and by whom?

Multimedia Resources

Audio/Visual

Substance Abuse: Everyone's Problem
Running time: 19 minutes
Purchase: $250
Rental: $70
To order: AJN Company, 555 West 57th St., New York, NY, 10019, Attn: Interactive Video Dept., or call 1-800-CALL-AJN, or FAX to (212) 944-9055.
DESCRIPTION: This video describes the signs of drug and alcohol abuse and the steps to take if a staff member is suspected of having these problems. Emphasis is placed on teaching the nurse manager how to help his/her employee acknowledge a substance abuse problem and get help.

Before Christmas: Alcoholism
Running time: 30 minutes
Purchase: $285
Rental: $70
To order: AJN Company, 555 West 57th St., New York, NY, 10019, Attn: Interactive Video Dept., or call 1-800-CALL-AJN, or FAX to (212) 944-9055.
DESCRIPTION: Shows the very positive role a nurse can play in the detection, assessment, and treatment of alcoholism. Depicts a married, adult male whose chronic alcoholism results in hospitalization for acute care. Concludes when the patient is physically well but just beginning the long task of recovery through a recognized treatment program.

Impaired Nursing Practice: Assessment and Intervention
Running time: 28 minutes
Purchase: $285
Rental: $70
To order: AJN Company, 555 West 57th St., New York, NY, 10019, Attn: Interactive Video Dept., or call 1-800-CALL-AJN, or FAX to (212) 944-9055.
DESCRIPTION: Designed to help nurses detect chemical abuse and take appropriate action. Explains why nurses may fail to recognize impaired practice. Describes the role denial plays. Explains ethical and legal reasons why action must be taken.

The Chemically Dependent Nurse (3 videos)
Purchase: $700 or $280 each
Rental: $50 for 10 days
To order: Concept Media Inc., PO Box 19542, Irvine, CA, 92713-9849, or call 1-800-233-7078, or FAX to (714) 660-0206.

The Nurse's Story
Running time: 20 minutes
DESCRIPTION: Describes the characteristics of nurses who become chemically dependent and discusses the high cost to health care facilities of such addiction. Uses Hutchinson's model of "trajectory toward self-annihilation" and discusses the process of chemical dependency in depth.

Identification and Response
Running time: 27 minutes
DESCRIPTION: Describes behaviors which are indicative of substance abuse in both nursing students and graduate student nurses, including problems at home, job shrinkage, and changes in attendance records. Describes different methods of drug diversion and ways of detecting it.

Nurse-to-Nurse: From Addiction to Recovery
Running time: 20 minutes
DESCRIPTION: Compiled from candid interviews with nurses in recovery, this provides a compelling look at the internal struggle of addiction and the challenging road to recovery. Emphasizes the importance of overcoming the stigma and denial common among care givers, and the disturbing tendency nurses have while taking care of others to overlook the care of themselves and their colleagues.

The What and Why of Co-Dependency
Running time: 22 minutes
Purchase: $175
Rental: $50 for 10 days
To order: Concept Media Inc., PO Box 19542, Irvine, CA, 92713-9849, or call 1-800-233-7078, or FAX to (714) 660-0206.
DESCRIPTION: Using a combination of mimes and family vignettes, the program gives an overview of the history of co-dependency. Describes current thinking regarding the disorder and its origins.

Characteristics of Co-Dependents
Running time: 23 minutes
Purchase: $175
Rental: $50 for 10 days
To order: Concept Media Inc., PO Box 19542, Irvine, CA, 92713-9849, or call 1-800-233-7078, or FAX to (714) 660-0206.
DESCRIPTION: Using vignettes of three individuals it discusses common characteristics of co-dependents, including being externally focused, overly responsible, controlling, rigid, and engaging in compulsive behavior.

Mosby's Nursing Care of Clients with Substance Abuse Video Series
Six Video Series
Running time: 20 to 25 minutes each
To order: Pat Newman, Mosby, Inc., 11830 Westline Industrial Dr., St. Louis, MO, 63146-9934, or call 1-800-426-4545, or FAX 1-800-535-9935.
DESCRIPTION: Includes substance abuse in the hospital, substance abuse in perinatal care, substance abuse in families, children, and adolescents, substance abuse in the community, substance abuse in chemical dependency treatment centers, and dual diagnosis. Each video includes documentary-style footage and clinical vignettes illustrating the collaborative role of the nurse with other health care professionals. Each video comes with an instructor's booklet, a pretest, posttest, and discussion questions.

Chapter 17

Delirium, Dementia, and Amnestic and Other Cognitive Disorders

Critical Thinking Questions

1. Differentiate between delirium, dementia, depression, and late-onset schizophrenia. Why would misdiagnosis of any of these conditions be critical? What part would the family's input regarding the history of onset play in the diagnosis? Would a complete physical examination and blood testing be essential? Explain your answers.

2. What is the relationship between confusion, confabulation, and disorientation? To which conditions do these manifestations relate? What are the overt behaviors of each symptom cluster? How would the nursing interventions differ for clients exhibiting one or another of these behaviors?

3. Discuss the prognosis for each of the cognitive disorders.

   If a person who develops Alzheimer's disease has no living relatives, who will care for him or her? Are there health insurance policies that make provision for the long-term care of the client with Alzheimer's disease?

Enrichment Activities

1. Have students contact the local chapter of the Alzheimer's Disease Association and ask if there is a caregiver of a live-in client with Alzheimer's disease who needs some respite. The caregiver may be elderly and not drive a car. Offer to drive the caregiver to the grocery store, to church, to a beauty parlor or barbershop, or to a physician's appointment, while another family member stays with the client with Alzheimer's disease. Interview the caregiver. Ask that person what their daily life is like, what their relative was like before becoming ill, and what help they need from others in the family and the community.

2. Students can visit a local nursing home and interview one of the clients who is slightly or moderately cognitively impaired. Students should encourage reminiscence. In reporting on the experience, the student should describe the differences noted in memory for recent and long past events. Note the client's orientation to time, place, and person (What aspect of orientation has deteriorated the least?) What was the elder's attitude toward the student? (Most nursing home residents are eager for company and attention; they may want to shift the conversation to what *you* have been doing!)

3. Another type of living arrangement for the elderly, confused client is the board and care facility or the residential facility for the elderly who are not physically ill. Have students visit one or the other, and note the living conditions there for the clients. Talk to the clients; what are their concerns? Some residences have excellent staffing patterns, good, nutritious meals, and enhancing environments; others are marginally staffed, have unappetizing meals, and are drab in appearance. What accounts for these differences? Who gives the medications the clients need at these facilities? Many persons are under the impression that Medicare takes care of payment for the elderly person in a residential facility. What really is the situation?

   This is a good learning experience for students, who may be faced at some point with making decisions about caring for an elderly parent or relative.

   Report to the class on this experience.

Multimedia Resources

Audio/Visual

Communication Strategies for Alzheimer's Patients
Running time: 30 minutes
Purchase: $285
Rental: $70
To order: AJN Company, 555 West 57th St., New York, NY, 10019, Attn: Interactive Video Dept., or call 1-800-CALL-AJN, or FAX to (212) 944-9055.
DESCRIPTION: Deals with behavioral changes which Alzheimer's patients and other cognitively impaired persons undergo. Discusses revitalization techniques to improve the effectiveness of communication and ways to maintain client's dignity and self-respect. Differentiates between mechanical use of language and meaningful use.

Alzheimer's Disease — Part I: Coping with Confusion
Running time: 28 minutes
Purchase: $285
Rental: $70
To order: AJN Company, 555 West 57th St., New York, NY, 10019, Attn: Interactive Video Dept., or call 1-800-CALL-AJN, or FAX to (212) 944-9055.
DESCRIPTION: Portrays several patients with Alzheimer's Disease in various stages of the disease process. Stresses specific interventions nurses might use to deal with common problems. Presents demographic and diagnostic background information.

Sonia
Running time: 53 minutes
Purchase: $350
Rental: $70
To order: AJN Company, 555 West 57th St., New York, NY, 10019, Attn: Interactive Video Dept., or call 1-800-CALL-AJN, or FAX to (212) 944-9055.
DESCRIPTION: A dramatic yet tender video about Alzheimer's Disease and the fragility of human existence. Sonia is a 58-year-old woman who experiences memory lapses that increase and are accompanied by confusion, irritability, and agitation. An excellent discussion tool on Alzheimer's Disease, its course, and means of coping.

Chapter 18

Disorders of Childhood and Adolescence

Critical Thinking Questions

1. Research and discuss the Roger O. case. As a consequence of this case, persons as young as ten years of age cannot be detained against their will if they are found to be competent. Previously, it was possible for parents to hospitalize minors simply because they were management or discipline problems in their homes. What, then, should be done to address the problem of the difficult-to-manage child or adolescent? (Education, family therapy, environmental adjustment are possibilities.)

2. How are the changing composition of the American family and the social pressures on the single parent affecting child mental health? How is society attempting to "fix" the problems of children born to single mothers on welfare, fathers who abandon their children, drug addicted mothers, etc? What do you think will be the effects of these proposed solutions on the children involved?

3. What are some of the characteristic concerns and behaviors of the adolescent developmental stage? What conflicts do these present for the adolescent, and what maladaptive responses may arise?

Enrichment Activities

1. Just as there are Residential Treatment Centers (RTC) for Adolescents (See enrichment activities, chapter 8), there are also facilities for children who are not able to live at home, or whose parents have deserted them. The staff makes every attempt to socialize the children to living in the community, in foster care situations. A students' visit to a center for emotionally disturbed children, particularly around the time of a holiday such as Christmas or Hanukkah, can be rewarding for both the children and the students. Have the students visit different centers and report on the festivities—a caroling trip is suggested.

2. Clinical assignment to a children's unit is usually a sought after experience for students. Because of the assistance of the students, the children or adolescents can be taken on outings. At Halloween, a trip to the pumpkin patch is enjoyable. For adolescents, consider an outing to a local nature park. Ask the students if they notice a difference in child or adolescent behavior when they are on an outing, as opposed to when they are on the unit. Do the clients try harder to control their behavior? Are they disappointed in themselves if they act out? Use this as an example to enforce the fact that mental illness really is not a condition that individuals can "snap out of"; their behavior may be out of their conscious control.

3. Nursing students can help the children who are in the school classroom on the unit. Their encouragement and one-on-one attention helps the child to build self-esteem. Have the students plan a teaching-learning activity with the children, with instructions as follows:
   a. Through observation, nursing students determine a learning need of a group of children. (For example, the children may need to learn the joy of giving and doing things for others.)
   b. Nursing students plan a project directed to this learning need. (For instance, the children could make paper flowers and decorate empty orange juice cans to put them in.) Students should consider the materials needed, time the project would take, and the arrangements necessary with staff. When finished, the children could be escorted to the older adult unit to give them to the clients.

c. Students write several behavioral objectives for the behavior expected by the children and the nursing students.
d. Students schedule the project with both the children's unit staff and the staff of the older adult unit.
e. After the project is completed, have the students write about the experience, describing the project, the rationale for the learning tool used ("flower vases"), the evaluation of the outcome, and what they might do differently "next time".

This experience is called teaching-learning, because not only do the children learn, but the nursing students are given the opportunity to both teach and learn!

Multimedia Resources

Audio/Visual

Detection and Treatment of Sexually Abused Children — Part 1 and Part 2
Running time: 28 minutes each
Purchase: $285 each
Rental: $70
To order: AJN Company, 555 West 57th St., New York, NY, 10019, Attn: Interactive Video Dept., or call 1-800-CALL-AJN, or FAX to (212) 944-9055.
DESCRIPTION: Part 1 defines sexual abuse and incest and shows nurses how to identify the physical and behavioral signs of abuse. Discusses basic assessment strategies in detail, along with appropriate nursing interventions. Part 2 explains the Accommodation Syndrome of child sexual abuse, which details common behaviors observed in victims. Describes the characteristic protective responses of such children. Features the nurse's role in encouraging victims to disclose sexual abuse and in protecting them from further trauma.

Chapter 19: Eating Disorders

Critical Thinking Questions

1. What are the societal pressures in the United States today that contribute to the emphasis on thinness? What is the ambivalent message being sent by the advertisers of various products? Describe the contradictory relationship between dieting and social activities. What connection is there with the high incidence of bulimia in women?

2. Identify some family patterns that may contribute to the development of anorexia nervosa. If an adolescent girl has strict, controlling parents, what can she control in her life?

   What is her relationship with the male members of the family?

   What is the level of self-esteem of the adolescent girl and the attitude of her family members toward her?

3. What are some of the personality characteristics attributed to the obese individual? Are these judgments based on sound evidence? What are the effects of rejection and stigmatization on the obese person?

Enrichment Activities

1. If nursing students live in a dormitory, discuss the importance of being on the alert for signs of bulimia. Sounds of gagging and smells of vomitus demand investigation, whatever the cause. A constant "sour smell" is a signal that someone may be suffering from an eating disorder. Report your observations and suspicions to the school nurse.

2. Have students attend a family group session for a client with anorexia. They should note the family dynamics, and report on the session to the class. Were there some problematic relationships among the family members? How did the therapist handle conflicts, the silent member of the group, and the authoritarian member? What "homework" was assigned to group members?

3. Have students attend a community support group such as Overeaters Anonymous or Weight Watchers. What is the difference in the philosophy of the two groups? Do all individuals who attend Weight Watchers believe that they have an *eating disorder*?

   What defense mechanisms do overweight persons use?

Multimedia Resources

Audio/Visual

Dying To Be Thin: Surviving Anorexia and Bulimia
Running time: 58 minutes
Purchase: $285
Rental: $70
To order: AJN Company, 555 West 57th St., New York, NY, 10019, Attn: Interactive Video Dept., or call 1-800-CALL-AJN, or FAX to (212) 944-9055.
DESCRIPTION: This tape explores the causes, symptoms, and dire results of anorexia and bulimia, the factors that contribute to their development, and reviews methods of detection, treatment, and prevention of these disorders.

Chapter 20

Sexual Disorders

Critical Thinking Questions

1. If a mental health professional has been accused of engaging in sexual misconduct with a client, what are the possible consequences for the professional? For the client? How reliable is the testimony of a mental health client? (For the professional, loss of license is a distinct possibility. For the client, psychological and social (family) damage is likely. Reliability is a large issue, dependent not only on the mental status of the client, but also often seen to be influenced by the client's gender, age, and ethnic background.)

2. Consider the various paraphilias described in the chapter. In your opinion, would any of these be considered normal sexual behavior? Would they be accepted in some cultures, but not in others? What potential physical or psychological harm to self or others originates with some form of sexual deviation?

3. What are some of the physiological causes of sexual dysfunction? What are some psychological factors involved? How would you answer a recovered heart attack victim who wants to know if he can engage in sexual intercourse, or if that activity will bring on another heart attack? What prescription medications may adversely affect sexual expression?

Enrichment Activities

1. Have a class discussion on the sexual revolution and the effects it has had on various age groups in society. Students who have watched Dr. Ruth Westheimer or other sex therapists on television can identify the common concerns of the public.

2. A type of discussion group that is useful for this chapter is the debate format. However, the strategy needs to be planned in advance, and some preparation must be done ahead of time. Have students plan a class debate on whether or not sex education should be taught in the fifth grade. (Average age of students is 10 to 11 years, early puberty.) Collect recent newspaper articles on this topic for rationale presented by persons on both sides of this issue. Divide the class in half, randomly, with two opposing teams in each half. Each team should have several presenters on the issue, with a rebuttal person who notes the arguments presented by the opposing team, and contradicts each point rationally, after both teams have presented. There will be two debates on the topic, one by each half of the class, so that while one half is presenting, the other half of the class will be observers (similar to a jury) who can offer critique and discussion points afterward. The topics for each half of the class can vary slightly. For example, one half of the class can argue the pros and cons of sex education in the fifth grade, and the other half of the class can discuss sex education in the tenth grade of high school (ages 15 to 16).

3. Seek out a local sex therapist, and ask him or her to your class to describe methods and results of sex therapy from his or her practice. If the school has honoraria for outside presenters, offer an honorarium. (If not, take the therapist to lunch.) Many therapists are interested in building up their practice, and realize that people have sexual problems they are often reluctant to share. Some of the students in the class may be struggling with this issue, or know of a friend or relative who is having difficulties, and will appreciate business cards that are distributed by the therapist to everyone in the class.

Chapter 21: Adjustment Disorders

Critical Thinking Questions

1. How does an adjustment disorder compare with the following: dysthymia, post-traumatic stress disorder, developmental disorder, a life crisis? Give specific examples of the distinguishing features of an adjustment disorder.

2. Why is knowledge of the various developmental theories so important in the assessment of clients who may be experiencing an adjustment disorder?

3. How do cultural, social, and psychological influence relate to adjustment disorders? How can nurses structure interview questions during the assessment phase that would address these influences?

4. How can nurses teach clients and their families or significant others to recognize symptoms of adjustment disorders and educate them about their roles in managing the treatment regimen? What about preventive practices?

Enrichment Activities

1. Have a class discussion on the implications of an adjustment disorder for persons who are not hospitalized and are not receiving treatment. Students may be able to draw from their own experiences or those of persons who are close to them. As a result of the student now being in the psychiatric mental health nursing class, friends and relatives may call upon them for help with these less serious but disturbing problems of adjustment. What symptoms are usually discussed with the helper? When would the student consider it necessary that the individual be referred for expert psychological or psychiatric help by a practitioner?

2. Relate the present economic conditions (downsizing, lack of opportunities for suitable employment, bankruptcy) to the possibility of an increase in adjustment disorders in the general public. How is it dangerous for individuals and for society if the economic problems or the adjustment problems are not addressed? Have a class discussion on this topic. Students can cite from newspaper articles about the effects of stressors on vulnerable individuals.

3. Students can be asked to list pros and cons on the issue of mandatory retirement at the age of 65. Despite the recent claim that a policy of mandatory retirement is unfair and discriminatory, employers often have many loopholes and strategies they can use to coerce employees to leave at age 65 or younger. What are some of these strategies? Why would an individual *not* want to, or not be able to retire at age 65 or younger? What are some problems that would occur if everyone were allowed to work as long as they wished? The instructor should look for and uncover misconceptions about aging, and hidden prejudices in this discussion.

Chapter 22: Interactive Therapies and Methods of Implementation

Critical Thinking Questions

1. How can nurses successfully develop therapeutic boundaries during nurse-client interactions, and why are well-defined boundaries so important in the therapeutic relationship?

2. What are several ways in which the nurse develops trust and safety with clients and significant others? How can trust and safety positively impact individual, group, family and milieu therapy?

3. What are some examples of transference and countertransference that can block the therapeutic process? What can nurses do to avoid or minimize this? Can such situations offer nurses insight into the therapeutic relationship? Explain how.

4. What are five examples of verbal techniques that can facilitate the therapeutic process? How can nonverbal gestures or responses positively impact the nurse-client interaction?

Enrichment Activities

1. Students should participate in open group meetings on the unit, such as community meetings, and ask permission to join other groups, such as process groups, or occupational therapy and recreation groups. There are often restrictions to attending ongoing therapy groups, because of the sensitive issues that are discussed there. The dynamics of the group change if new members are added, and an us-versus-them feeling can be generated if students try to enter a small group. If students are welcome to join a group, they should sit randomly in the room, not next to the therapist, who will prepare them in advance concerning contributions and responses that are appropriate in the meeting. There are treatment facilities that are fortunate to have one-way glass and speaker phone systems, which permit students to observe therapy groups without being seen or intervening in the process. Group participants are told they are being observed by nursing students who are learning therapeutic techniques. Following the group meeting, the therapist debriefs the students and answers any questions.

2. While on clinical rotation, students should plan and co-lead a group experience that will last for two or three sessions. Support groups, teaching-learning experiences, and community meetings are appropriate for this assignment. To prepare for the assignment, it is useful to have each student complete a co-leader's self-inventory, addressing the following concerns, which can then be discussed with the instructor:
   a. Explain how involvement in a group can be helpful to the individual client.
   b. List several expectations of what might happen in a group that you would be co-leading. Identify the best and worst things that could happen.
   c. Consider what is negotiable for you as a co-leader. What behaviors would you not tolerate in your partner? What would your expectations of your co-leader's behavior be?
   d. What would your typical responses to the following incidents be? Consider how an effective leader would handle these situations:
      i. Someone in the group is talking too much.
      ii. There is a long period of silence.
      iii. Someone begins to cry.
      iv. Clients begin to discuss sexual feelings about you or others.
      v. Clients are excessively polite; not willing to confront each other.
      vi. There is conflict in the group.
      vii. A client begins to verbally attack another client.
   e. What makes you most uncomfortable in a group?

Following each group session, each student should evaluate the results in terms of the goals that were set and whether or not they were achieved, their ability to handle situations that arose, and effectiveness in working with their co-leader. The instructor can fish-bowl the groups and later share with students an analysis of the group's dynamics, examples of how they handled unexpected occurrences and facilitated ongoing interactions, their application of theory, their demonstration of insight, and their cooperation with the co-leader. Were they able to see a change and some progress in the last session of the group as opposed to the first session?

3. If the clinical nursing specialist on the unit is conducting family therapy, or knows of someone who is doing that in the day treatment center, permission may be obtained for the student to fish-bowl one of these sessions. The dynamics are quite different from those observed in therapy groups on the unit, because of the uniqueness of each family and the long associations among the members. Patterns of communication that have been reinforced over the years, and may be not within the family's conscious awareness, can be seen by an objective individual such as the therapist or the observing student. Families are often in pain and unable to nurture each other, due to faulty communication patterns, and it is instructive for the students to see how the therapist facilitates nurturing behavior.

Chapter 23
Psychopharmacology and Other Biologic Therapies

Critical Thinking Questions

1. As a nurse in a psychiatric mental health facility what behaviors or situations require the use of antipsychotic medications? What are the therapeutic effects you would expect from those medications? What are possible non-therapeutic effects? What serious or adverse effects might occur?

2. How would you describe the behavior of a client who is expressing anticholinergic effects after being given initial doses of tricyclic antidepressant medications? When would you expect therapeutic results to occur?

3. What are several nursing interventions for clients experiencing adverse effects of psychiatric medications; e.g: anticholinergic, extrapyramidal, cardiovascular? What are some preventive measures? How can assessment questions be structured to reflect familial history of medication responses? How can this knowledge impact clients?

4. What are important aspects nurses need to consider for clients who are candidates for electroconvulsive therapy (ECT), e.g., historical data, physical considerations, communication and teaching techniques, treatment safety factors, post-ECT interventions and care?

5. How can nurses structure a course or class for clients and significant others that addresses their roles in medication administration and assessment? What types of teaching techniques would nurses include? What about handouts or articles? How would a nurse involve a pharmacologist in the class discussion? What useful information could the pharmacologist add to the course?

6. What criteria indicate that ECT is a treatment of choice for a particular client? What is the rationale for this criteria? Where are considered contraindications for ECT as a treatment alternative? What is the rationale for this? What is the nurse's role in ECT?

Enrichment Activities

1. While students are on the clinical unit, ask the hospital pharmacologist to explain and discuss the newer psychotropic medications with students. Textbooks contain information on the most commonly used medications and those that have been on the market for a longer period of time. However, the pharmacologist can enrich the student learning experience by introducing the newer medications or discussing the rationale for other indications for use, of commonly used substances.

2. Psychiatric mental health nurses are often the best persons to dispel the myths and fears of the general public about electroconvulsive therapy (ECT). Therefore, it is important for nursing students to observe a session of ECT, with the permission of the client, the attending physician, and the physician who will be administering the ECT. The physician administering will usually be quite willing to explain the procedure and its effects to students in the session. The students can be quite helpful and supportive to the client in the disorientation phase that occurs following treatment.

3. Using unlabeled colored picture cards, have the students identify the various commonly used psychotropic medications, indications for use, side effects, and nursing implications.

Chapter 24

Alternative Therapies

Critical Thinking Questions

1. What impact has the current trend toward alternative therapies had on the public's choices for health care?

2. Why are alternative therapies currently popular in the United States and Canada?

3. How does a person's philosophy of wellness and disease affect choices for health care?

4. What are the benefits of traditional medicine?

5. How do the benefits from acupuncture compare with the benefits from medications?

6. Why does pet therapy seem to be effective with hospitalized individuals?

7. What client teaching is necessary in traditional therapy? In alternative therapy?

8. How does the interaction of mind-body-spirit affect a person's actual and perceived well-being?

Enrichment Activities

1. Have students interview a practitioner of health care, using the same tool with questions that are prepared by students. This will necessitate discussion to determine questions that the group thinks are important. Health care practitioners may be selected from the following suggested list or from many other sources: nurse practitioners; hospice nurses; psychiatrists; homeopathic physicians; pharmacist in psychiatric settings; acupuncturists; biofeedback therapists.

Questions must be unbiased and focus on practitioner's opinions of both traditional and alternative therapy. Students will avoid giving their own opinions during interviews.

Sample questions include the following:
(1) If you have a choice between traditional and alternative therapy for yourself, which do you tend to choose?
(2) Why do you choose your answer in #1?
(3) What has influenced your preference in health care choices?
(4) What do you think the public's preference for health care will be in the year 2004?
(5) What are the pros and cons of traditional medicine and alternative therapy?

2. Have each student select an alternative therapy and arrange to observe a session between a therapist and a client. Report to the class in a scheduled period to educate rather than to change the opinions of others. By class consensus, opinions may or may not be voiced.

3. Interview clients who engage in alternative therapies. Report findings and clients' opinions to classmates in a scheduled time period.

Multimedia Resources

Alternative Medicine: Expanding Your Horizons
Description: Provides overview of several alternative methods of delivery of health care.
Running time: 29 minutes
Purchase: $179
To order: Insight Media, 2162 Broadway, PO Box 621, New York, NY 10024.
e-mail cs@insight-media.com
Internet www.insight-media.com

Why People Don't Heal and How They Can
Description: Challenges fundamental ideas about health and healing and addresses peoples confrontation with cultural obstacles to getting well.
Running time: 76 minutes
Purchase: $89
To order: Same as above. See Insight Media.

Alternative Medicine
Description: Discusses gradual integration of alternative therapies in America, and gives overview of several types of therapy.
Running time: 29 minutes
Purchase: $129
To order: Films for the Humanities and Sciences, PO Box 2053, Princeton, NJ 08543, or call 800-257-5126.
e-mail:custserv@films.com
Internet: http://www.films.com

Healing The Whole: The Promise of Holistic Medicine (NEW)
Description: Describes interplay between physical and psychological factors and discusses strategies from different disciplines for certain disorders.
Running time: 30 minutes
Purchase: $129 (may be rented)
To order: Same as above. See Films for the Humanities and Sciences.

Chapter 25

Crisis Intervention

Critical Thinking Questions

1. As a nurse in a community mental health center, how would you manage a homeless client who presents in a crisis situation? What initial assessment tools would be useful? Would you employ the generic or individual approach to this client? Why?

2. How would you recognize a client's or family's adaptive coping skills in a crisis situation? Which behaviors would reflect maladaptive coping responses? What steps would you take in promoting more effective coping methods? What is your rationale for this intervention?

3. How would you construct a brief course or class that teaches clients and families about the types of crises, the phases of a crisis, and steps that can be taken to reduce the impact of a crisis? What teaching techniques would be useful? Which teaching aids would you employ? What group of clients would be an appropriate audience?

4. What type of crisis is mental illness considered? How can a nurse minimize a client's response to such a crisis? What can be done to help families or significant others understand the pervasive impact of mental illness? How can they be helped to anticipate feelings about this crisis and work toward more therapeutic adaptive responses?

5. Why is crisis theory important for nurses and other health care givers to learn? How can it be applied to clients in a variety of health-threatening situations? How can it be used as a preventive measure? In what ways can it assist home care and community based nurses?

Enrichment Activities

1. Assign students to visit, individually or in pairs, the crisis intervention line (911) center. Students should find out who staffs these lines, what psychological characteristics are essential, and what training staff receives. Early in the training process, a supervisor will listen in on calls received by a trainee, and intervene if the trainee is hesitant or cannot handle the situation adequately. Allowing a student to listen in (but not intervene) can provide valuable insights on handling emergency situations. Students may decide to volunteer some of their time to the crisis line.

2. In some communities, there is an organization of empathic citizens that the police department will call in the event of a crisis, such as an automobile crash or other accident. One organization is called Helping Other People in Emergencies (HOPE). Individuals in the organization come to the scene of the accident and help those who have not been injured to cope with the emotions, make telephone calls, arrange for transportation from the scene of the accident, and follow up on support persons for continuing care. Students need to know of this valuable resource, and may want to join one of these organizations.

3. The American Red Cross offers valuable training to meet adventitious crises. When one occurs, all medical and nursing personnel, whether licensed or in the student stage, are needed. Have students contact the local chapter of the American Red Cross or the Salvation Army and state that they are available when a call for help is issued. On graduation, the Red Cross training is an essential, to meet the community service obligation that is incumbent on all nurses and physicians.

Multimedia Resources

Audio/Visual

Crisis Intervention: Families under Stress
Running time: 28 minutes
Purchase: $285
Rental: $70
To order: AJN Company, 555 West 57th St., New York, NY, 10019, Attn: Interactive Video Dept., or call 1-800-CALL-AJN, or FAX to (212) 944-9055.
DESCRIPTION: Outlines important supportive actions for staff nurses in acute care. Urges nurses to develop empathy by identifying what their needs would be if a member of their family was hospitalized. Stresses trusting in the staff, privacy, timely information, and hope as essential needs of the family under stress. Outlines steps of crisis intervention and illustrates successful and unsuccessful outcomes.

Chapter 26: Activity Therapies

Critical Thinking Questions

1. What are the goals of adjunct therapy for clients with mental and emotional disorders? How do the objectives of occupational therapy differ from those of recreation therapy?

2. What is the nurse's role in managing clients who are involved in adjunct therapy activities facilitated by an occupational therapist, a recreation therapist, and a therapist specializing in art, music, and dance?

3. What important steps are taken by nurses who facilitate a task-oriented activity for a group of clients diagnosed with depression, mania, Alzheimer's disease, or schizophrenia? How would the nurse structure this activity to accommodate each group of clients?

4. What diagnostic group of clients would be more likely to benefit from occupational therapy versus recreation therapy during an acute phase of the disorder? Consider the structure of each therapeutic activity and their focus.

5. What diagnostic group of clients would benefit from psychodrama? Why? Which diagnostic group of clients are not appropriate for psychodrama? Why not?

Enrichment Activities

1. Poll the group of students to see who plays a musical instrument, and who has experience singing in a choir. Encourage students to arrange a participatory musical session with the clients, and discuss the results in the class afterward.

2. Occupational therapy is a useful modality to prepare chronically mentally ill clients for a day hospital or a sheltered workshop program. Students should be encouraged to visit the occupational therapy shop with clients. The students will learn how occupational therapy is used for diagnostic as well as therapeutic purposes. Student presence in occupational therapy will expose them to a valuable resource to assist the mentally ill, will encourage clients, and will build their self-esteem.

3. Students can aid depressed clients by helping them to plant a small garden of flowers or vegetables on the hospital grounds, or in flower pots in the client's room. Also, keeping and caring for a small animal or a tank of fish is therapeutic. It gives clients a sense of worth to be responsible for another living creature, and something positive to look forward to every day. Pets give unconditional love, and inspire hope for the future.

Chapter 27
Survivors of Family Violence

Critical Thinking Questions

1. What types of situations are categorized as violent? How does this impact the responsibility of nurses and other health care givers?

2. How would you intervene in a situation where spousal abuse was suspected involving a client in a mental health facility, in a psychiatric-home care situation, in a local community mental health center?

3. How would you respond to suspected child abuse as a nurse in a child and adolescent psychiatric facility? What steps would you take that complied with current statutes?

4. Can nurses and other health care workers offer information that would help communities understand situations such as domestic violence, incest, child neglect, and abuse? Why is this information so critical to families and communities?

5. How would you structure a course or class that discusses violent behavior patterns, etiologies of violence, influences of violence and methods of intervention? Include preventive strategies.

Enrichment Activities

1. Have students attend a parents anonymous presentation, to learn about factors which may indirectly incite violent behavior.

    Also, they should observe a parent effectiveness training program.

2. Schedule visits for students (a few at a time) to a shelter for battered women. Caution them that the location of these shelters is confidential, so that abusers do not gain access to them.

3. Invite an officer from the domestic violence division of the police department to talk to the class about his or her experiences. Every nurse, as a health professional, must report cases of suspected abuse or neglect. Have the officer review the state mandatory reporting law with the class: what to report, to whom, and when.

Multimedia Resources

Audio/Visual

Elder Abuse: A Family Secret
Running time: 28 minutes
Purchase: $285
Rental: $70
To order: AJN Company, 555 West 57th St., New York, NY, 10019, Attn: Interactive Video Dept., or call 1-800-CALL-AJN, or FAX to (212) 944-9055.
DESCRIPTION: The video focuses on the victims and on the various agencies designed to help them. Describes the conflict that arises when the abused elder rejects help for their physical and emotional pain and explains how their entrenched feelings of shame, love, and fear often immobilize them and perpetuate the "cycle of abuse."

Domestic Violence—Part 1 and 2
Running time: 56 minutes
Purchase: $285
Rental: $70
To order: AJN Company, 555 West 57th St., New York, NY, 10019, Attn: Interactive Video Dept., or call 1-800-CALL-AJN, or FAX to (212) 944-9055.
DESCRIPTION: This video defines domestic violence and describes methods of nursing intervention. Part I explains and defines domestic violence in detail and explores and clarifies realities and myths. Part 2 gives additional facts and focuses on methods of helping the victim and the family.

Understanding and Treating the Rape Victim
Running time: 60 minutes
Purchase: $285
Rental: $70
To order: AJN Company, 555 West 57th St., New York, NY, 10019, Attn: Interactive Video Dept., or call 1-800-CALL-AJN, or FAX to (212) 944-9055.
DESCRIPTION: Guidelines for managing the rape victim admitted to an emergency unit are presented. The emphasis of the program is on the nurse's role in treating and documenting injuries sustained in the attack, collecting evidence of recent sexual intercourse, and assessing the victim's degree of acute stress reaction or rape trauma syndrome. One video, two parts.

Child Abuse
Running time: 28 minutes
Purchase: $285
Rental: $70
To order: AJN Company, 555 West 57th St., New York, NY, 10019, Attn: Interactive Video Dept., or call 1-800-CALL-AJN, or FAX to (212) 944-9055.
DESCRIPTION: Emphasizes the need to understand why child abuse and neglect occur. Focuses on prevention, detection, and management. Examines the nurse's role, the team approach, legal responsibilities, group support, and therapeutic programs.

Focus on Women: Childhood Legacy
Running time: 30 minutes
Purchase: $175
Rental: $50 for 10 days
To order: Concept Media Inc., PO Box 19542, Irvine, CA, 92713-9849, or call 1-800-233-7078, or FAX to (714) 660-0206.
DESCRIPTION: Discusses specific factors in a woman's past, especially the influence of childhood environment and the relationship with parents, which negatively affect her emotional status and make it difficult for her to function effectively and achieve success and happiness in adult relationships. Issues include being placed in adult roles as children, sexual abuse, and family and societal factors which make it difficult to identify and express feelings.

In Our Best Interest: Part I
Running time: Approximately 65 minutes
Purchase: $200
To order: National Training Project, 206 West Fourth St., Duluth, MN, 55806, or call (218) 722-2781.
DESCRIPTION: Thirteen, three- to five-minute scenes depicting a batterer using one or more abusive tactics on the Power and Control Wheel against his partner. A manual is included ($20) that facilitates the use of the themes used in the video. Poster of the Power and Control Wheel are also available ($6), as well as Audio Cassettes ($6 each).

In Our Best Interest: Part II
Running time: Approximately 1$^{1}/_{2}$ hours
Purchase: $60
To order: National Training Project, 206 West Fourth St., Duluth, MN, 55806, or call (218) 722-2781.
DESCRIPTION: Four, 20- to 25-minute lectures including Tactics of batterers, cultural facilitators of battering, "Why do I feel crazy," and women's rage. The manual, Process for Personal and Social Changes, is a facilitator ($20).

A Matter of Culture
Running time: 17 minutes
Purchase: $25
To order: National Training Project, 206 West Fourth St., Duluth, MN, 55806, or call (218) 722-2781.
DESCRIPTION: The video examines the nature of violence in society by looking at seven men and women whose victimizations appeared to be individual but were, in fact, interconnected. It encourages the viewer to participate in creating a culture based on life-sustaining and nurturing values.

The Duluth Curriculum for Facilitating Men's Groups Power and Control: Tactics of Men Who Batter 1 and 2, and Using the Control Log
Purchase: $550 for entire series
To order: National Training Project, 206 West Fourth St., Duluth, MN 55806, or call (218) 722-2781.
DESCRIPTION: The first video depicts abusive tactics used by abusers against their partners. A book is included along with a facilitator handbook ($29). The second video is a woman's perspective and features six formerly battered women who discuss how each tactic on the Power and Control Wheel was used against them and the impact of their abuse on their children, their relationships, and themselves. The third video, using the Control Log, is an edited video of a men's group in Duluth. This video is used for training facilitators on the use of the Control Log.

The Rites of Violence
Running time: 23 minutes
Purchase: $85
To Order: National Training Project, 206 West Fourth St., Duluth, MN, 55806, or call (218) 722-2781.
DESCRIPTION: A documentary shows the policies and procedures guiding the intervention of domestic assault cases by police, jailers, probation officers, judges, counselors, shelter workers, and the Duluth Domestic Abuse Intervention Project. A dramatization shows the handling of cases in the Duluth system.

Chapter 28: Suicide

Critical Thinking Questions

1. How are such factors as age, gender, ethnicity, etc., related to suicidality, and what are other key factors that can determine suicidal behaviors?

2. What critical steps are involved in conducting a suicide assessment for clients experiencing depression? What key responses should the nurse consider as prerequisites for suicidal precautions that provide safety for clients?

3. What are the key elements (risk factors) in the assessment of suicide risk, and how can nurses and other caregivers use preventive measures for clients who demonstrate these elements?

4. It is generally agreed that depression is the single best indicator of suicidal risk; but what are some other disorders that are known to contribute to suicidal behaviors and why?

5. How would a nurse deal with a client who expressed suicidal ideation during a task oriented group activity? What would the nurse communicate to the client and to other group members? What is the rationale for the nurse's choice of interventions?

6. Can confidentiality be subject to certain considerations? For example, suppose a client reveals that he has AIDS? Or that she intends to commit suicide, in a specific, well-planned way?

Enrichment Activities

1. Acquaint students with the American Association of Suicidology, whose mission is to study predictors and effects of suicide. If they are interested in the topic as a professional pursuit, student memberships are available at greatly reduced rates. The association holds annual conferences. When the conference is held in a nearby location, encourage students to attend.

2. Students may be reluctant to assess suicide potential with direct interviewing techniques, since these seem invasive and are contrary to the usual nondirective approaches used in the therapeutic relationship. To desensitize students to using direct interviewing techniques, pair them and have them role play (reversing roles, also) the types of questions to ask:
   a. Are you thinking of hurting or killing yourself?
   b. How would you do that? Describe the details.
   c. When do you plan to do this?
   d. Is anyone else around at that time?
   e. Who do you usually talk to when you have a problem?

   Debrief students following this class exercise and ask them what difficulties they had in role playing the interviews.

3. Identify a community agency that supports the survivors who are victims of a suicide in the family or circle of close friends. Have students plan a visit to this support group, and share experiences with others in a subsequent class session.

Multimedia Resources

CAI Software

Care of the Suicidal Client
Purchase: $275
To order: Computerized Educational Systems, PO Box 536905, Orlando, FL, 32853-6905, or call 1-800-275-1474, or (407) 541-6230.
DESCRIPTION: This program lets you simulate care of the suicidal client, recognize selected clues indicating increased suicide risk, use a suicidal intention scale to assess suicide risk, select appropriate levels of suicide precautions, describe features of a therapeutic milieu for suicidal clients, apply the nursing process in the care of the client receiving tricyclic antidepressants, apply cognitive therapeutic interventions, and differentiate facts from myths about suicide. A posttest assesses understanding and documents competency.

Clinical Simulations in Nursing, Psychiatric Nursing Simulations I, 2/e
Purchase: $150 each or $450 for set of four units
To order: Medi-Sim/Williams and Wilkins, Electronic Media Division, 428 E. Preston St., Baltimore, MD, 21202, or call 1-800-527-5597, or (410) 528-4223.
DESCRIPTION: Five units cover a suicidal adolescent, a chronic patient, a patient with psychosis and mania and a patient with pain and anxiety. You select how to interact, how to assess, and how to help the patient cope.

Chapter 29: Grief and Loss

Critical Thinking Questions

1. What are some important assessment skills that would assist the nurse in determining a client's response to grief or loss? Which responses would suggest the need for more in-depth interventions? Why?

2. How would you assist survivors to go through the grief work that is part of the grief process? Why is grief work so critical to the grief process? What are factors that could complicate or inhibit grief work?

3. How might you use your own grief experiences to assist clients and families experiencing grief without blurring boundaries between you and them? Why is it so important to remain objective while still conveying empathy?

4. As a nurse, how can you assess a grieving client's need for spiritual guidance during the grief process? What steps would you take to offer such assistance? What would your options be in a hospital situation, a home care setting, or a community agency?

5. How would you facilitate a group of day treatment clients who are experiencing various stages of grief and loss? How would your focus differ with clients experiencing chronic sorrow? What major points would you cover for each group? What would be your short term goals for each group? How would client's age, past grieving experiences and value-belief system impact their responses in the group discussion?

Enrichment Activities

1. Have students identify and visit local support groups for families who have suffered loss of a member through death. (A hospice group is a possibility.) Look for examples of supportive help through sharing, extending offers of tangible help, and togetherness. Did all members of the group participate? What physical and psychological behaviors were helpful in the group? Have students report to the class on these experiences.

2. Suggest to students that they help a grieving person or family they know to develop an album biography of the deceased member's life, to help with grief work and affect closure. The album could include pictures of the deceased with family and friends, letters written to or by the deceased, notes from friends on hearing of the death, newspaper clippings, school or college yearbooks—whatever fits the individual situation. Encourage the family to talk about the things the deceased person did to make the lives of others more enjoyable. Help them express anger at the fate that deprived them of their loved one. Use touch and hugs when appropriate, and do not be afraid to show your own sadness. This helping process is best timed for a month or two after the death, when others have said their condolences and gone on their way.

   If the bereaved is a widow or widower, continue to invite him or her to social gatherings.

3. To understand what the experience of chronic ongoing grief means to parents, attend a support group for parents of Down syndrome children, or other mental retardation syndrome. The American Association for Retarded Children and Adults hosts support meetings, Special Olympics, and other events for families with a retarded member.

Multimedia Resources

Audio/Visual

A Child Dies
Running time: 28 minutes
Purchase: $275
Rental: $60
To order: AJN Company, 555 West 57th St., New York, NY, 10019, Attn: Interactive Video Dept., or call 1-800-CALL-AJN, or FAX to (212) 944-9055.
DESCRIPTION: Designed to inform and fortify nursing staff and students to meet the challenge of supporting a family after the death of a child. Describes the common feelings, stages, and many forms of grief. Stresses the importance of allowing clients to express themselves completely as part of the healing process.

The Grieving Family
Running time: 28 minutes
Purchase: $275
Rental: $60
To order: AJN Company, 555 West 57th St., New York, NY, 10019, Attn: Interactive Video Dept., or call 1-800-CALL-AJN, or FAX to (212) 944-9055.
DESCRIPTION: Gives nurses a checklist of actions they can take to aid a family grieving the death of a child; help parents and siblings find ways to say good-bye, arrange for the funeral, resolve decisions brought on by the crisis, and how to give each other support. Urges nurses to prepare by striving for self-awareness and competence in managing their own feelings.

Letting Go
Running time: 29 minutes
Purchase: $285
Rental: $70
To order: AJN Company, 555 West 57th St., New York, NY, 10019, Attn: Interactive Video Dept., or call 1-800-CALL-AJN, or FAX to (212) 944-9055.
DESCRIPTION: This video shares the experiences of parents and nurses who have lived through the death of a child. The child's point of view is shown, offering the opportunity to understand the child's feelings which may be very different from the adults.

Interactive Video

Bereavement Counseling: Theoretical and Clinical Perspectives— Part I and 2
Purchase: $1,195 each
To order: AJN Company, 555 West 57th St., New York, NY, 10019, Attn: Interactive Video Dept., or call 1-800-CALL-AJN, or FAX to (212) 944-9055.
DESCRIPTION: Bereavement Issues' Part 1, provides background information and experiential preparation essential to bereavement counseling. Part 2 teaches support strategies that span the course of the grief process. A reference book section provides a bibliography, glossary of terms, review of concepts, and a listing of organizations and groups providing bereavement assistance.

Chapter 30

Persons With HIV/AIDS

Critical Thinking Questions

1. What are the physical and psychosocial needs of clients experiencing the HIV virus or AIDS? What are the needs of their families and significant others? How can crisis theory be useful in these situations? How can the nurse use grief and loss theory to help these clients and their loved ones?

2. How does the nurse's role interact with public health officials regarding clients' initial diagnosis of AIDS or HIV virus? Why is this a critical public health threat? What are the implications of non-reporting to the Public Health Department?

3. Knowing how HIV/AIDS is contracted, how can nurses prepare themselves as agents who help prevent this life-threatening disease from occurring or being transmitted to others? What precautions can nurses and other health care workers take to protect themselves against the threat of AIDS?

4. How would you develop a course or class for clients, families and students that addresses HIV and AIDS? How would you select an appropriate audience for this course? What would be your course objectives, teaching techniques, and audio-visual equipment?

5. As a nurse working with clients with HIV or AIDS, how would you use self-talk strategies to manage your own feelings, fears and self-doubts? How would you help other co-workers deal with their feelings and emotions? How could you help separate myth from reality regarding AIDS transmission?

Enrichment Activities

1. A class exercise to help the students assess their attitudes and beliefs about persons with AIDS follows. After completing the anonymous questionnaire, the instructor collects the papers and uses them as a discussion vehicle to clarify misperceptions, and to help students assume a more open-minded stance on HIV-related diagnoses. How are attitudes and beliefs likely to effect the plan of care for a client with AIDS? Students should check only one answer for each item.

   a. A nurse should have the right to refuse to care for an AIDS client.

Strongly Agree	Agree	Disagree	Strongly Disagree
____	____	____	____

   b. It is difficult to understand why people persist in homosexual behaviors when they realize the connection with AIDS.

Strongly Agree	Agree	Disagree	Strongly Disagree
____	____	____	____

   c. Transfusion recipients and children are the only innocent victims of AIDS.

Strongly Agree	Agree	Disagree	Strongly Disagree
____	____	____	____

   d. It is difficult to be empathic with IV drug users who get AIDS.

Strongly Agree	Agree	Disagree	Strongly Disagree
____	____	____	____

   e. Women do not usually get AIDS, unless their significant other infects them.

Strongly Agree	Agree	Disagree	Strongly Disagree
____	____	____	____

   f. Persons with an HIV positive diagnosis are certain to get AIDS within a year or two.

Strongly Agree	Agree	Disagree	Strongly Disagree
____	____	____	____

g. AIDS clients displaying dementia are the exception rather than the rule.

Strongly Agree	Agree	Disagree	Strongly Disagree
___	___	___	___

h. There is no relationship between AIDS and malignancy.

Strongly Agree	Agree	Disagree	Strongly Disagree
___	___	___	___

i. There is no treatment available for babies who are born HIV positive.

Strongly Agree	Agree	Disagree	Strongly Disagree
___	___	___	___

j. Persons who are at risk for HIV usually go for testing as soon as possible.

Strongly Agree	Agree	Disagree	Strongly Disagree
___	___	___	___

2. Discuss the shock, disillusionment, and anticipatory grief usually suffered by families and victims of AIDS. What are some ways nurses can help to preserve the social networks needed at this time? How can nurses help the client to maintain some control over quality of life and cope with physical decline? Are some sublimation activities available for the client to avert hopelessness and boost self-esteem? What precautions must be observed in treating the physical manifestations of the illness?

3. Invite a community psychiatric-mental health nurse who is caring for clients with AIDS in the community to talk to the class about his or her caseload and the therapies and precautions which must be addressed. What is the role of the pharmaceutical company, and how does it interface with the nursing role? What self-help and supportive groups are available for the client?

Multimedia Resources

Audio/Visual

AIDS: Caring for the Caregiver
Running time: 28 minutes
Purchase: $285
Rental: $70
To order: AJN Company, 555 West 57th St., New York, NY, 10019, Attn: Interactive Video Dept., or call 1-800-CALL-AJN, or FAX to (212) 944-9055.
DESCRIPTION: Explores the psychosocial stressors which affect the caregiver of patients with AIDS. Creative coping strategies to promote growth and ensure optimal patient care are presented.

AIDS and the Health Care Provider
Running time: 19 minutes
Purchase: $250
Rental: $60
To order: AJN Company, 555 West 57th St., New York, NY, 10019, Attn: Interactive Video Dept., or call 1-800-CALL-AJN, or FAX to (212) 944-9055.
DESCRIPTION: Reduces fear about AIDS, which can interfere with and prevent appropriate patient care. Clarifies the recommended precautions from the CDC. Provides personal perspectives.

Now That You Know: Living Healthy with HIV (4 videos)
Purchase: $50
Rental: $50 for 10 days
To order: Concept Media Inc., PO Box 19542, Irvine, CA, 92713-9849, or call 1-800-233-7078, or FAX to (714) 660-0206.

Coping with the News
Running time: 49 minutes
DESCRIPTION: Takes the viewer from receiving notice of a positive HIV status to developing a support system. The program reveals a range of shared feelings and behaviors while offering the viewer some very practical ways of moving through the initial stage of discovery.

Understanding HIV
Running time: 34 minutes
DESCRIPTION: Designed to give the viewer an understanding of how the virus works and how to monitor one's own health. The program explores the emotional, as well as the practical aspects of taking care of one's health.

Lifestyle Choices and Changes
Running time: 51 minutes
DESCRIPTION: Explores how the viewer can maintain good health both physically and emotionally by examining one's current lifestyle and deciding what changes to make. Offers insight into how and why people have made such changes and the significance to them.

Understanding Treatment
Running time: 63 minutes
DESCRIPTION: Designed for those experiencing symptoms. Discusses the full range of symptoms, opportunistic infections, and the treatments currently available.

HIV+/AIDS: The Facts and the Future
3-Modules series
Purchase: $325 or $139 each Individual Module
Participant Manuals: $29.95 each
AIDS Map: $.65 each
To order: Mosby Great Performance, Order Dept., 11830 Westline Industrial Dr., St. Louis, MO, 63146, or call 1-800-433-3803, or FAX 800-535-9935.
DESCRIPTION: The three Modules include: Overcoming Fear, Disease Overview, and Protecting Yourself. The series explores the special needs of patients with AIDS and addresses the skills and attitudes required to interact with AIDS patients safely and compassionately. The Documentary-style video covers the course of the disease and psychological, emotional, ethical, and legal issues. Participative classroom exercises and activities reinforce key concepts. Detailed teaching guides ease the instructor's task. These teaching and learning tools comply with OSHA guidelines and Joint Commission and RN relicensure requirements.

Facing AIDS: Stories of Health Care Workers
Running time: 28 minutes
Purchase $175 (NLN member's price: $157.50)
Rental: $100 for 10 days
To order: Customer Service, Publications/Video Order Unit, National League for Nursing, 350 Hudson St., New York, NY, 10014, or call 1-800-669-9656, ext. 138, or FAX to (212) 989-3710.
DESCRIPTION: This provocative documentary features interviews that are candid, allowing for a fresh understanding of the impact of HIV and AIDS in the workplace. Includes free 20-page Video Discussion Guide with current information on HIV/AIDS and tuberculosis.

HIV/AIDS: The Facts and the Future, Parts I, II, and III
To order: Pat Newman, Mosby, Inc., 11830 Westline Industrial Dr., St. Louis, MO, 63146-9934, or call 1-800-426-4545, or FAX to 1-800-535-9935.
DESCRIPTION: This complete series comes with OSHA, JCAHO, and RN relicensure requirements and is perfect for any health care worker who requires HIV/AIDS education. Part I — Overcoming Fear; Part II — Disease Overview; Part III — Protecting Yourself and the Patient. Also includes Instructor's Manual and 12 transparencies (sold separately).

Chapter 31

Psychologic Aspects of Physiologic Illness

Critical Thinking Questions

1. What is meant by the mind-body connection and how does it affect wellness, health promotion and illness?

2. Why is "hardiness" such an important quality in preventing illness resulting from the mind-body relationship?

3. What is the definition of "holistic" health care and its emphasis on health, wellness, and illness prevention? What are your thoughts regarding "holistic" health care practices?

4. How does a client manifest behaviors that reflect a "sick role", based on society's expectations? What is the nurse's role in helping both the client and society?

Enrichment Activities

1. Have students consider the relationship between stress and physical illness. Assign small groups to examine a particular physiological condition that is related to a personality type: migraine headache, asthma, hypertension, skin conditions, cardiac disease, etc. Ask each group to construct a chart of stressful situations that might possibly trigger a physiological reaction in the client having a tendency to react in a certain way to stressors. Rationales should be included.

2. Using small groups of students, have them focus on a specific environment—home, school, workplace, or neighborhood—and list the potential stressors and environmental hazards in that environment. This will raise the awareness level of the students to recognize the potential triggers of psychophysiological illnesses. Student groups will report their results to the class for discussion.

3. Pair students for a role-playing situation in which one student role-plays a client with a physical condition who is having psychological difficulty with adjustment to the disease. The other student will play the psychiatric mental health nurse who is approached by the client for help in the situation. For example, one student role-plays the client who has had a colostomy six months ago and is having difficulty coping in social relationships. Or, a student could role-play the wheelchair bound individual with a recent leg amputation, whose friends are having problems relating to him as they usually did. After the role-plays, the class will discuss ways to help these clients, friends, and significant others to adjust.

Multimedia Resources

Audio/Visual

Mental Health in Nursing: Caring for Body and Mind
Running time: 28 minutes
Purchase: $250 (NLN member's price: $225)
Rental: $100 for 10 days
To order: Customer Service, Publications/Video Order Unit, National League for Nursing, 350 Hudson St., New York, NY 10014, or call 1-800-669-9656, ext. 138, or FAX to (212) 989-3710.
DESCRIPTION: This program begins with a curriculum discussion for faculty where leading nurse educators debate a range of issues, including whether mental health should be integrated throughout the curriculum and how to overcome negative attitudes toward the mentally ill. It explores the delicate balance between mind and body and highlights innovative mental health treatment models.

Chapter 32

Persons With Chronic Mental Illness

Critical Thinking Questions

1. What are three major psychosocial problems demonstrated by clients with chronic mental illness that impact the clients, their families and the community? How can nurses help manage these problems?

2. How do the behaviors commonly manifested by clients with chronic mental illness interrupt their ability to function autonomously as family or community members? How can nurses assist families and communities to understand?

3. How does the process of institutionalization affect clients with chronic mental illness as compared to brief acute care or more infrequent mental health treatment? What are your thoughts on these different approaches?

4. What behaviors are exhibited by young adults with chronic mental illness that result in severe, overt pathology. How is pathology expressed by these young clients? How can nurses intervene?

5. Mental illness is one of the most costly health conditions one can have. How should priorities for spending the health care dollar be set? Should one consider the possibility of whether or not the health condition is curable? Remediable? Fatal? How do such variables as age, gender, income, etc. fit into the picture? If there was a choice between building a half-way house or fixing the streets in *your* neighborhood, what would you choose? What might your neighbors choose?

Enrichment Activities

1. Divide the class into several small groups (3 to 4 persons), and have each group design a plan for a client with a chronic mental illness, who will be returning to the community. (Leave the choice and description of the illness up to each group.) What functional goals can be set with the client? How will socialization be accomplished? Who will be the client's support persons in the community, and where will the client go for follow-up care, medication monitoring, etc.? Set a time for each group to report out to the class, and combine unique aspects of each separate plan into one major plan for a discharged client with chronic mental illness.

2. Arrange a class visit to a state hospital for the chronically mentally ill who are unable to live in the community. How do clients in that environment differ from the clients seen in acute care and private hospital situations? What factors in the environment contribute to the depersonalization and institutionalization of the chronically mentally ill? Does the large state institution seem to have a culture of its own?

3. Invite a nurse from a long-term care facility, such as a hospital for the chronically mentally ill clients, to talk to the class regarding:
   a. his or her reasons for choosing the challenging clientele,
   b. changes seen in the past several years in the treatment and prognosis of the chronically mentally ill,
   c. frustrations and rewards in working with the chronically mentally ill, and
   d. expectations of society for the client with chronic mental illness.

This presentation can be followed by a thoughtful review of the concepts of stigma, the role of family and society in the development of chronicity, and the recent advances in medical science potentially affecting prognosis in mental illness.

Multimedia Resources

Audio/Visual

The Homeless Mentally Ill
Running time: 28 minutes
Purchase: $285
Rental: $70
To order: AJN Company, 555 West 57th St., New York, NY, 10019, Attn: Interactive Video Dept., or call 1-800-CALL-AJN, or FAX to (212) 944-9055.
DESCRIPTION: Focuses on the third of the homeless population that is mentally ill. Portrays typical behaviors and symptoms of hallucinations, delusions, depression, and mania. It illustrates efforts of local clinics and hospitals to solve the problem through transitional programs such as three-quarter or halfway houses and city support services.

Chapter 33

Community Psychiatric Mental Health Nursing

Critical Thinking Questions

1. How can psychiatric home care meet the needs of mentally ill clients who do not qualify for inpatient care or partial hospitalization programs? What roles can nurses play in psychiatric home care?

2. What is the role of case management on an interdisciplinary level in psychiatric home care or community based programs? How can the disciplines best work together to serve these clients?

3. What are the roles of family members and significant others in managing the home care environment for mentally ill clients? How can these roles be expanded?

4. How can local community centers help meet the special needs of clients with psychiatric diagnoses and their loved ones? How can their services be improved?

Enrichment Activities

1. The Veterans Administration has an outreach program in which teams comprised of an advanced practice nurse and a psychiatric social worker go into the community, locate mentally ill homeless veterans, and offer them treatment and other types of tangible help. It is possible to offer students the experience of going with these professionals for one clinical day, for first-hand knowledge psychiatric-mental health nursing practice.

2. Have students visit a community mental health agency that is run as a follow-up clinic. They can then report to the class on the goals and functions of the agency, the population served, strengths and limitations of the service, role of nursing in the agency, and how clients are referred to the service. If they or a member of their family needed the service, would they feel comfortable using it?

3. Contact an agency in the community that supplies psychiatric mental health nurses who make visits to the clients' homes. If possible, arrange to have a nursing student assigned to go with the nurse to a client's home. Students should report to the class on the educational preparation and psychiatric mental health experience of the nurse. What services does the nurse provide? (Physical and psychological assessment? Individual and family service?) What are some problems the nurse has encountered? Is there collaborative nurse/physician practice?

Multimedia Resources

Audio/Visual

Patient and Care Giver Education in the Home: Teaching Techniques for Home Health Nurses
Running time: 25 minutes
Purchase: $195
Rental: $70
To order: AJN Company, 555 West 57th St., New York, NY, 10019, Attn: Interactive Video Dept., or call 1-800-CALL-AJN, or FAX to (212) 944-9055.
DESCRIPTION: Actual demonstrations, filmed in a patient's home, portray a variety of teaching techniques. Cognitive, affective, and psychomotor learning are discussed. Stresses the importance of communication between health team members regarding the patient's learning progress, requirements for teaching plans, and reimbursement.

Home Health Nursing: Nursing Diagnosis in the Home Health Setting
Running time: 40 minutes
Purchase: $195
Rental: $70
To order: AJN Company, 555 West 57th St., New York, NY, 10019, Attn: Interactive Video Dept., or call 1-800-CALL-AJN, or FAX to (212) 944-9055.
DESCRIPTION: An overview of the entire nursing process is reviewed in the context of an initial visit of a home health nurse to a patient's home. Topics covered include taking an accurate patient history, setting goals, performing a physical assessment, teaching the caregiver, and assessing the environment.

Coping with Feelings
Part of the Home Care Training Videos
Running time: 28 minutes
Purchase: $125 (NLN member's price: $112.50)
Rental: $60 for 10 days
To order: Customer Service, Publications/Video Order Unit, National League for Nursing, 350 Hudson St., New York, NY 10014, or call 1-800-669-9656, ext. 138, or FAX to (212) 989-3710.
DESCRIPTION: It covers differentiating between physiological and psychosocial needs, communicating effectively with patients, handling patient's feelings of helplessness and depression, and coping with feelings that patients and aides experience.

Chapter 34 Spirituality

Critical Thinking Questions

1. What critical concepts do nurses need to know concerning their views and biases about spirituality that would enhance their role in addressing the spiritual dimension of clients with mental disorders?

2. How can the nurse's awareness of each client's "stages of faith" help determine the client's spiritual needs and goals and result in effective nursing interventions? Stages of faith include the following:
   a. The impartial individual
   b. The institutional individual
   c. The individual seeker
   d. The integrated individual

3. What is the nurse's role in assisting the chaplain to address the spiritual needs of the following clients:
   a. The client experiencing guilt
   b. The client experiencing delusions
   c. The client experiencing hallucinations
   d. The client experiencing dementia

4. How does culture play a role in an individual's spirituality and value-belief system? How can cultural differences influence the client's view of mental illness and the nurse's spiritual assessment?

Enrichment Activities

1. Conduct a spiritual workshop for the nursing staff and other members of the mental health treatment team. Invite the chaplain to lead a discussion about the purpose and role of spiritual care for clients with psychiatric disorders. Discussion should include the following:
   a. Definitions of spirituality, religion, and faith
   b. Explanation of the spiritual dimension of individuals
   c. The stages of faith (see Chapter 34, Spirituality, for descriptions of the stages of faith)

2. Develop a spiritual assessment tool, individualizing each client's special spiritual needs and goals. Utilize the chaplain's background and knowledge in constructing the tool. (See Chapter 34, Spirituality, for an example of a spiritual assessment tool.)

3. Invite staff members of various cultures and spiritual beliefs to an interactive meeting that promotes a discussion about each person's culture and belief. Determine the differences and similarities among the different cultural groups. Relate these experiences to the role of the nurse in addressing the spiritual needs of the diverse patient population.

4. Identify the predominant cultures in your facility, and determine their spiritual needs and goals. Emerging majority cultures may include the following:
   a. African
   b. Asian
   c. Hispanic
   d. Native Americans

5. Introduce cultural competence classes in your facility, and discuss the spiritual and value-belief system of the predominant cultures in your community and mental health environment. Cultural competence education and training are currently mandated or strongly recommended by specific managed care organizations. Mental health nurses and other disciplines are encouraged to increase their awareness of the diverse cultures and spiritual beliefs of the patients who they serve, in order to provide quality and holistic care.

6. Invite the chaplain to treatment team meetings on a regular basis, and address the spiritual needs of the clients, with input from the nurses and other members of the multidisciplinary mental health team.
   a. Discuss the psychiatric diagnoses of each client and determine how the symptoms may affect the spiritual assessment. Identify spiritual interventions that would best meet client needs.
   b. Construct a spiritual assessment plan for each client who requires or requests spiritual care, and individualize special spiritual needs and goals.

Strategies for Teaching Psychiatric Mental Health Nursing

Preparing the Syllabus

A well-prepared syllabus is the students' best resource for understanding what the course will offer, what is expected of the students, and how they will be evaluated. Instruct the students to keep their syllabi for every course they take. Other educational institutions often rely on the contents of the course syllabus for evaluation of transfer credit or as a suitable preparation for graduate school.

Usually, a course in psychiatric mental health nursing will have two sections to the comprehensive syllabus. One section will contain the course outline and items related to the didactic portion of the course, while the other section will be related to the clinical experience in the particular agency to which the student is assigned. The enrichment activities section of this manual contains many suggestions for unique and reinforcing clinical experiences.

The clinical portion of the syllabus will specify clinical days and hours, location of the clinical facilities, and mandatory assignments to be completed while in clinical. These will probably include charting, journals, fieldwork activities, process recordings, care plans, mandatory inservice offerings, teaching-learning, and group work projects. There will also be an explanation of the policy of the agency as it relates to nursing students, the dress code, a section that identifies the interdisciplinary staff on the units, and the schedule of daily activities for the clients in the agency.

The comprehensive syllabus will have the name and location of the college or university, the division or department, the title of the course, the course number, and the semester and year. The placement level of the course, number of units assigned, and prerequisite or co-requisite courses should also appear. Most important is the course description, exactly as it appears in the school catalog. The name and credentials of the instructor(s), their office hours, and how they can be reached in an emergency must also be included. Furnish each clinical agency with a copy of the syllabus, so the staff will know what experiences the students are seeking.

The course outline will vary according to whether the course is a 5-week, 8-week, or a 16-week course. Suggested content for each structure is provided in this manual. With the sequential outline for each class topic, and each clinical day, the instructor should provide information concerning the topic to be covered, the assignments that are due on that date, and the reading that students are expected to do in preparation for class, or as a review of the material presented. A sample from a 5-week course outline is shown on page 62.

Note conscientious inclusion of important aspects of psychiatric mental health nursing that cannot be part of classroom lecture/discussion sessions due to the abbreviated nature of the course. The video demonstrates the relationship between physical and mental illness, and the paper the students are assigned to write necessitates brief research into the concept of anxiety. With careful planning, it will be possible to include concepts of mental health nursing, other than the major ones presented and discussed in class, in a succinct format.

Other themes in the syllabus are:
Learning objectives for each class
Teaching strategies you will use
Grading policy and how students will be evaluated
Required and recommended textbooks and other readings
Attendance policy, tardiness policy, and participation
Quality expected in written and oral presentations
Grading sheets to objectively record each criterion
Test policy
Appendixes, which may contain recent articles, handouts

Class	Day & Date	Lecture/Discussion Topic	Readings
6	Mon. 03/04	Ch. 13: *Mood Disorders: Depression and Mania* Discussion and Enrichment Activity I *Video:* Uncovering depression in the medically ill client **DUE: Paper on effects of anxiety**	Fortinash & Holoday-Worret, Ch. 13

Tests in the Course

For the undergraduate nursing student, either the mixed objective test or the multiple choice test is usually used. Unless the class is very large and the course is truncated, the mixed objective test is preferred. This test contains true/false, multiple choice, matching, completion, and possibly some short answer questions, such as "List three reasons . . ."

A small number of true/false questions at the beginning will enhance student confidence to continue with the test. Multiple choice is a format students are familiar with and is the type of question used on the state board examinations. Matching is a little more challenging, forcing students to make fine distinctions between concepts. Completion depends on recall memory, a little more difficult to summon than recognition memory. Finally, the short answer questions demand critical thinking responses.

Usually, course tests consist of a mid-term and a final, but there are good reasons for choosing another alternative. In the 5-week course, one does not have much choice, and the mid-term and final structure is usual, with about 75 questions in each, taking about an hour to complete.

In the 8-week course, one might try giving three exams, one at the end of the third week, one in the middle of week six, and one at the end of the course. The rationale is that such an arrangement allows the course to be absorbed in more manageable chunks: it reduces the anxiety about any particular exam; except for the final, exams fall on a date when the students are not also taking mid-terms in other subjects, and it provides both students and instructor with valuable feedback on students' ability and instructor's effectiveness in teaching the course, and on the quality and clarity of the test itself.

In the 16-week course, four tests could be scheduled. Of course, the more tests, the fewer questions needed per test, and the less time it will take for students to complete the test. To lower test-taking anxiety, see Enrichment Activity 1 for Chapter 12. If a student has extreme test-taking anxiety, two or three short, individual anxiety-reducing exercises supervised by the instructor may produce gratifying results. On one occasion, a student raised her average test-taking grades by a full GPA point!

In this same context, it is helpful to relieve the fear of the unknown by giving students a short, five- to ten-question multiple choice, ungraded "sample" test they can test themselves with. In addition, it is advisable to have several alternate forms of the same test, in case a student has to make up an examination because he or she was ill the day of the test. Finally, it is advisable to use a different form of the same test in other semesters.

Teaching the Course

Getting Students' Attention

Stage presence is the key to getting the attention of the class. Stage presence is the art of making your presence known to your audience, by announcing your arrival in clear, unequivocal terms. Stride to the front of the classroom, and announce "Good morning" with a smile. "I'm Dr. Jones, welcome to your first Psychiatric-Mental Health Nursing class." It helps if you are tall; tall people are viewed as being in command. However, if you are not tall, *think tall*, and you will be perceived as being taller than you are. Your self-esteem will show and invite others to use you as a role model.

Start by going over the day's agenda. It helps if you have arrived a few minutes early so you can have the agenda posted on the board. A timed agenda is recommended. This helps you and your class to track the ongoing activities—lecture, discussion, BREAK, exercises, demonstrations, video, etc. First, take care of any "housekeeping" details: attendance, distribution of hand-outs, general announcements, questions from students. Head the agenda with the title of the day's topic: for example, "Ethical and Legal Issues."

In a topic such as ethical and legal issues, students may be preconditioned to think of the subject as of little interest to them—they are in an ethical profession, but they are not lawyers. However, in today's malpractice-conscious society, it is important for every nurse to have a working knowledge of the law as it pertains to the mental health client, and as it pertains to the nurse as a part of the treatment team. Therefore, such a topic can challenge the instructor to generate and hold the interest of the class.

It is often useful to begin by relaxing the class, showing a humorous overhead transparency. Try to relate it closely to the topic of the day. If the topic concerns the move from hospital treatment to the community, use a "Drive-through brain surgery" transparency as the most ridiculous extension of the idea. To continue with the example of ethical and legal issues cited above, use the Johari window, and relate the different aspects of awareness to the ethical and legal problems individuals experience in their relations with one another. Why is the open domain the easiest to live with? Have the class cite from their own experiences how it felt when a confidence was violated (private domain), or how surprised he or she felt when the blind domain was exposed by another. Has anyone had the experience of stumbling into the closed domain—for example, finding out how one would react in an earthquake, by actually *experiencing* an earthquake? How might this domain figure in acts of violence?

Holding Students' Attention

The key to holding students' attention is variety. Keep your energy level high, and involve the students as you go, by approaching them and walking around the classroom when they are involved in a group activity. Plan out a timed agenda: lecture for 30 minutes, break into a group activity for 15 minutes, discuss and exchange what was accomplished in each group for 10 minutes, then revert to lecture again. Handouts that relate to the practices in *your* particular state are especially useful, since only general principles can be covered in the text, and practices differ from one region to another. For example, consider the child abuse reporting requirement. Although reporting is mandatory, each locality has a slightly different way of doing that.

Transparencies during lecture are a good way to emphasize important points, and serve as visual aids, avoiding "How do you spell that?" and "What was that again?" Transparencies allow you to move around and to avoid turning your back to the class. While chalkboards are useful for some exercises, like brainstorming for ideas, transparencies give immediacy to the lecture. Colored transparencies are particularly attention-getting. You can be creative and design your own transparencies, either black and white or colored, highlighting key points of the lecture. Be sure you use a large font, so the display can be seen from the back of the class. Be alert for cartoons that embody certain ideas, such as one which shows a physician telling a client, "You are making good progress, but of course a complete recovery depends on your insurance company." Mosby's Psychiatric Nursing Transparency Acetates, both first and second editions, are excellent sources for supplemental transparencies.

Multimedia. Interspersing lecture time with an audio-visual presentation is another way to hold class interest. There are many excellent videotapes and CAI materials on the market, which are annotated and discussed elsewhere in this manual. Videotapes are useful for classroom presentation, while CAI materials can be made available to students in the school library. Occasionally an audiotape, especially one which has been made by a psychiatric clinical nursing specialist, will have considerable teaching potential. The author is reminded of one made in her practice, in which the anonymous client, a functional man with schizophrenia living and working in the community, was retelling a particularly vivid hallucinatory experience. Students will have the opportunity to learn from persons with a variety of mental illness diagnoses, including individuals they may not encounter in institutions.

Discussion groups help students with active learning and critical thinking. A particularly engaging type of discussion group is the debate format. This strategy needs to be planned and prepared in advance. In the topic on sexual disorders, for instance, there are many issues that would be interesting to debate. The debate could take the form of the one described in the enrichment activities section for Chapter 20: Sexual Disorders. Or, in teaching legal-ethical issues, one side of the issue may argue that the "guilty but mentally ill" plea is not effective or is cruel and unusual punishment, because prisons are not suitable treatment centers for the mentally ill. The other side of the issue may argue that the plea decreases the number of insanity defense cases, in which the capacity of the accused to understand the wrongdoing is difficult to establish and justice may be thwarted.

The critical thinking section for each chapter in this manual presents critical thinking questions for each chapter of the text, which will help to keep student involvement high. In general, discussions work better when the class has had a chance to come together through one or two class sessions, to establish some trust, and to learn one another's names. But rapport can be instituted rapidly through the use of some ice-breaking techniques in the first lecture, as described below:

Have students count off by fours: 1, 2, 3, 4, 1, 2, 3, 4, etc. Ask the ones to pair with the threes, and the twos with the fours. This will prevent close friends, who sit near one another, from being paired. If there is a leftover person, pair with him or her. If not, use the next five minutes to check your lecture notes, etc. The instructions to the class are:

Starting with students one and two in the pairs, the student will introduce himself or herself to the partner, and tell of the "best day of my life" for the next two minutes. Call "Switch" at the end of the two minutes, and the other partner in the pair will go through the introduction and the "best day of my life."

After the second one in the pair has reported for two minutes, call "Time." Then each student will introduce his or her partner to the class and describe what the partner's best day was like. This exercise is not only fun and entertaining, but helps bring to awareness the importance of good listening skills, for psychiatric-mental health nursing. Make this connection for the class, and compliment them on their performance. Self-disclose to the students about your own "best day" too, of course.

Ideas for discussion can come from the students themselves, or they can be presented as brief case studies from the experiences of persons in the mental health field. Throughout the text, there are many case studies which make excellent discussion topics. The critical thinking questions in this manual are other examples.

Breaking the class into small groups of three or four persons for discussions promotes participation from all, and allows for whole class sharing and response. When forming groups, it is best to do it by the "counting off" method, to avoid the same persons always getting into the same group of close friends, and encouraging class members to get to know others as well.

Suggested Readings. Instructors usually have a reference inventory that they include with the syllabus, listing the most recent articles on particular topics, as well as classical works with which every student should be familiar. These suggested readings are excellent resources for students when they are assigned to write a paper on a special topic.

Classroom behavior. When giving a lecture, use gestures for emphasis, and do not let your voice lapse into a monotone. Be involved: smile frequently, use humorous anecdotes and ask for comments from students. Students learn better when the instructor enjoys teaching the class and demonstrates enthusiasm.

When fielding questions, ask "*What* questions do you have?" (using an open stance and a smile), rather than "Does anyone have a question?" Move toward the person asking a question, and reward the behavior by your presence or by verbally affirming, "Good question."

Letting the class know that there is interest in hearing from each individual, not only from those eager to speak, is paramount. Invite passive students to contribute: "What are your thoughts on that, John?" Controlling dominant individuals is also difficult, but can be managed by setting limits and enlisting their aid in involving other members of the class.

Since classes can vary in the length of time allocated to each, according to the master schedule, the instructor must be creative in varying the activities and allowing breaks. Monitor the time carefully to ensure that you cover the material intended. It is a good idea to let students know when break time occurs for the classes, because otherwise students get restless after an hour and a half to two hours into a long class, and may leave the room earlier. Break time can be negotiable, but inform students that the class continues immediately after the scheduled break ends. Explain to students why a certain number of minutes in each class session is mandatory under the conditions of accreditation of the program.

Closing the Class
A summary before closing the class is essential, especially when discussion has been a part of the learning experience. Students may work on developing structured notes during a lecture, but seldom understand how the main points of a discussion fit into the application of theory that the lecture has presented. Consequently, the instructor may either recount the main points of the discussion to the students, or have students identify the purpose of the discussion and link it to the concepts presented in the lecture. Paraphrase student comments to emphasize and reinforce their contributions. Have a different student report out each time there is a discussion period, to develop their presentation skills and to avoid the burden of group management falling to a few of the most capable.

There will be many times when not all of the material in the text gets covered in class. This is to be expected, and the students do need to take responsibility for their own learning. Reading all parts of the text, even those of lower priority than the parts dealt with in class, will add to and enrich the educational experience.

Suggestions for Behavior in the Clinical Setting

As explained in Chapter 2: Clinical Experiences: Rewards, Challenges, Solutions, new students are often uncomfortable with the idea that they will be having a clinical experience in a psychiatric hospital. They may fear being hurt, or hurting a client by saying "the wrong thing." Reassure them that you are there to help and support them, and that the staff and clients will welcome their arrival. Clients in the mental health system many times have been the victims of uncaring or heartless persons, and students' genuine expression of caring will attract them and enable the students to do therapeutic work. Express your own enthusiasm for working with the mentally ill, and indicate the rewards of this wonderful specialty in nursing.

Usually, what helps students most during their first days of clinical are concrete, practical directives they can count on. A few of these follow:

1. **At first, keep a low profile.** Observe, talk with the clients, and read their charts. Watch how staff works with them. Ask questions about tactics you do not understand in post-conference. What may seem like client abuse at first glance, may actually be a therapeutic maneuver. But do not take anything for granted, either. Client abuse rarely occurs in well-run institutions today, but it does happen, and questionable incidents need to be checked out with the instructor.

2. **Follow the care plan,** and work with the client as the care plan directs. Only by all care providers working together in the same direction, will progress be made. Develop your own method of keeping track of goals and interventions; some students keep a small pocket notebook. Your learning depends on your own effort.

3. **Treat clients with dignity and respect.** Realize that their way of thinking and doing things makes sense *to them*. You don't have to agree with their delusions, but you can respect their interaction with you, and express that although you know the client believes a certain way, you see things differently.

4. **Give clients their privacy.** Knock before entering, and ask permission to come into the room. If you need to clean out a client's locker or night stand, do it in his or her presence.

   Allow a client his or her personal space; remember personal space can be culturally determined.

5. **Be trustworthy.** Do not make promises you cannot fulfill. Many mentally ill persons have been betrayed, manipulated, or lied to. Explain inconveniences honestly, and admit your own errors if a mistake is made.

Also, some caveats—

1. **Don't take things personally.** Realize that you are "OK," and that the client may be trying to gain power over you by zeroing in on your real or imagined shortcomings.

2. **Don't get into a power struggle.** Think of creative ways you can encourage compliance with the treatment plan, without insisting rigidly that certain things must be done in only one way, and *now.*

3. **Don't try to become a client's personal friend.** This can be very hard to avoid, especially if the client is a small child, or a vulnerable adult who reminds you of someone you know and love (the counter-transference issue). Get help from your instructor if you find yourself wanting to adopt a child client, date an adult client, or invite a client to your home.

4. **Be careful about giving choices.** Instead of saying, "Do you want a piece of fruit?" (yes/no question), say, "Would you rather have an apple or an orange?"

5. **Don't assume a client can't accomplish things, or is stupid.** Slow responses may be a part of the client's symptoms, or the result of medication he or she is taking. Assume the client wants to be functional, like others. Give simple and direct instructions, and pitch in to help the client, giving praise for the effort made.

6. **Never give up on people.** Keep an open mind, and focus on the client's strengths. They are all they, and you, have to build upon. Focus on infinitesimal gains and encourage, encourage, encourage. Keep your eyes on the stars, and give yourself a pat on the back for a job well done.

Suggested Course Outlines

The following course outlines are provided as suggestions for adapting the book's chapters to courses of varying lengths. Suggestions are for a 5-week, an 8-week, and a 16-week course.

5-Week Course

Week 1
Chapter 1: Foundations of Psychiatric Mental Health Nursing
Chapter 3: Theoretic Perspectives

Week 2
Chapter 7: The Nursing Process
Chapter 8: Principles of Communication

Week 3
Chapter 23: Psychopharmacology and Other Biologic Therapies
Chapter 13: Mood Disorders: Depression and Mania

Week 4
Chapter 14: The Schizophrenias
Chapter 16: Substance-Related Disorders

Week 5
Chapter 17: Delirium, Dementia, and Amnestic and Other Cognitive Disorders
Chapter 18: Disorders of Childhood and Adolescence

8-Week Course

Week 1
Chapter 1: Foundations of Psychiatric Mental Health Nursing
Chapter 3: Theoretic Perspectives

Week 2
Chapter 6: Cultural Issues
Chapter 7: The Nursing Process

Week 3
Chapter 8: Principles of Communication
Chapter 12: Anxiety and Related Disorders

(Continued)

Week 4
Chapter 4: Psychobiology
Chapter 23: Psychopharmacology and Other Biologic Therapies
Chapter 13: Mood Disorders: Depression and Mania

Week 5
Chapter 14: The Schizophrenias
Chapter 16: Substance-Related Disorders

Week 6
Chapter 17: Delirium, Dementia, and Amnestic and Other Cognitive Disorders
Chapter 18: Disorders of Childhood and Adolescence

Week 7
Chapter 19: Eating Disorders
Chapter 25: Crisis Intervention

Week 8
Chapter 32: Persons With Chronic Mental Illness
Chapter 33: Community Mental Health and Home Care

16-Week Course

Week 1
Chapter 1: Foundations of Psychiatric Mental Health Nursing
Chapter 2: Clinical Experiences: Rewards, Challenges, and Solutions

Week 2
Chapter 6: Cultural Issues
Chapter 3: Theoretic Perspectives

Week 3
Chapter 5: Legal-Ethical Issues
Chapter 7: The Nursing Process

Week 4
Chapter 8: Principles of Communication
Chapter 9: Children and Adolescents

Week 5
Chapter 10: The Adult
Chapter 11: The Elderly

Week 6
Chapter 4: Psychobiology
Chapter 12: Anxiety and Related Disorders
Chapter 13: Mood Disorders: Depression and Mania

Week 7
Chapter 14: The Schizophrenias
Chapter 15: Personality Disorders

(Continued)

Week 8
Chapter 16: Substance-Related Disorders
Chapter 17: Delirium, Dementia, and Amnestic and Other Cognitive Disorders

Week 9
Chapter 18: Disorders of Childhood and Adolescence
Chapter 19: Eating Disorders

Week 10
Chapter 20: Sexual Disorders
Chapter 21: Adjustment Disorders

Week 11
Chapter 25: Crisis Intervention
Chapter 22: Interactive Therapies and Methods of Implementation
Chapter 24: Alternative Therapies

Week 12
Chapter 23: Psychopharmacology and Other Biologic Therapies
Chapter 26: Activity Therapies

Week 13
Chapter 27: Survivors of Family Violence
Chapter 28: Suicide

Week 14
Chapter 29: Grief and Loss
Chapter 30: Persons With HIV/AIDS

Week 15
Chapter 31: Psychologic Aspects of Physiologic Illness
Chapter 32: Persons With Chronic Mental Illness

Week 16
Chapter 33: Community Psychiatric Mental Health Nursing
Review of Course

Student Worksheets

Chapter 1

Foundations of Psychiatric Mental Health Nursing

Name _____

Briefly discuss the following questions.

1. Identify the five principles and guidelines for developing a nurse-client relationship.
   a.

   b.

   c.

   d.

   e.

2. Identify both the typical client responses and the nurse's role for each stage of the therapeutic relationship.
   a. Preorientation stage
      Client responses   Nurse's role

   b. Orientation stage
      Client responses   Nurse's role

   c. Working stage
      Client responses   Nurse's role

   d. Termination stage
      Client responses   Nurse's role

3. Read the signs of unhealthy boundaries listed in Box 1-6 in the text. Discuss five of these that might present a challenge to you in working with a client who is experiencing these signs of unhealthy boundaries.
   a.

   b.

   c.

   d.

   e.

4. Review the conscious and unconscious defense mechanisms listed in Box 1-1 and Box 1-8 in the text. View the film *Safe Passages,* and identify the defense mechanisms used by members of the Singer family as they respond to a crisis situation.

For items 5 to 14, identify the level of prevention described in Chapter 1 (primary, secondary, tertiary) by using the letters P, S, or T.

_____ 5. Participate in a program that identifies the elderly in the community, who are isolated.

_____ 6. Volunteer in the community center to help do crafts with children of working mothers, after school.

_____ 7. Form a discussion group on use of medications at home, with clients who are preparing for discharge from the psychiatric hospital.

_____ 8. Refer a new mother who reports feeling overwhelmed, to a stress reduction workshop.

_____ 9. Lead a group of student nurses to identify signs and symptoms and steps to intervene with college freshmen who are abusing drugs.

_____ 10. Assist a client and her family in the home, with a schedule to administer medications.

_____ 11. Teach parenting classes to pregnant women and their spouses.

_____ 12. Review skills for socialization and activities of daily living with clients who have chronic mental disorders.

_____ 13. Report an incident of child abuse to authorities.

_____ 14. Be the nurse in charge on a psychiatric intensive care unit in a hospital.

Chapter 2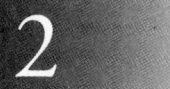

Clinical Experiences: Rewards, Challenges, and Solutions

Name _____

Critical Thinking Activity

Nurses who are helping clients cope with mental health/psychiatric issues will benefit from becoming aware of their responses to some typical situations that may arise and formulating an approach to these situations.

Read about each challenge in Chapter 2. Write about your thoughts and feelings concerning each challenge, then identify the approach you would plan to use if this situation were to arise during your nursing experience.

1. CHALLENGE: Fear of entering the psychiatric setting
   Self-awareness: What images do I have about the psychiatric patient? What are my major concerns about this clinical experience?

   Planned solution:

2. CHALLENGE: Performance inadequacy
   Self-awareness: What abilities do you feel confident in when caring for clients? Are you concerned that you will say the wrong thing in response to a client?

   Planned solution:

3. CHALLENGE: Concern over own mental health
   Self-awareness: What are your personal experiences with stress and mental illnesses?

   Planned solution:

4. **CHALLENGE:** Understanding the nurse's role in psychiatric/mental health practice
   Self-awareness: What do psychiatric nurses do? What is a psychiatric unit like?

   Planned solution:

5. **CHALLENGE:** Focus on client strengths versus client problems
   Self-awareness: How do you think you would be viewed if you were a client? Identify your own strengths and how these help you in a stressful situation.

   Planned solution:

6. **CHALLENGE:** Prioritizing nursing diagnoses and nursing interventions
   Self-awareness: What client problems are of a safety or health nature? What medical problems may be influencing the client situation?

   Planned solution:

7. **CHALLENGE:** Making inferences rather than observations
   Self-awareness: Are my interpretations of the client's behavior based on my personal opinions or my objective observations?

   Planned solution:

Chapter 3

Theoretic Perspectives

Name _____

Match each concept with its description.

_____ 1. cerebellum

_____ 2. extrapyramidal system

_____ 3. dopamine

_____ 4. hypothalamus

_____ 5. serotonin

_____ 6. synapse

_____ 7. gamma-aminobutyric acid (GABA)

_____ 8. peripheral nervous system

a. This is the area of contact between neurons where impulses cross.

b. This structure generates and coordinates emotion through the integration of endocrine and motor responses.

c. The staggering gait, clumsiness, and slurred speech of acute alcohol states are symptoms of malfunction in this structure.

d. It regulates stereotyped reflex movement of muscle tone and control of body movements, as in walking.

e. A build-up of concentrations of this increases the heart beat, raises blood pressure, and constricts key blood vessels.

f. It includes twelve pairs of cranial nerves and thirty-one pairs of spinal nerves and their branches.

g. This neurotransmitter is implicated in depression and sleep disturbances.

h. When an individual is anxious, it is thought that there is a change in balance between this inhibitory neurotransmitter and the excitatory transmitter acetylcholine.

Below is a list of procedures used to examine brain structure and activity. For items 9 to 14, select the best answer (abbreviation) from the list.

magnetic resonance imaging (MRI)
computerized tomography (CT)
brain electrical activity mapping (BEAM)
electroencephalography (EEG)
positron emission tomography (PET)
cerebral blood flow (CBF)

_____ 9. This examination identifies the metabolism of oxygen and glucose in the brain.

_____ 10. Slices or segments of the brain are revealed, allowing the complete study of brain structures and density.

_____ 11. This is a method of scanning physiologic and biochemical functions as they occur in live tissue.

_____ 12. The brain's electrical activity is monitored.

_____ 13. A radio frequency pulse is applied that results in an electronic signal yielding a superior image to those observed in CT scans.

_____ 14. A form of electrical activity mapping records spontaneous brain activity, and the data at each electrode site are categorized via spectral properties.

Chapter 4

Psychobiology

Name _____

Match each brain structure with its function.

_____ 1. axon

_____ 2. cerebrum

_____ 3. dendrite

_____ 4. sulcus

_____ 5. limbic system

_____ 6. hypothalamus

_____ 7. frontal lobe

_____ 8. corpus callosum

_____ 9. hippocampus

_____ 10. extrapyramidal system

a. Responsible for involuntary motor function

b. Bundles of matter; connects right and left sides of cerebrum

c. Shallow grooves in cerebrum between gyri

d. Responsible for memory, higher thought, judgment

e. Transmits signals from neuron cell body to other neurons

f. Part of neuron that collects incoming signals

g. Interacts between memories and reproduction of emotion

h. Regulates the basic human drives—hunger, sex, the sleep pattern, body temperature

i. Modulates instincts, drives, needs, emotions

j. Largest structure in the brain

Match the disorder with its implicated neurotransmitter.

_____ 11. Alzheimer's disease

_____ 12. anxiety disorders

_____ 13. schizophrenia

_____ 14. depression

a. dopamine

b. serotonin

c. GABA

d. acetylcholine

15. Name and describe two indicative anatomical changes that occur in the brain of a client with Alzheimer's disease.

16. Name the mental disorder associated with abnormal cortisol levels in the blood.

17. Students are aware that abnormalities in anatomy and/or physiology are implicated in mental disorders.
    a. Make a list of diagnostic studies that may aid in making diagnoses.
    b. Add a list of available current biological treatments for these disorders.
    c. Discuss students opinions of diagnostic methods, and biological treatments.

Chapter 5

Legal-Ethical Issues

Name _____

For items 1 to 7, select the answers from the list provided.

insanity
clear and convincing evidence
commitment
involuntary
competency to stand trial
privileged communication
permanent

liberal treatment
least restrictive alternative
emergency
duty to warn
informed consent
confidentiality
brief

1. Legally, _____ refers to a court order certifying that an individual is to be confined to a mental health facility for treatment.

2. _____ is given when the client agrees to treatment after being told about side effects, significant risks, and available alternatives.

3. The concept of _____ means providing mental health in a way that does not prevent a client from exercising his or her constitutional rights without clearly justified reasons.

4. _____ means that information about clients must not be disseminated either verbally or in writing without the written permission of the client or guardian.

5. There are three types of commitment in each of the states: _____ commitment, voluntary commitment, and _____ commitment.

6. The standard of proof that must be offered to uphold a commitment proceeding is _____.

7. The legal mandate for a mental health professional to notify an intended, identifiable victim is _____.

Define the following concepts related to malpractice.

8. Expert witness

9. Sexual misconduct

10. Wrongful death

11. Primum no nocere

Critical Thinking Activity

12. How many of the NLN Nursing Standards of Care can you describe in detail? If you were called to testify as an "expert witness" student nurse, what would be your response?

Chapter 6 Cultural Issues

Name _____

Critical Thinking Activity

1. Do you believe that you identify with a traditional background?

2. Read and complete the heritage assessment tool from Chapter 6, Box 6-3 in the text.

Heritage Assessment Tool

1. Where was your mother born?

2. Where was your father born?

3. Where were your grandparents born?

   a. Your mother's mother?

   b. Your mother's father?

   c. Your father's mother?

   d. Your father's father?

4. How many brothers and sisters do you have?

5. What setting did you grow up in?

   a. urban

   b. rural

   c. suburban

6. What country did your parents grow up in?

   a. father

   b. mother

7. How old were you when you came to the United States?

8. How old were your parents when they came to the United States?

9. When you were growing up, who lived with you? (ask this way)

   a. nuclear family
   b. extended family
   c. single parent family
   d. other

10. Have you maintained contact with:

    a. aunts, uncles, cousins?   (1) yes   (2) no

    b. brothers and sisters?   (1) yes   (2) no

    c. parents?   (1) yes   (2) no

    d. your own children?   (1) yes   (2) no

11. Did most of your aunts, uncles, and cousins live near to your home when you were growing up?

    a. yes
    b. no

12. Approximately how often did you visit your family members who lived outside of your home when you were young?
    a. daily
    b. weekly
    c. monthly
    d. once a year or less
    e. never

13. Was your original family name changed?

    a. yes
    b. no

(Continued)

Student Worksheets 83

Copyright © 2000 by Mosby, Inc. All rights reserved.

Heritage Assessment Tool—cont'd

14. Do you have a religious preference?

    a. yes (if yes, please specify)
    b. no (1 point for yes, but 0 for no)

15. Is your spouse the same religion as you?

    a. yes
    b. no

16. Is your spouse the same ethnic background as you?

    a. yes
    b. no

17. What kind of school did you go to?

    a. public (0)
    b. private
    c. parochial

18. As an adult, do you live in a neighborhood where the neighbors are the same religion and/or ethnic background as yourself?

    a. religion   (1) yes   (2) no
    b. ethnicity   (1) yes   (2) no

19. Do you belong to a religious institution?

    a. yes
    b. no

20. Would you describe yourself as an active member?

    a. yes
    b. no

21. How often do you attend your religious institution?

    a. more than once a week
    b. weekly
    c. monthly (0)
    d. special holidays only (0)
    e. never

22. Do you practice your religion in your home?

    a. yes (please specify, 1 point each example)
    b. praying
    c. bible reading
    d. diet
    e. celebrating religious holidays
    f. no

23. Do you prepare foods of your ethnic background?

    a. yes
    b. no

24. Do you participate in ethnic activities?

    a. yes (please specify, 1 point for each)
    b. singing
    c. holiday celebrations
    d. dancing
    e. festivals
    f. costumes
    g. other
    h. no

25. Are your friends from the same religious background as you?

    a. yes
    b. no

26. Are your friends from the same ethnic background as you?

    a. yes
    b. no

27. What is your native language (the language your parents may have spoken other than English)?

28. Do you speak this language?

    a. prefer
    b. occasionally (0)
    c. rarely (0)

29. Do you read this language?

    a. yes
    b. no

The greater the number of yes answers, the more likely the client is to strongly identify with a traditional heritage. (The one no answer that indicates heritage identity is "Was your name changed?") This assessment may be scored 1 point for each yes from question 10, except where noted (0), and 2 points for no if the person's family name was not Americanized. Again, a high score, usually greater than 15 points, is indicative of identification with a traditional background.

From Spector RE: *Cultural diversity in health and illness*, ed 4, Norwalk, Conn., 1996, Appleton & Lange.

3. What is your ethno-cultural heritage, and what role does this play in your life?

4. How does your ethno-cultural heritage affect your identity as a professional nurse?

5. Explore the impact of culture on the health-related issues listed below.
    a. Communication

    b. Attitude toward treatment

    c. Nutrition

    d. Compliance with medication regimen

    e. Experience of pain

Chapter 7

The Nursing Process

Name _____

Match the following items with their best descriptions.

_____ 1. Factors associated with the nursing process or which contribute to the diagnosis to the extent that the cause can be determined

_____ 2. Highly specific, measurable indicators that are used by nurses to determine whether the diagnosis has been resolved or reduced, or no longer is a risk

_____ 3. The nurse interprets data collected and applies standardized labels to client's health problems.

_____ 4. The nurse makes specific recommendations after comparing the client's current mental health state with that described in the outcomes and focused upon during interventions

_____ 5. Nursing interventions with rationale are selected based on the client's identified risk factors and defining characteristics

_____ 6. A two-part diagnostic statement composed of a possible nursing diagnosis and the factors which make this a concern

_____ 7. The psychiatric nurse accumulates data focused on the client's behavior, psychic strength, vulnerability, coping skills, and ego defenses

_____ 8. These are made evident by observable, measurable manifestations of client's responses

a. defining characteristics

b. outcome identification

c. assessment

d. evaluation

e. nursing diagnosis

f. planning

g. risk diagnosis

h. etiology

Critical Thinking Activities

9. Defend or disagree with the following statement: Nursing orders or nursing prescriptions are the most powerful pieces of the nursing process.

10. What is a common problem with nursing interventions, and how is it remedied?

11. What is the difference between a nursing diagnosis and a medical diagnosis?

Chapter 8
Principles of Communication

Name _____

1. Describe the six components of communication.
   a.
   b.
   c.
   d.
   e.
   f.

Critical Thinking Activities

2. Briefly describe the factors that influence communication and give examples of each.
   a.

   b.

   c.

   d.

   e.

   f.

   g.

3. Analyze part of a conversation using the structure indicated below.

Conversation	Nonverbal Communication	Interpretation
Client said		
Nurse said		

4. Discuss three therapeutic techniques and three ineffective therapeutic responses that you find challenging. Role play situations using these techniques and responses with a partner.

Chapter 9 Children and Adolescents

Name _____

Define the following concepts and the theory from which they originate.

1. Ego

2. Industry versus inferiority

3. Self-system

4. Instrumentality

5. Internal working models of self

6. Modeling

7. Compare the developmental issues as explained by psychosocial theory and interpersonal theory.

Psychosocial Theory	Interpersonal Theory
0 to 1 year	0 to 2 years
1 to 3 years	

Psychosocial Theory	Interpersonal Theory
3 to 6 years	2 to 6 years
7 to 11 years	6 to 10 years
12 to 18 years	10 to 13 years
	13 to 17 years
	17 to 19 years

Chapter 10

The Adult

Name _____

For items 1 to 5, select the answers from the list provided.
rites of passage
interpersonal
psychosocial
mid-life transition
generativity

1. Each of Erikson's _____ stages are organized around a critical developmental issue for the individual self in its relation to the social world.

2. _____ includes the ability to evaluate and appreciate one's past life, embrace the future, assume new responsibilities and new relationships, and acknowledge and utilize one's creativity.

3. Daniel Levinson's group in *The Seasons of a Man's Life* focused less on changes occurring within the person and more on the interface between the self and the _____ world.

4. _____ occurs during the years between the late thirties and early forties and is marked by struggles within the individual and the external world and the beginning of expected biological changes.

5. For each event in life there are _____ whose essential purpose is to enable the individual to pass from one defined position to another equally defined position.

For items 6 to 12, choose T for true or F for false.

_____ 6. Estrogen appears to be the most potent of the gonadal hormones affecting monoamine oxidase levels.

_____ 7. Women are most affected by losses of an ideal or goal, whereas men tend to become depressed with the loss of close relationships.

_____ 8. The term "meganeeds" refers to the yearnings for affection, intimacy, and establishing relationships with others.

_____ 9. Individuals with met safety needs perceive their world as trustworthy and are more self-directed, autonomous, and interested in others.

_____ 10. Love and intimacy needs include a desire for adequacy, self-respect, competence, independence, and freedom.

_____ 11. The final need to emerge, and the desire for self-esteem and respect is defined as the ongoing actualization of potentials, capacities, and talents.

_____ 12. Psychosocial strength depends on a total process that regulates the individual's life cycles, the sequence of generations, and the structure of society simultaneously.

Chapter 11 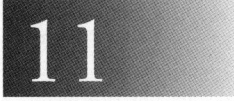 The Elderly

Name _____

Respond to the following questions.

1. Compare and contrast the terms *life expectancy* and *life span*.

2. Think about your personal and professional experience with elderly individuals. What aspects of your background affect your attitudes about caring for elderly clients?

3. Describe the biological theories of aging.

4. Briefly discuss the sociological theories of aging.

5. Considering the research findings on the sexual activity of elders, what creative nursing actions can you design to support an elderly client's sexual functioning?

For items 6 to 13, select the answers from the list provided.

ageism
transferring
cognitive
self-esteem
suicidal ideations
dystonic
I.A.D.L.
role transition

6. Erikson described the individual stage of development as maintaining a balance between a state of stability and a _____ state of disorder.

7. Maslow's hierarchy of needs includes physiological stability, safety and security, sense of belonging, _____ , and self-actualization.

8. The Katz index of ADLS is a valid objective tool which measures six areas of functioning: 1) bathing, 2) dressing, 3) toileting, 4) _____ , 5) continence, and 6) feeding.

9. _____ include transportation, shopping, preparing meals, and housework.

10. Researchers are finding that intellectual decline is avoidable or possibly reversible in healthy elderly persons with interventions focusing on development of _____ skills.

11. Retirement implies a major _____ for many elderly.

12. An older person may state that he or she has no _____, but appearance may indicate self-neglect, and behaviors may include withdrawing from social networks and accumulating drugs.

13. _____ is the process of systematic stereotyping and discrimination against people because they are elderly.

Chapter 12

Anxiety and Related Disorders

Name _____

Match the anxiety-related disorders theory with the best description.

_____ 1. One of the great tasks of psychology is to discover the generation of anxiety in response to relationships.

_____ 2. A method derived from learning theory in which the relaxed client is exposed to a graded hierarchy of phobic stimuli.

_____ 3. Three types of anxiety are identified: reality anxiety, moral anxiety, and neurotic anxiety.

_____ 4. The hypothalamus, pituitary, and the central nervous system have a reciprocal relationship relating to the "fight-or-flight response."

a. Freud-Psychodynamic

b. Wolpe-Systematic Desensitization

c. Selye-Biological

d. Sullivan-Interpersonal Model

For items 5 to 11, choose T for true and F for false.

_____ 5. The prominent feature of a fugue state is that the client experiences panic attacks in response to particular situations.

_____ 6. Clients with post-traumatic stress disorder are drawn to stimuli associated with the trauma.

_____ 7. Obsessions are recurrent and persistent ideas, impulses, or images experienced as intrusive or inappropriate.

_____ 8. Compulsions are images or mental processes which cause the client to relive the trauma experienced at an earlier time.

_____ 9. It is important to prevent the client with OCD from performing their rituals or compulsions.

_____ 10. A conversion disorder causes the client to develop deficits that affect voluntary motor or sensory function.

_____ 11. Dissociative identity disorder is diagnosed when the individual demonstrates a personality state resembling a famous person.

Respond briefly to the following question.

12. What causes anxiety for you as an individual? Try a new coping technique described in this chapter and record your results.

Chapter 13

Mood Disorders: Depression and Mania

Name _____

Critical Thinking Activity

Read the following situation and respond to the questions below.

Mr. Pollack, who has a history of bipolar I disorder is a 46-year-old accountant who has come to the community clinic with obvious pressured speech and agitation. His concerned friend brought him to the clinic because he has been unable to sleep in the past week, has refused several major business accounts, and insists that he will become a famous artist even though he has never had an interest in art. To pursue his art career, he has purchased over $900 of supplies.

1. What information would be important to assess immediately upon seeing Mr. Pollack?

2. What additional questions would the nurse consider when evaluating Mr. Pollack?

3. Mr. Pollack is recommended to resume lithium as part of his treatment. What information about this medication will be included in the health teaching plan?

Chapter 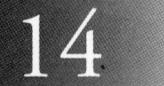 The Schizophrenias

Name _____

Critical Thinking Activity

Read the following case study and respond briefly to the questions.

Jeffrey is a 20-year-old man with a 4-year history of paranoia, hearing voices, and believing that his brain is controlling the subway system. He was hospitalized because he barricaded himself in his apartment with an assault rifle and threatened to shoot all "secret agents trying to regain control over the subway."

1. Given the information in the case study, what does Jeffrey's behavior indicate?

2. What level of restrictiveness should Jeffrey be placed upon?

3. What medications would be selected for this client?

4. Identify the side effects you would be vigilant for as you evaluate Jeffrey's response to his medications.

5. How would you approach Jeffrey's delusional beliefs?

Chapter 15

Personality Disorders

Name _____

Critical Thinking Activity

Read this case study from the textbook and respond to the questions that follow.

Angela is a 29-year-old single female who became suicidal after her boyfriend, Al, told her their relationship was over. She started to drink and use Valium to calm down after Al told her they were through. The relationship had become stormy, with frequent threats from Al that he would stop seeing her. Angela became vengeful, went to Al's parents' house where he was staying, and threw a rock into their living room window, shouting that she loves Al and cannot live without him. She then ran into the street in front of an oncoming car. The driver slammed on the brakes and hit Angela enough to knock her down and cause a pelvic fracture. She was admitted to the local hospital, still vowing to harm herself if Al did not return to her.

1. Using the DSM-IV general criteria for personality disorders, cite evidence that Angela is experiencing symptoms of a personality disorder. Identify the corresponding nursing diagnoses.

DSM-IV Personality Disorder Criteria	Nursing Diagnosis
a.	
b.	
c.	
d.	

2. What would be the priority of Angela's primary nurse?

3. What discharge criteria would be appropriate for Angela?

Chapter 16

Substance-Related Disorders

Name _____

Respond briefly to the following questions.

1. Identify the risks to a fetus that may develop as a result of maternal alcohol or drug abuse.

2. What are the common signs of adolescent drug use/abuse?

3. Compare and contrast the causes, symptoms, and nursing care alerts related to the syndromes listed below.

Syndrome	Cause	Symptoms	Nursing Care Alert
a. Acute alcoholic hallucinosis			
b. Wernicke's syndrome			
c. Korsakoff's syndrome			
d. Substance withdrawal delirium (delirium tremens or DTs)			

Chapter 17

Delirium, Dementia, and Amnestic and Other Cognitive Disorders

Name _____

For items 1 to 7, choose T for true or F for false.

_____ 1. Delirium is a disorder that involves global impairment of cognitive functions; it is usually progressive and interferes with normal functional abilities of the client.

_____ 2. Alzheimer's disease (AD) impairs short-term memory first, then progresses to deteriorate intellectual abilities such as speech, reading, writing, and comprehension.

_____ 3. Alzheimer's disease can be reversed if treated during stage one.

_____ 4. Neuritic plaques of Alzheimer's disease can be diagnosed using positron emission tomography (PET) scans, thus confirming presence of the disorder.

_____ 5. Approximately 80% of dementias are caused by degenerative disease and are termed primary dementias.

_____ 6. One out of three families with a member 65 years or older will include a person with Alzheimer's disease.

_____ 7. The most common cause of death in clients with Alzheimer's disease is aspiration pneumonia.

Match the following terms with the correct descriptions.

_____ 8. Pick's disease

_____ 9. Parkinson's dementia

_____ 10. Vascular dementia (multi infarct dementia)

_____ 11. Cerebrovascular accidents

_____ 12. Creutzfeldt-Jacob disease

_____ 13. Down syndrome dementia

a. This results from the occlusion of small arteries or arterioles in the cortex of the brain caused by an increased number of vascular wall cells.

b. Beginning with the insidious onset of confusion, depression, and altered sensation, this progresses in weeks or months to dementia, ataxia, sometimes cortical blindness, and palsy.

c. This degenerative process of nerve cells, usually frontal and temporal lobe, causes changes in personality, deterioration of social skills, emotional blunting, behavioral disinhibition, and language abnormalities.

d. About 50% of individuals over 40 years old with a characteristic congenital genetic problem develop this illness, which is first manifested by memory loss.

e. Cerebrovascular amyloid deposits either block the vessel or cause it to rupture, producing a cerebral hemorrhage. This occurs in the gray matter and therefore does not result in paralysis.

f. Associated with this is involuntary tremulous motion, muscle weakness, stiffness, immobile face, and mumbling speech.

14. What information will you give a family that requests information about the warning signs of Alzheimer's dementia?

Chapter 18
Disorders of Childhood and Adolescence

Name _____

Read each statement and write the best response in the space provided.

1. _____ associated with _____ disorder manifests itself by: impatience, impulse control problems, interrupting others to the point of social, academic, or occupational problems.

2. _____ is repeated passage of feces into inappropriate places whether involuntary or intentional.

3. Mild mental retardation constitutes _____% of individuals with mental retardation.

4. _____ presents mainly with a repetitive and persistent pattern of behavior that violates the basic rights of others or major age-appropriate societal norms or rules.

5. _____ is characterized by marked impairment of social and cognitive abilities and is the most common pervasive developmental disorder.

6. Most common tics in _____ involve the head and the torso and limbs. Vocal tics include clicks, grunts, barks, sniffs, snorts, and coughs.

For items 7 to 12, choose T for true and F for false.

_____ 7. Older children and adolescents with separation anxiety disorder may experience a racing and pounding heart, dizziness, and faintness.

_____ 8. When a child over 9 years old has an episode of voiding in inappropriate places, consistent punishment is the preferred response.

_____ 9. Encopresis is the repeated voiding of urine into bed or clothes.

_____ 10. Approximately 5% of public school students have an identified learning disorder.

_____ 11. Children and adolescents with learning disorders drop out of school at a rate of nearly 20%.

_____ 12. The most common method of adolescent suicide is firearm use.

13. Identify the common risk factors for adolescent suicide.

Chapter 19

Eating Disorders

Name _____

1. Describe the etiology of eating disorders using the following categories:
   A. Biological factors
      1.
      2.
   B. Psychological factors
      1.
      2.
      3.
   C. Sociocultural factors
      1.
      2.
      3.
   D. Family factors
      1.
      2.
      3.
      4.
      5.

2. Anorexia nervosa and bulimia nervosa are distinct diagnostic categories and yet have many overlapping features. List clinical symptoms for each of these disorders and star overlapping features. In the second column identify the corresponding nursing diagnosis.

Anorexia Nervosa	Nursing Diagnosis
A.	
1.	1.
2.	2.
3.	3.
4.	
B.	
1.	1.
2.	2.
3.	3.
4.	4.
5.	5.
C.	
1.	1.
2.	2.
3.	3.
4.	4.
5.	5.
	6.
	7.
	8.

Bulimia Nervosa	Nursing Diagnosis

A.
    1.
    2.
	1.
	2.
	3.

B.
    1.
        a.
        b.
        c.
    2.
        a.
        b.
        c.
    3.
        a.
    4.
        a.
        b.
        c.
        d.
        e.
    5.
        a.
        b.
        c.
        d.
	1.
	2.
	
	1.
	2.
	
	1.
	2.
	3.
	
	1.

C.
    1.
    2.
    3.
    4.
	1.
	2.
	3.
	4.
	5.
	6.
	7.
	8.

Chapter 20

Sexual Disorders

Name _____

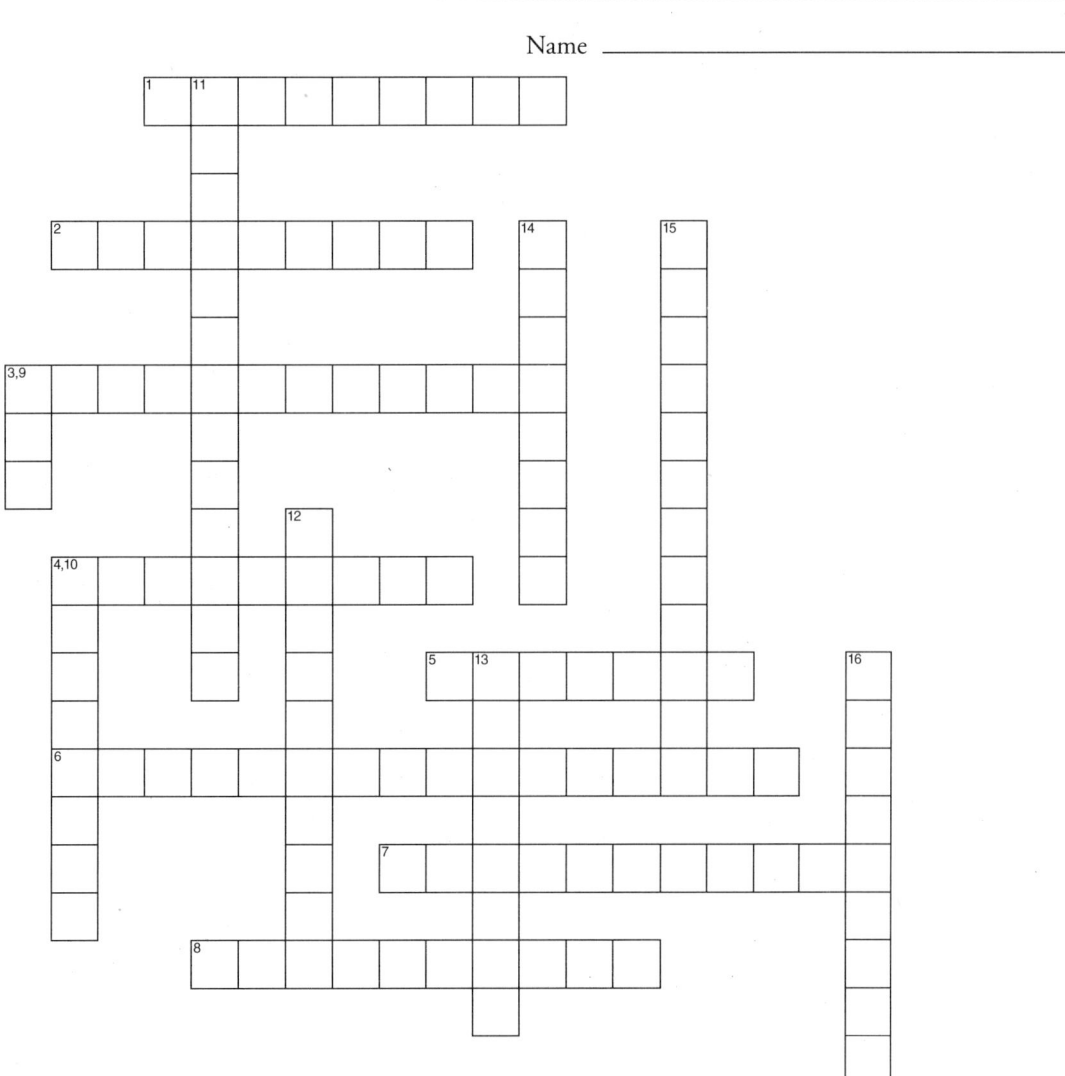

Across
1. Use of objects for purposes of sexual arousal.
2. An alpha-adrenoreceptor blocker that may facilitate blood flow to the genitalia and therefore improve arousal, especially in men.
3. The tendency to monitor one's own sexual activity, thus distracting from the actual experience.
4. Involuntary contractions of the perineal muscles upon penetration.
5. A personal image that depicts the idealized lover and lovemaking activities.
6. The nonfunction of testicles in relation to production of sperm.
7. Genital pain associated with sexual intercourse.
8. A group of behaviors commonly accepted by the clinical description of sexual deviations.

Down
9. Disease acquired during sexual intercourse with an infected partner.
10. A device used intravaginally to produce erotic stimulation.
11. Exposing the genitals to another person in inappropriate situations.
12. Sex offender.
13. The ability to experience the state of physical and emotional excitement that occurs at the climax of sexual intercourse.
14. Stimuli that heighten unacceptable sexual cravings.
15. An agent that stimulates sexual desire.
16. Endocrine testing for females only, that may reflect level of desire.

Chapter 21

Adjustment Disorders

Name _____

1. List below the five criteria used to define an adjustment disorder.
   a.
   b.
   c.
   d.
   e.

2. What categories of behavioral symptoms and mood and affect data can be used by the nurse during initial assessment?

3. Identify helpful questions to ask during assessment of the client with an adjustment disorder.
   a.
   b.
   c.
   d.

4. Describe the health teaching appropriate for a client or family experiencing an adjustment disorder.

For items 5 to 10, choose T for true and F for false.

_____ 5. Adjustment disorders represent transient episodes in the lives of otherwise mentally healthy individuals.

_____ 6. Stress-adaptation theory suggests a psychological response to stress called the general adaptation syndrome.

_____ 7. A nurse who expects a client from another culture to resolve grieving in the way that the dominant culture favors is showing cultural advocacy.

_____ 8. There are six sub-types of adjustment disorder, which include depressed mood, anxious mood, mixed anxiety and depressive mood, disturbance of conduct, mixed disturbance of emotions and conduct, and unspecified.

_____ 9. People experiencing adjustment disorders are not at risk for violence, self-directed or other directed.

_____ 10. A community care nurse is an ideal member of the health team to supply long-term therapy and support to clients with adjustment disorders.

11. List the typical nursing diagnoses used for treating clients with adjustment disorders.

Chapter 22

Interactive Therapies and Methods of Implementation

Name _____

Define the following terms related to the therapeutic relationship.

1. Self-reflection

2. Client centered

3. Countertransference

4. Goal directed

5. Objectivity

6. Transference

7. Boundary

8. Read the following situation and identify important leadership tasks for the nurse group leader.

    A group of six clients are attending the health education group. Each of these clients has a history of chronic mental health problems. The skills that will be fostered in this group are participation in a group activity, development of trust, successfully maintaining appropriate boundaries, and learning about a health-related topic.

Chapter 23

Psychopharmacology and Other Biologic Therapies

Name _____

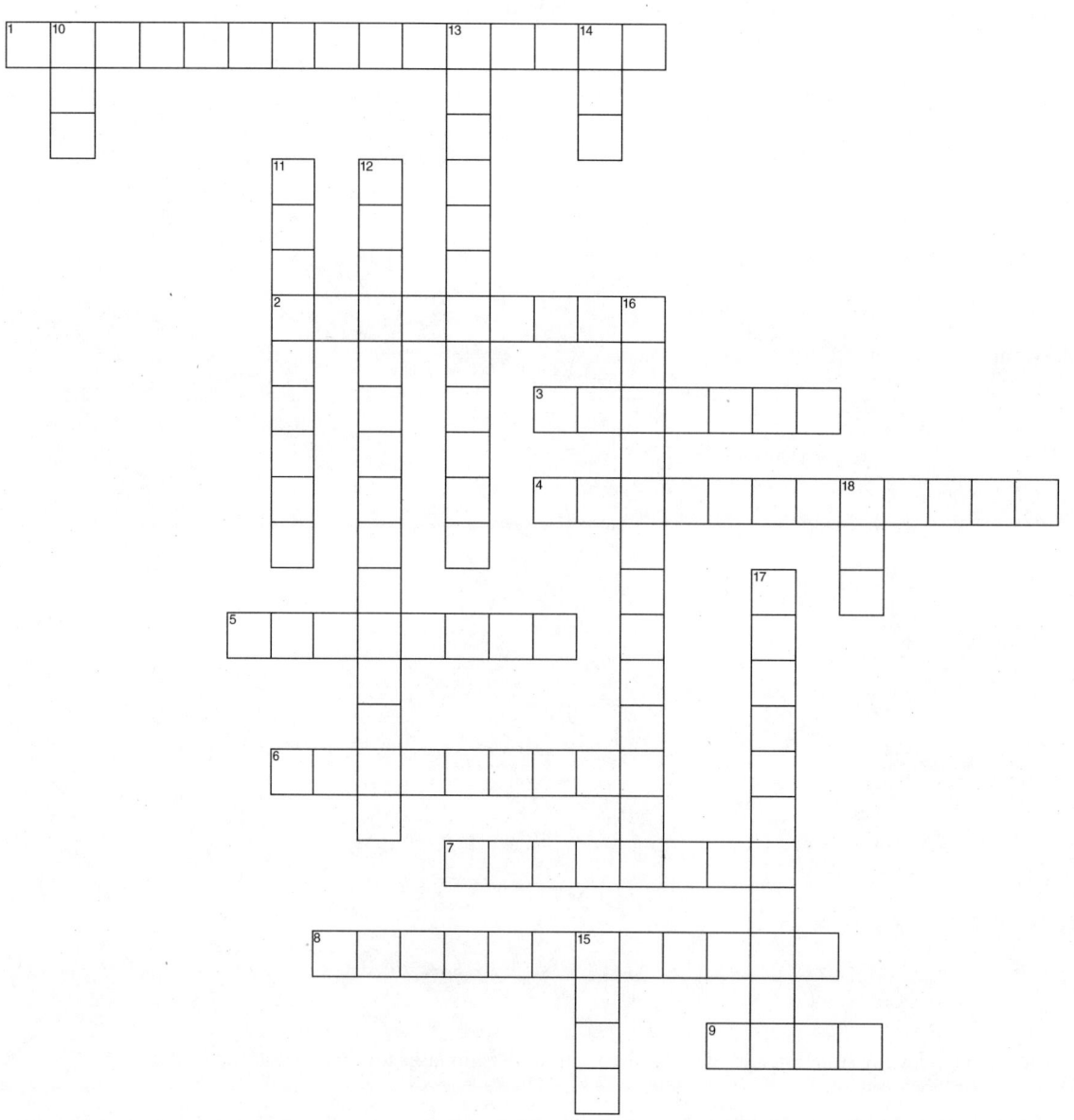

Across
1. Valium is one, but buspirone is not.
2. Motor restlessness, pacing, rocking, and foot tapping.
3. Used to treat bipolar disorder.
4. A crisis reaction to dietary tyramine.
5. Blepharospasm, torticollis, and oculogyric crisis.
6. Used to treat attention deficit disorder.
7. A client taking lithium experiences vomiting, diarrhea, and course tremors due to
8. Breast development resulting from increased prolactin as a side effect of a phenothiazine.
9. Prozac.

Down
10. Somatic treatment for depression.
11. Prolixin and Haldol can both be given as monthly or biweekly injections in this form.
12. A side effect that develops in approximately 1% of clozapine-treated clients.
13. A treatment for seasonal affective disorder.
14. Dystonia, akathesia, and akinesia.
15. Nardil, Marplan, and Parnate are examples of this category.
16. A neuroleptic drug is categorized as one.
17. Used for management of tension, sedation, and insomnia.
18. Characterized by muscle rigidity, hyperthermia, altered consciousness, and autonomic dysfunction.

Chapter 24

Alternative Therapies

Name _____

Match the following descriptions with the items to which they refer.

_____ 1. The use of specific body postures, breath control, and directed meditation

_____ 2. The utilization of laughter in this therapy is believed to enhance healing

_____ 3. Practice of balancing body energy by use of insertion of small needles

_____ 4. The body is viewed as a pharmacy that can make its own natural drugs to heal itself

_____ 5. Dilute solutions of a drug that can produce the same symptoms of a person's illness are used to heal the illness

_____ 6. Manipulation of soft tissue and joints to correct malalignment and affect health

_____ 7. Use of things in nature (roots, tree bark, herbs,) to treat ailments

_____ 8. Massage of the feet to relax and stimulate corresponding body parts

_____ 9. Identification and removal of molds, chemicals, and dust in the work place that may cause illness

_____ 10. A method of communication with a superior being, believed to enhance or restore health

a. prayer
b. reflexology
c. yoga
d. Ayurveda
e. herbal medicine
f. osteopathy
g. humor
h. homeopathy
i. acupuncture
j. environmental medicine

Chapter 25

Crisis Intervention

Name _____

For items 1 to 5, choose T for true and F for false.

_____ 1. From his experience in treating the survivors of the 493 people who perished in the Coconut Grove Fire, Eric London began to evolve concepts that lead to crisis intervention techniques.

_____ 2. Certain situations like bereavement and childbirth produce crisis for all persons experiencing them.

_____ 3. When customary problem-solving techniques cannot be used to meet the daily problems of living, a crisis response may ensue.

_____ 4. Typical to a crisis is the experience of a decrease in inner tension, increased organization, and emotional numbness.

_____ 5. Crisis is characteristically self-limiting and usually occurs for four to six weeks.

6. Identify the phases of crisis.

7. Identify the three balancing factors that are important to consider for the client in crisis.

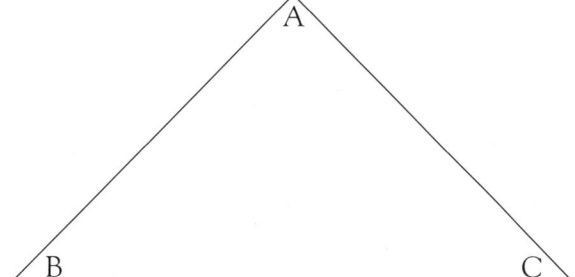

Critical Thinking Activity

8. In the film *Ordinary People* a family is thrown into crisis by the drowning of the older son, Buck, while sailing in a storm. The younger son, Conrad, who is sailing with him, is unable to save his brother. Conrad subsequently develops the following symptoms: flash backs, suicidal ideation, altered sleep patterns, isolation, anger, and acting out.

   Describe the category of crisis Conrad is experiencing and detail the priority nursing diagnoses, interventions, and outcomes.

   Category _____

Nursing Diagnoses	Outcomes	Interventions

Chapter 26

Activity Therapies

Name _____

Match the adjunct therapy with its best description.

_____ 1. movement/dance therapy
_____ 2. recreational therapy
_____ 3. occupational therapy
_____ 4. psychodrama
_____ 5. music therapy

a. This requires a double who operates as the "inner voice" expressing repressed thoughts, feelings, and conflicts.
b. Using body-focused movements to promote increased awareness of the body and changes in feeling states.
c. The applications of goal-directed purposeful activity in an effort to support optimum functioning of individuals with physical or developmental disabilities.
d. The use of music to provide a variety of listening and participatory experiences.
e. The use of games or play to stimulate activity, enhance socialization and increase enjoyment of life.

Identify the nurse's role for each of the adjunct therapies listed below.

Adjunct Therapy	Nurse's Role
6. Occupational	
7. Recreational	
8. Movement/dance	
9. Music	
10. Psychodrama	

Chapter 27

Survivors of Family Violence

Name _____

Fill in the blanks with the statistics related to survivors of violence.

50%	20%	17%
7%	84%	20%
10%	50%	90%

1. Between _____ and _____ of all women are abused by their intimate partners at least once.

2. In _____ of rape cases, the victim is acquainted with the offender.

3. _____ of psychiatric clients have histories of physical and sexual abuse.

4. _____ to _____ of pregnant women experience physical abuse by their partners.

5. Only one in _____ to _____ of rapes are reported to the police.

6. _____ of college women are raped at some time during their college career.

7. Over _____ of rape victims are women.

8. Briefly describe the battered partner and identify the forms of battering.

9. What is the most important focus for the nurse treating a woman who is in a relationship with a violent man?

For items 10 to 15 choose T for true and F for false.

_____ 10. Physical abuse of a child may include inflicted injury to the child, where psychological abuse might involve behaviors toward the child that are rejecting, degrading, terrorizing, exploiting, isolating, and demonstrate unreliable parenting.

_____ 11. Typical reactions of the nurse to child abuse include horror, denial, and attempting to rescue the child.

_____ 12. Hospitals and agencies that provide care to victims of abuse are encouraged by nursing organizations to provide ongoing treatment and referral.

_____ 13. A random sample of 953 women showed one-third of the women were sexually abused as children.

_____ 14. The symbolic offender is a perpetrator of incest who is socially immature and has difficulty relating to adults.

_____ 15. Survivors of sexual abuse often report recurring physical problems for which no organic cause can be found.

Chapter 28

Suicide

Name _____

For items 1 to 6, choose T for true and F for false.

_____ 1. The suicide rate for the elderly population is growing faster than for any age group.

_____ 2. In his psychoanalytic theory, Freud described suicide and self-destruction as hostility directed outward toward the externalized love object.

_____ 3. Medications that regulate serotonin levels are effective in the treatment of mood disorders that often accompany suicidal ideation.

_____ 4. Temporal lobe dysfunction is thought to be related to feelings of hopelessness and worthlessness.

_____ 5. Cognitive flexibility and the ability to identify problems has been hypothesized as a factor when suicide is accompanied by stress.

_____ 6. Schneidman defined suicide as a "response to an inner decision that the pain is unendurable, intolerable and unacceptable."

Match the terms with their corresponding psychological commonality of suicide.

_____ 7. perceptual state
_____ 8. stressor
_____ 9. purpose
_____ 10. action
_____ 11. cognitive state
_____ 12. goal
_____ 13. consistency
_____ 14. interpersonal act
_____ 15. emotions

a. Frustrated needs, such as achievement, affiliation, aggression, autonomy, dominance, harm avoidance, shame avoidance, nurturance order, or play
b. Cessation of consciousness
c. Communication of intention
d. Helplessness and hopelessness
e. Seek a solution to a problem
f. Aggression or exiting the scene
g. Lifelong patterns of failure, stress, duress, and threats to self-esteem
h. Ambivalence
i. Constriction with pain, frustration of needs, and helplessness

Respond briefly to the questions below.

16. Name and define the five levels of suicidal thought.

17. Identify potential risk factors in the following situation:

Miss Lewis, a 19-year-old white woman with a history of alcoholism, gave birth to her first child 3 weeks ago. The child died within 2 days from a congenital heart defect. You see her for a postpartum checkup and observe that she has lost 25 pounds. She claims to be undisturbed by the loss but complains of insomnia and you note a theme of hopelessness in her conversation.

Chapter 29

Grief and Loss

Name _____

Critical Thinking Activity

Mrs. Tanner is a mother and homemaker. Her oldest son, Joshua (17 years old) was killed in a car crash one year ago. Mrs. Tanner's youngest son Sandy (15 years old) was recently hospitalized because of attempted suicide. Mrs. Tanner states she was unable to visit Sandy in the hospital because "she had the flu."

During a home visit, the nurse notices that Joshua's room is still intact. All of his trophies are freshly dusted and his bed is made. When the nurse inquires about this room, Mrs. Tanner becomes agitated and asks the nurse to leave, saying that she and her husband cannot bear to sort through Joshua's things.

1. What assessment factors are important for the nurse to identify?

2. What nursing diagnosis would be applicable to this situation?

3. Describe some strategies that a nurse could use in approaching this case.

4. What community resources would be available to this family?

Chapter 30

Persons With HIV/AIDS

Name _____

For items 1 to 7, choose T for true and F for false.

_____ 1. Prevention and treatment of HIV should be more focused on the culture-specific needs of the Native American and African-American groups, who are most disproportionately represented in the AIDS community.

_____ 2. In a study of persons with AIDS enrolled as patients at the Gay Men's Health Crisis Center in New York, it was found that there were low rates of current mood disorders or psychiatric distress.

_____ 3. Women with AIDS have been found to have a decreased survival rate compared with men with AIDS.

_____ 4. HIV can cause a sub-acute encephalopathy, which leads to AIDS-Bend Alzheimer's Syndrome.

_____ 5. People who believe that they are at risk for HIV but have not gone for testing are termed the "worried well."

_____ 6. The CD4 lymphocyte count (T 4 cell count) is often extremely elevated in individuals suffering from full-blown AIDS.

_____ 7. Declining physical health status and grief reactions both enhance suicide risk.

8. Name three common psychiatric disorders found among patients with AIDS.
   a.

   b.

   c.

9. Identify the common HIV related problems observed during psychiatric hospital admissions.
   a.

   b.

   c.

Chapter 31

Psychologic Aspects of Physiologic Illness

Name _____

Match the following items with their best description.

_____ 1. General inhibition syndrome
_____ 2. Adaptation
_____ 3. Secondary appraisal
_____ 4. Psychoimmunology
_____ 5. Primary appraisal
_____ 6. Hardiness
_____ 7. General adaptation syndrome

a. A field that examines the impact of emotional and psychological disturbances on neural and organic function, as well as the promotion of wellness through mind-body techniques.
b. Alarm reaction, resistance, and the stage of exhaustion.
c. Stress is a reflection of an imbalance between the parasympathetic and sympathetic components of the autonomic nervous system.
d. A sense of mastery or self-confidence needed to appraise and interpret health stressors.
e. In this phase of Lazarus' theory, stressors are classified as irrelevant, benign-positive, or stressful.
f. Ongoing process involving both cognitive and physiological neural-chemical-endocrine processes.
g. During this phase, coping methods are chosen.

For items 8 to 14, choose T for true and F for false.

_____ 8. Therapeutic touch is based on a theory that the release of excess energy from the healer helps the client restore healthful energy patterns.

_____ 9. Norman Cousins described therapeutic touch as a treatment for ankylosing spondylitis in *Anatomy of an Illness, a Patient's Perspective*.

_____ 10. In studies by Spiegal, group therapy and self-hypnosis were found to double the life expectancy of women with metastatic breast cancer.

_____ 11. Ayurvedic medicine uses a combination of meditation, massage, herbs, aroma therapy, and biofeedback.

_____ 12. Homeopathic medicine is based on the belief that a drug that will produce specific disease symptoms in a healthy person can provide a cure for a client experiencing symptoms of the disease.

_____ 13. Individuals with chronic illnesses may use their illness for the primary gains of receiving attention or gaining control over other people.

_____ 14. Chronic physiological diseases often cause depression and suicidal behavior.

15. Imagine being told that you have cancer. Of the treatments described in this chapter, which would you choose as coping methods?

Chapter 32

Persons With Chronic Mental Illness

Name _____

Critical Thinking Activity

Identify the prominent psychologic and behavioral manifestations of chronic mental illness and the corresponding nursing actions.

A. **Psychologic manifestations**   **Nursing actions**

   1.   1.

   2.   2.

   3.   3.

   4.   4.

B. **Behavioral manifestations**   **Nursing actions**

   1.   1.

   2.   2.

   3.   3.

   4.   4.

   5.   5.

Chapter 33

Community Psychiatric Mental Health Nursing

Name _____

For items 1 to 5, select the best answer from the list below.

correctional
psychotropic medications
families
V.N.A.
deinstitutionalization
ethnomethodologic
H.M.O.
aggregates

1. Community care for clients with symptoms of mental illness become more prevalent after development of _____ and _____.

2. _____ approaches are inductive qualitative methods of studying people in their environment—the home.

3. Finding the right balance between custody and caring is difficult in a _____ setting.

4. The community health nurse focuses upon _____ or _____ as the unit of care while the home health nurse focuses upon the care of an individual at home.

5. Provider agencies in home care may originate from a hospital, a _____, a _____, or a health department.

6. Identify the functions of the nurse at each level of prevention.
   a. Primary prevention

   b. Secondary prevention

   c. Tertiary prevention

7. Describe the typical phases of a home visit.
   a.

   b.

   c.

   d.

   e.

8. What categories are included in a cultural assessment?

Chapter 34 Spirituality

Name _____

1. Define briefly the following terms:
   a. Spirituality

   b. Religion

   c. Faith

2. Describe the Stages of Faith.
   a. The impartial individual
   b. The institutional individual
   c. The individual seeker
   d. The integrated individual

3. List one nursing intervention for clients experiencing each of the following Stages of Faith.
   a. The impartial individual
      Intervention _____
   b. The institutional individual
      Intervention _____
   c. The individual seeker
      Intervention _____
   d. The integrated individual
      Intervention _____

Critical Thinking Activities

4. Nurses working with chaplains in addressing the spiritual needs of clients with psychiatric disorders will greatly benefit from a self-assessment of their own attitudes, biases, and strengths related to spirituality. After reading Chapter 34, write about your personal views and perceptions about the spiritual dimension of individuals and your feelings and thoughts about addressing the spiritual needs of clients with mental disorders.

5. List three qualities you possess that will assist your role in managing the spiritual goals and needs of clients with mental disorders.
   a.

   b.

   c.

6. List three challenges that may become obstacles in your path as you attempt to address the spiritual dimension of your clients. List a plan next to each challenge that will help you overcome that challenge.

   Challenge   Plan
   a.

   b.

   c.

7. Develop a spiritual treatment plan for a client with a predominant culture in your facility. Select one of the Stages of Faith that the client may be experiencing and incorporate that in your treatment plan. (See Chapter 34, Spirituality, for assistance.)

Match the Stages of Faith with their best descriptions.

_____ 8. Faith is internalized and religious rules are strictly obeyed   a. Individual seeker

_____ 9. Formal rules of religion are challenged   b. Impartial individual

_____ 10. "Good person/bad person" view of spirituality   c. Integrated individual

_____ 11. Minimal involvement in the faith community   d. Institutional individual

Student Worksheets Answers

Chapter 1

1. a. The relationship is for therapeutic purposes, rather than social purposes.
   b. The focus is directed consistently toward the client and the client's issues rather than the nurse or other issues.
   c. The relationship is purposeful and goal-directed.
   d. The relationship is objective, not subjective, in quality.
   e. The relationship has a clearly-defined time frame and is time-limited.

2. a. Preorientation stage
      Client responses
      (none)

      Nurse's role
      1. Gather data about the client, his or her condition and situation.
      2. The nurse engages in self-awareness about his or her thoughts, feelings, perceptions, and attitudes regarding this particular client.

   b. Orientation stage
      Client responses
      1. Build trust and rapport.
      2. Strengths, limitations, and problem areas are identified.
      3. Testing the relationship.
      4. Questions about confidentiality.

      Nurse's role
      1. Establish a contract.
      2. Be dependable.
      3. Establish outcome criteria.
      4. Formulate a plan of care jointly with the client.

   c. Working stage
      Client responses
      1. Client may take responsibility for behavior change.
      2. Secondary gain.
      3. Manipulation.
      4. Transference.

      Nurse's role
      1. Prioritize client needs.
      2. Separate provocative content from actual process and growth.
      3. Aid client in identifying problems.

   d. Termination stage
      Client responses
      1. Establish boundaries of relationship—may want to contact nurse outside the facility inappropriately.
      2. Identify changes toward growth.
      3. Express feelings and thoughts about the ending of the relationship.
      4. Acting-out or grieving behaviors may occur.

      Nurse's role
      1. Begin in orientation stage to inform client of length of relationship.
      2. Encourage client to clarify boundaries of relationship.
      3. Encourage the planning for termination and review of the relationship.
      4. Help client express feelings and views about ending relationship.

3. Students' responses will vary.

4. Examples of defense mechanisms portrayed in the film *Safe Passages:*
    a. Reaction formation—The mother's overprotection of her children prevents awareness of her own frustration and anger at being controlled and limited by family responsibilities.
    b. Displacement
        1. The father's anger and loss of temper when on the phone with the Marine Corps.
        2. The mother's anger about her husband leaving his teabags in the sink.
    c. Sublimation—The family garage cleaning episode (ending in Alfred acting-out his anger and frustration by setting fire to the pile of trash).
    d. Regression—The mother playing loud music and lying on the sofa with a pillow over her head.
    e. Omnipotence—The mother running off the football field carrying her son to medical attention and also the scene where she tackles the dog.

5. S

6. P

7. T

8. S

9. S

10. T

11. P

12. T

13. S

14. S

Chapter 2

Self-Awareness:

Student's personal response

Possible Planned Solutions:

1. a. Read about the nursing management of the behaviors that concern you (i.e., impulsive behavior, violence, suicidality and psychotic behavior).
   b. Learn about the psychiatric diagnoses and read case studies that include nursing care plans.
   c. Become familiar with unit policies and role expectations.
   d. Talk openly with instructor, fellow students, and nursing staff about your concerns and their approach to these situations.
   e. Interact with clients.

2. a. Read case studies that include verbatim accounts of what nurses say in response to client's comments.
   b. Learn and use therapeutic communication techniques.
   c. Role play situations you are concerned about with another student and together devise a good response.
   d. Imagine the worst thing you could say or do, then think of the best thing you could say or do. How do you picture the client responding to you in both situations?

3. a. Read over the Chapter 1 content about personal boundaries.
   b. Talk with your instructor and experienced psychiatric nurses. Supervision is an important component of competent psychiatric nursing care.
   c. Explore the possibility of seeking counseling to support yourself in working on personal issues.
   d. Form a stress reduction plan that includes:
      1. some form of physical exercise
      2. eating and drinking comforting healthful food and fluids
      3. practicing relaxation techniques and positive affirmations

4. a. Engage in an orientation to your unit and make a check list of things you want to get an understanding of early in your experience.
   b. Identify your usual way of getting comfortable in a new environment and apply that to this situation.
   c. Find a way to use your strengths to enter this new experience comfortably.
   d. Make daily objectives and validate these with an instructor and experienced nurse.

5. a. Get in the habit of looking for what others do well as opposed to the things which are difficult for them.
   b. Practice identifying ways to use these strengths in the psychiatric setting and encourage these.
   c. Put yourself in the place of a client you are working with. How would you want to be viewed?

6. a. Safety and health issues are cared for first.
   b. Practice systematic psycho-social assessment by designing a care plan for a client and discuss prioritization with faculty and fellow students. This should include assessment of client's physical, psychological, social, spiritual, and developmental status.

7. a. Focus on behaviors and facts not the person.
   b. Remain neutral without being indifferent and use care to avoid taking the behavior or comments of a client personally.
   c. Avoid evaluative statements and use statements of recognition.

Chapter 3

1. c

2. d

3. e

4. b

5. g

6. a

7. h

8. f

9. CBF

10. CT

11. PET

12. EEG

13. MRI

14. BEAM

Chapter 4

1. e

2. j

3. f

4. c

5. i

6. h

7. d

8. b

9. g

10. a

11. d

12. c

13. a

14. b

15. Neurofibrillary tangles; neuritic plaques; brain atrophy; brain vacuoles

16. Major depression

17. Answers will vary from class to class because of the wide range of choices.

Chapter 5

1. commitment

2. informed consent

3. least restrictive alternative

4. confidentiality

5. emergency, involuntary

6. clear and convincing evidence

7. duty to warn

8. Using an identified expert in the same specialty of nursing practice to testify as to the standards of a reasonably prudent nurse.

9. Some states have mandatory reporting laws about awareness of sexual contact between a therapist and a client.

10. Malpractice suits and wrongful death actions can be filed for a homicide client's injury to a third party and death from suicide.

11. "First do no harm."

12. Personal answer of student. Refer to NLN Standards for each specialty.

Chapter 6

1-4. Personal response of student.

5. a. People from various cultural backgrounds communicate using widely different paralinguistic cues and language. In order to give culturally competent care a nurse must learn the specific meaning of these nonverbal cues and language. Use of interpreters must be closely monitored for misunderstandings.
    b. It is necessary to understand bicultural variations in health and illness as well as the impact of culturally rooted values and beliefs upon the patient's attitude toward treatment.
    c. Nurses must familiarize themselves with their own dietary beliefs and practices as well as those of other cultures. Awareness of culturally determined meal patterns and acceptability of specific foods is an important nursing tool.
    d. Compliance with prescribed medication is dependent upon the patient's understanding of their illness, availability of financial or insurance coverage, attitudes of significant others (including traditional healers), etc.
    e. Perception, tolerance, and expression of pain very greatly among individuals of different cultures. In order to accurately assess pain and alleviate it, the nurse needs specific knowledge of the patient's cultural heritage.

Chapter 7

1. h
2. b
3. e
4. d
5. f
6. g
7. c
8. a

9. During this part of the process the treatment approach to a health problem is implemented.

10. They are weak, vague, and nonspecific. They must prescribe a course of action and not simply support the existing regimen.

11. A nursing diagnosis is a multiple part statement that describes a standard health problem and identifies its possible cause(s) or risk factors and clearly delineates any particular manifestations of this problem the client is experiencing. A medical diagnosis is a compilation of the distinguishing features of a disorder. Various disciplines within mental health refer to the DSM-IV in order to apply consistent diagnostic names to the specific distinguishing features of each disorder.

Chapter 8

1.
   a. Stimulus—reason for communication.
   b. Sender—individual who initiates the transmission of information.
   c. Message—the information being sent, such as feelings or ideas.
   d. Medium—the method by which the method is sent.
   e. Receiver—receives and interprets the message that has been sent.
   f. Feedback—a continual process in which a response to the message occurs and provides a new stimulus. The original receiver then becomes the sender of the next message and sender and receiver continue to reverse roles throughout the communication.

2.
   a. Environmental factors that control the effectiveness of communication include time, place, noise, privacy, comfort, and temperature.
      Timing—counting to ten when angry.
   b. The relationship of the people involved can affect the communication process. Some communication can occur from two different sources and be responded to very differently (e.g., Both an intimate friend and the President of the U.S. call you to ask your opinion on an issue).
   c. The context or place must be appropriate to the type of interaction. Meeting with a client while sitting in his or her room on the bed can generate a sense of invasion of privacy or sexual responses between the client and the nurse.
   d. Attitude determines how one person generally responds to another person and includes the level of openness and acceptance experienced in relation to the interaction. An intimate social attitude on the part of the nurse can be frightening and confusing to a client.
   e. Learning that occurs socially within family and culture influences the patterns and types of communication used. In some traditional Native American families, it is considered a sign of respect to lower the eyes when speaking with a member of the opposite sex or elder.
   f. Knowledge differences can cause imbalance in levels of understanding. Nurses using medical jargon can confuse and frighten clients. The statement, "I'll take your vital signs" could be interpreted as a threat to perform a life-risking procedure by a client who does not understand the meaning of the phrase.
   g. Perception is an individual's subjective experience related to the communication. Misperceptions can create problems in communication. A client who is told they are being admitted to a locked unit may be fearful of never being released or of being harmed while on the unit.

3. Individual student response.

4. Students and partners should refer to Table 7-4 "Ineffective Responses" and Table 7-5 "Therapeutic Responses."

Chapter 9

1. The individual's sense of reality which mediates between id and superego. This is from Freud's psychosexual theory.

2. At age 7 to 11 years of life the child develops skills in peer interactions and academic performance. This is from Erikson's psychosocial theory.

3. The child develops a sense of "good me," "bad me," or "not me," in relation to the responses of nurturers to cope with anxiety and need gratification. This is from Sullivan's interpersonal theory.

4. The discovery of how actions can lead to outcomes which develop through trial and errors. This is from Piaget's cognitive theory.

5. The infant develops a generalized expectation about the caretaker responses and the infant's own role in producing these reactions. This is from Bowlby's adaptation theory.

6. Learning and development proceed not merely from reinforcement or consequences but more from the influence of observing the actions of others and the consequences of their actions. This is from Albert Bandura's cognitive social learning theory.

Psychosocial Theory

0 to 1 year
Satisfaction of basic needs develops trust in self and world versus mistrust.

1 to 3 years
Satisfaction of needs for autonomy and free choice. Development of impulse control. Under controlling or overcontrolling parental behaviors result in shame and doubt of abilities.

3 to 6 years
Learns to plan tasks, join with others in cooperation, and pretend play. Accepts responsibility and is enthusiastic about helping. If family responds with increased conflict, guilt develops.

7 to 11 years
Focus on learning and mastery of academic skills and peer interaction. Success leads to self-assurance, failure to inferiority, and hesitance to try new things.

12 to 18 years
Concerned with how others view him or her. May make occupational choices. Develops self-esteem and emotional stability or poor self-confidence, alienation, and acting out.

Interpersonal Theory

0 to 2 years
Infant learns to differentiate from self and others and connects comfort or discomfort to caregiver. Develops self-system "good me" from positive parental feedback, "bad me" from negative parental feedback, and "not me" from extreme parental disapproval with severe anxiety.

2 to 6 years
Language takes on symbolic function of communication. Self-system continues development with expression of impulses in socially acceptable ways or development of a feeling of living among enemies.

6 to 10 years
Develops conscience. Able to distinguish fantasy and reality and develop syntactic communication.

10 to 13 years
Works with peers toward a common goal and develops a sense of oneness. Is emotionally attached to same-sex friend.

13 to 17 years
Sexual attractions encourage adolescent to try intimate relationships. Will feel insecure and lonely if severely discouraged.

17 to 19 years
Genuine intimacy achieved by integrating needs of society without excessive insecurity or anxiety. Failure to achieve personality integration can result in regression and egocentrism.

Chapter 10

1. psychosocial
2. generativity
3. interpersonal
4. mid-life transition
5. rites of passage
6. T
7. F
8. F
9. T
10. F
11. F
12. T

Chapter 11

1. a. Life expectancy, which is the number of expected years of life, is affected by gender, race, and environmental conditions.
   b. Life span refers to the maximum length of survival that is genetically fixed for each species.

2. Personal response of student.

3. **Genetic theory**—Juvenescent genes promote and maintain growth and vigor during the adult years, while senescent genes, which are active in middle adult years, initiate the process of decline and deterioration. The biological clock theory suggests that an organism's development and decline are regulated by a programmed internal genetic clock.
   Immunologic theory—The appearance of autoantibodies signals a decline in the immune system function. Immune function declines with age.
   Cross link theory—Collagen bonds change with aging and cause tissue to be more rigid and fragile.

4. **Disengagement theory**—Process of mutual withdrawal naturally occurs between the aging individual and society, which is inevitable and universal.
   Continuity theory—As one ages, he or she attempts to maintain continuity and consistency of habits, beliefs, norms, values, and other aspects of personality.
   Activity theory—Maintaining an active lifestyle and social roles affects the negative effects of aging.

5. Physical changes in the elderly such as decreased mobility, pain associated with intercourse, and impotency are challenging to the elderly client with active sexual needs. A creative nurse can provide opportunities for discussion of positioning, use of mechanical aids, monitoring of medications that may impact sexuality, and increased need for lubrication.

6. dystonic

7. self-esteem

8. transferring

9. Instrumental activities of daily living (IADL)

10. cognitive

11. role transition

12. suicidal ideation

13. ageism

Chapter 12

1. d

2. b

3. a

4. c

5. F (Phobias instead of fugue state.)

6. F (They avoid these stimuli.)

7. T

8. F (Substitute flashbacks for compulsions.)

9. F (This decreases gradually with medication and therapeutic intervention.)

10. T

11. F (Person develops more than one distinct personality.)

12. Students' responses will vary.

Chapter 13

1. In view of Mr. Pollack's sleeplessness and impaired judgment, the nurse must assess his recent intake of fluid, food, and medication and evaluate his physiological stability. Suicidal risk must also be evaluated thoroughly. Is there history of suicidal behavior, current suicidality, or a plan for suicide?

2. a. Are there situational stressors which have provoked this recurrence of symptoms?
   b. Has he ever been treated for bipolar I disorder successfully?
   c. What members of the client's support system are available to collaborate with the treatment team and encourage Mr. Pollack to participate in treatment?
   d. Is he willing to accept treatment?

3. a. Before beginning lithium treatment, laboratory tests are done to assess functioning of the heart, kidneys, thyroid gland, and body chemistry.
   b. It is important to take the medication regularly to maintain a steady blood level. It is necessary to have your blood drawn regularly to check the lithium blood levels. This is done about eight hours after the last dose of lithium.
   c. Common side effects of lithium are thirst, fine tremors, weight gain, muscle weakness, and increased urine output.
   d. Toxic side effects of lithium which can be life-threatening include nausea and vomiting, diarrhea, course tremors, lack of coordination, muscle twitching, confusion, seizures, and coma.
   e. It is important to maintain adequate fluid and sodium intake, especially during exercising, illness, or hot weather.
   f. Do not combine over-the-counter medications with lithium without consulting with the professional who prescribed it. Diuretics, ibuprofen, and verapamil can elevate the blood lithium level.
   g. In a pregnant female client, lithium could interfere with normal fetal development if taken during the first trimester. Adequate birth control and monitoring for potential pregnancy are important.

Chapter 14

1. This acutely psychotic and potentially violent client is demonstrating behavior, which reflects panic level anxiety, disordered thinking, hallucinations, and delusional beliefs.

2. He should be constantly observed to prevent injury to self or to others. Initially, he will be secluded with constant staff observation. Restraint may be necessary if he experiences periods of violence.

3. Antipsychotic medications, antiparkinson medications.

4. Orthostatic hypotension, extrapyramidal side effects (dystonia, akinesia, akathisia), tardive dyskinesia, neuroleptic malignant syndrome

5. Focus upon establishing trust initially. Do not challenge his delusion. Assure the client that he won't be harmed. Offer concern and protection to prevent harm to self and others.

Chapter 15

1. DSM-IV Personality Disorder Criteria / Nursing Diagnosis

   A. Enduring pattern of inner experience that deviates markedly from the expectations of the individual's culture.
      a. cognition—dysfunctional thinking
      b. affectivity—dysfunctional emotions
      c. interpersonal dysfunction
      d. lack of impulse control

   Risk for altered thought processes
   Self-concept disturbance
   Ineffective individual coping
   Impaired social interaction
   Risk for violence,
      self-directed
      other-directed
   Social isolation
   Self-care deficit
   Sleep pattern disturbance

   B. Maladaptive pattern of behavior that spans a range of personal and social situations

   Impaired social interaction
   Self-care deficit
   Altered nutrition

   C. Distress and functional impairment

   Risk for injury

   D. Drug and alcohol abuse

Evaluate for abuse vs. dependence

2. Evaluate client's degree of risk for suicide:
   a. Possible warning signs: increasing agitation, labile mood, theme of self-deprecation, violence or hopelessness in conversation or artistic expression
   b. Admission of thoughts to harm self; evaluate lethality of imagined method
   c. Admission of intent to harm self; evaluate lethality of method chosen
   d. Concreteness and detail of suicide plan
   e. Available resources

3. *Angela identifies a safety plan for future suicidal ideation.
   *Angela is able to talk about the end of the relationship with Al without suicidal thoughts.
   *Angela participates in an ongoing treatment program to maintain sobriety (AA, sponsor, day treatment, or other structured support).
   *Angela discusses her loss with peers and family to complete her grief process.
   *Angela plans ongoing supportive therapy

Chapter 16

1. Intrauterine drug exposure is associated with low birth weight; physical and congenital malformations (the 2nd to the 8th week of gestation is the highest risk period for teratogenic effects of substances); withdrawal effects including irritability, tremors, seizures, hypertonia, abdominal distention, increased respiration, and vomiting; and central nervous system damage resulting in neurobehavioral effects.
   Intrauterine alcohol exposure is associated with fetal alcohol syndrome, including low birth weight; certain facial characteristics such as small head circumference, low nasal bridge, epicanthal folds, short eyelid tissues, short nose, small midface, indistinct infranal depression, and a thin upper lip; and neurological abnormalities.

2. Sudden behavioral changes
   Sweating, especially at night
   Needle marks (anticulsitol fosa, between toes, under tongue)
   Inebriation
   Change in nutritional intake
   Nasal congestion
   Rhinorrhea, with cocaine use
   School problems

3.

Syndrome	Cause	Symptoms	Nursing Care Alert
a. Acute alcoholic hallucinosis	Prolonged period of drinking	Threatening auditory hallucinations, delusions (still oriented to time and place), threatening behavior	Constant observation, monitor safety and potential for violence
b. Wernicke's Syndrome	Years of excessive alcohol intake	Neurobiological disturbances; ataxia, ophthmoplegia, nystaginus,	Early intervention with large doses of parenteral thiamine to prevent chronicity

c. Korsakoff's Syndrome	Years of excessive alcohol intake B vitamin deficiency: riboflavin, thiamine, and folic acid	Amnestic syndrome: amnesia, disorientation to time and place, falsification of memory (confabulation), severe peripheral neuropathy	confusion and need for custodial care Replacement of B vitamins: thiamine, folic acid, monitor safety, prevent causing severe pain when moving client (secondary to peripheral neuropathy), prevent foot drop
d. Substance withdrawal delirium (delirium tremens or DTs)	In severe alcohol withdrawl, this occurs 24-72 hours after the last drink for 5% of those hospitalized for alcoholism.	Confusion and disorientation regarding time and place, visual and auditory hallucinations that are accusatory and threatening, illusions (reptiles and insects are common), severe agitation, profuse sweating, tachycardia, tachypnea, possible grand mal seizure activity	Safety precautions, seizure precautions, rehydration, preparation for emergency medical intervention

Chapter 17

1. F
2. T
3. F
4. F
5. T
6. T
7. T
8. c

9. f

10. a

11. e

12. b

13. d

14. Seek medical care if you observe the following:
    1. Shopping difficulty, tasks involved correlating lists, remembering, and calculating money
    2. Driving problems (e.g., accidents, losing car, or getting lost)
    3. Missed social engagements or appointments
    4. Difficulty with finances (e.g., balancing checkbook, paying bills)
    5. Pacing or wandering away from home
    6. Misidentifying friends or family
    7. Inability to accomplish common household tasks.

Chapter 18

1. Hyperactivity, attention deficit/hyperactivity

2. Encopresis

3. 85%

4. Conduct disorder

5. Autism

6. Tourette's disorder

7. T

8. F (no punishment—only evaluation)

9. F (eneuresis)

10. T

11. F (40%)

12. T

13. a. Psychiatric diagnosis
       depression and anxiety
       personality disorder
       substance abuse
       disruptive disorders
    b. Psychosocial stressors
       dysfunctional family
       chronic stress
       suicide of family member or friend
       history of physical or sexual abuse
       substance abuse

Chapter 19

1. A. Biologic factors
     1. Biologic tendency toward being overweight may increase the body dissatisfaction and dieting behavior which fuels an eating disorder.
     2. There is a connection between depression and eating disorders.
   B. Psychologic factors
     1. Self-esteem is lower in individuals diagnosed with eating disorders than in other diagnostic groups.
     2. Dichotomous thinking, erroneous control issues, and personalization are disordered thinking patterns which occur in clients with eating disorders.
     3. Personality traits that occur frequently among clients with eating disorders include perfectionism, social insecurity, affective instability, immaturity, compliance, perceived ineffectiveness, and inability to identify and respond to bodily sensations correctly.
   C. Sociocultural factors
     1. Cultural focus on eating, dressing, and exercising to look thin and "beautiful."
     2. The equating of food with pleasure, comfort, and love.
     3. Use of food in childrearing practices to nurture, punish, or reward. Unsuccessful struggle to balance societal expectations.
   D. Family factors
     1. Tension
     2. Rigidity
     3. Poor boundaries
     4. Poor conflict resolution skills
     5. Overemphasis on social acceptance and achievement.

2. **Anorexia Nervosa**

   Nursing Diagnosis

   A. Behavioral symptoms
     1. Self-starvation
     2. Rituals or compulsive behaviors toward eating or weight loss
     3. Self-induced vomiting, laxative and exercise abuse
     4. Weight is 15% or more below that expected for height and frame

   1. Risk for self-mutilation
   2. Altered nutrition less than body requirements
   3. Impaired social interaction

   B. Physical symptoms
     1. Amenorrhea
     2. Decreased pulse and body temperature
     3. Cachexia
     4. Lanugo present
     5. Constipation

   1. Sexual dysfunction
   2. Altered growth and development
   3. Risk for altered body temperature
   4. Fluid volume deficit
   5. Perceived/actual constipation

   C. Psychological
     1. Denial of low weight
     2. Body image disturbance
     3. Irrational fear of weight gain
     4. Impaired self-concept
     5. Preoccupation with food preparation

   1. Anxiety
   2. Ineffective denial
   3. Body image disturbance
   4. Self-esteem disturbance
   5. Powerlessness
   6. Ineffective coping
   7. Hopelessness
   8. Ineffective family coping

Bulimia Nervosa
A. Behavioral symptoms
 1. Binge eating
 2. Self-induced vomiting, abuse of laxatives, diuretics, diet pills, ipecac, enemas, exercise, or fasting
B. Possible physical symptoms
 1. Fluid and electrolyte disturbance from purging
  a. Hypokalemia
  b. Alkalosis
  c. Dehydration
 2. Cardiovascular instability
  a. Hypotension
  b. Arrhythmia/dysrrhythmia
  c. Cardiomyopathy
 3. Endocrine
  a. Menstrual dysfunction
 4. Gastrointestinal
  a. Constipation/diarrhea
  b. Gastroparesis
  c. Esophageal reflux
  d. Esophagitis
  e. Mallory-Weiss tears
 5. Eye/ear/nose/throat
  a. Enamel erosion
  b. Gum irritation and bleeding
  c. Parotid gland enlargement
  d. Halitosis
C. Psychologic symptoms
 1. See body as unrealistically fat
 2. Persistent focus on weight, shape, and proportions
 3. Striving for the perfect body
 4. Self-concept unduly influenced by perceived body weight and shape

Nursing Diagnoses

1. Risk of self-mutilation
2. Knowledge deficit regarding nutrition: side effects of bulimic behavior
3. Noncompliance with treatment

1. Altered nutrition: less than body requirements
2. Fluid volume deficit

1. Altered peripheral, cardiopulmonary, cerebral, and renal tissue perfusion
2. Sexual dysfunction

1. Constipation/diarrhea
2. High risk for self-mutilation
3. Knowledge deficit: disease process and treatment reflux esophagitis

1. Knowledge deficit: complications of bulimia

1. Anxiety
2. Body image disturbance
3. Self-esteem disturbance
4. Powerlessness
5. Helplessness
6. Social isolation
7. Impaired social interaction
8. Ineffective individual coping

Chapter 20

Across
1. fetishism
2. yohimbine
3. spectatoring
4. vaginamus
5. lovemap
6. aspermatogenesis
7. dyspariunia
8. paraphilia

Down
9. STD
10. vibrator
11. exhibitionism
12. victimizer
13. orgasmic
14. triggers
15. aphrodisiacs
16. estradiol

Chapter 21

DSM IV Criteria

1. a. The reaction to an identifiable psychosocial stressor that has occurred with three months of the stressor.
   b. Symptoms of distress are marked and in excess of expected response.
   c. Axis I or II disorder criteria are not met by this disturbance.
   d. This diagnosis is not used when symptoms represent bereavement.
   e. Symptoms of the disorder must resolve within six months of the creation of the stressor. Subtypes specify the nature of prominent symptomotology.

2. a. Sensory perceptual
   b. Thinking disturbances—both process and content
   c. Feeling disturbances
   d. Behavioral and relating disturbances

3. a. What has happened in your life in the recent past?
   b. In what way did that event affect you?
   c. What has helped you to cope with similar events in the past?
   d. Tell me about your family and friends and their roles in this event?

4. Teach the client or family:
   a. To identify the symptoms of the adjustment disorder.
   b. Management techniques such as relaxation, exercise, visualization.
   c. Symptoms should be reported to the case worker.
   d. To rely upon coping methods which have succeeded in the past.
   e. Signs of depression and suicidality and safety plan.
   f. Dosage, frequency and effects of medications.

5. T

6. F (physiologic response)

7. F (cultural bias)

8. T

9. F (common problem)

10. F

11. a. Risk for violence, self-directed or directed at others
    b. Anxiety
    c. Ineffective individual coping
    d. Spiritual distress
    e. Impaired adjustment
    f. Dysfunctional grieving
    g. Self-esteem disturbance
    h. Impaired social interaction

Chapter 22

1. Nurses continually assess their values and attitudes. It is useful to explore judgmental attitudes, responsibility, and potential for human growth, as well as the need to be liked.

2. A therapeutic relationship is focused upon the client and his or her goals, reactions, coping strategies, and personal growth.

3. The feelings a nurse has toward the client (both positive and negative).

4. The purpose of the relationship. The specific ways in which the therapeutic relationship is used to help the client move toward health and self responsibility.

5. An analytical approach to subjective experience is used to separate personal feelings and reactions to clients and allow the focus to remain upon therapeutic interaction.

6. The feelings a client has toward the nurse and the therapeutic relationship.

7. The definition and separation of the self from others. Acting in ways that are appropriate to the role and the circumstances.

8. a. Plan an appropriate, well-structured activity like "Nutrition Bingo" (foods printed on cards in lieu of numbers, etc.).
   b. Prepare clients for group by announcing the time and location in plenty of time for them to get ready. Make 1:1 contact with group members to increase comfort.
   c. Orientation to the time limit and goal of the group.
   d. Discuss confidentiality, highlighting the need for group discussion to be kept confidential where private matters are concerned.
   e. Encourage discussion of topic and refocus people if they wander onto unrelated issues.
   f. Help group members contribute and maintain comfort and gain feedback.
   g. Summarize the group achievements at the end of the group time and end group.

Chapter 23

Across
1. benzodiazepines
2. akathisia
3. lithium
4. hypertensive
5. dystonia
6. stimulant
7. toxicity
8. gynecomastia
9. SSRI

Down
10. ECT
11. decanoate
12. agranulocytosis
13. phototherapy
14. EPS
15. MAOI
16. antipsychotic
17. anxiolytics
18. NMS

Chapter 24

1. c
2. g
3. i
4. d
5. h
6. f
7. e
8. b
9. j
10. a

Chapter 25

1. F (Lindeman)
2. F (only those vulnerable to the particular stress)
3. T
4. F (rise in tension, disorganization, and emotional turmoil)
5. T
6. a. Rise in tension as stimulus continues and discomfort is ongoing.
   b. Coping response is ineffective and discomfort continues.
   c. Tension increases sharply mobilizing internal and external resources.
   d. Disorganization occurs if problem is not solved or avoided.
7. A—Perception of Event
   B—Coping Mechanism
   C—Available Situational Supports
8. Category: Situational
   Nursing diagnosis—High risk for violence: self-directed, related to unresolved grief for brother as evidenced by thoughts of cutting his wrists.
   Outcomes—Conrad will verbalize an absence of suicidal ideation, intent, plan.
   Interventions—Assess clients suicide risks at regular intervals, contract for safety, check client and room for potentially dangerous items, observe for any secretive behavior.

Chapter 26

1. b
2. e
3. c
4. a
5. d

Adjunct therapy	Nurse's role
6. Occupational	Frequent contact with client in order to provide reality testing in self-care/maintenance tasks, role modeling, support and encouragement.
7. Recreational	Demonstrating and applying techniques to encourage clients in developing interests in leisure skills that they consider enjoyable and rewarding.
8. Movement/Dance	Participate in exercise or responses to music and encourage clients with feedback and discussion of response to activities.
9. Music	To provide nonjudgmental validation of feelings, model healthy behavior and address anxiety as it becomes apparent.
10. Psychodrama	Assist, participate in, and encourage clients to share their responses.

Chapter 27

1. 25% and 50%
2. 84%
3. 50%
4. 7% to 17%
5. 10% to 20%
6. 20%
7. 90%
8. a. Women who have been battered by those with whom they have been intimate.
   b. Economic abuse, sexual abuse threats and intimidation, forced isolation, constant demeaning and insulting, and breaking things to scare her.

9. If she has current injuries, they need to be assessed. She must be treated with the knowledge that seeking help places her in more danger of retaliation by her partner. Availability of safe houses and anonymous shelters can provide her with a safe haven in which to recover and plan her future.

    If a woman returns to her violent partner, she should do so with a clearly formulated emergency plan and identified resources for a quick escape when a new episode of battering occurs.

10. T

11. T

12. F (mandated to provided treatment by Joint Commission of Accreditation of Health Organization)

13. T

14. F (symbiotic offender)

15. T

Chapter 28

1. T

2. F (inward direction toward internalized love object)

3. T

4. F (frontal lobe)

5. F (cognitive rigidity; the inability to identify problems)

6. T

7. i

8. a

9. e

10. f

11. h

12. b

13. g

14. c

15. d

16. a. Suicidal ideation—thoughts or fantasies of suicide expressed verbally or through writing or art, without definite intent to act
    b. Suicidal threat—direct verbal or written expression of intent to commit suicide, but without action
    c. Suicidal gestures—self-destructive actions that result in no injury or minor injury

d. Suicide attempt—serious self-directed actions that may result in minor or major injury by persons who intended to end their lives or cause serious harm to themselves
   e. Successful suicide—death of person who ended his or her life by his or her own means

17. Risk factors:
   a. Suicide rates for whites are twice as high as those for nonwhites.
   b. Youths age 15 to 24 and people 65 and older are the persons most at risk for suicide.
   c. Medical problems that involve pain, debilitation, and acute physical stress offer a special concern for suicide risk (particularly vulnerable are postpartum women).
   d. Loss—unresolved grief reactions can lead to depression and suicide.
   e. Alcohol and drug abuse—the history of substance abuse combined with increased stress can be dangerous. Alcohol lowers inhibition, heightens depression, and increases impulsivity.
   f. Physical and emotional symptoms—significant changes in weight, serious sleep disturbance, and feelings of hopelessness are often signs of depression, which is often a precursor to suicidal behavior.

Chapter 29

1. Assessment of Mrs. Tanner for signs of depression and suicidality is critical. Note her thought pattern and identify the themes in her conversation. Assess her suicide potential directly and thoroughly.
   Clarify Sandy's status as to depression and suicidality.

2. Unresolved grief
   Ineffective family coping

3. Identify a safety contract when suicidality is present and construct a plan to follow if suicidality emerges. Support Mrs. Tanner and her family to begin to grieve the loss of their family member.
   Engage the whole family in treatment of this unresolved grief. Coordinate the family sessions with son Sandy's treatment plan.

4. Support groups focused upon loss can supply validation of the Tanners' current experience of loss and an environment conducive to healing. At school, Sandy has available counseling and teen supports, which are important outlets that could reconnect him with his peers.

Chapter 30

1. F

2. T

3. T

4. F

5. T

6. F

7. T

8. a. Major depressive episode
   b. Psychoactive substance abuse
   c. Adjustment disorders with anxious or depressed mood

9. a. Anxiety and depression over deteriorating physical health
   b. Social rejection related to HIV seropositive status
   c. Increased drug use as a response to HIV seropositivity

Chapter 31

1. c
2. f
3. g
4. a
5. e
6. d
7. b
8. T
9. F
10. T
11. T
12. T
13. F
14. T
15. Personal response of student

Chapter 32

A. Psychologic manifestations	Nursing actions
1. Altered thought process	1. Assess client for safety risk and ability to perform skills basic to survival. Monitor response to medications.
2. Chronic low self-esteem	2. Assist client in locating acceptable opportunities for socialization and work (e.g., community based social club for people affected by mental illness and sheltered workshops).
3. Loneliness/hopelessness	3. Encourage client's participation in structured treatment setting (day treatment) or club or sheltered workshop. Encourage contact when client withdraws.
4. Depression	4. Assess client for safety risk, evaluate consistently for symptoms of depression.

B. **Behavioral manifestations**

1. Inconsistent ability to perform activities of daily living
   a. self-maintenance skills
   b. social interaction difficulty

2. Inconsistent ability to living independent

3. Inconsistent ability to maintain employment or attend school

4. Inconsistent ability to live with family or friends

5. Risk for inappropriate sexual boundaries

Nursing actions

1. Evaluate client's ability to function regularly and make emergency contact available. Provide structured setting when necessary (day treatment or hospitalization).

2. Offer structured living situation if needed (e.g.; professionally supervised apartments or halfway houses).

3. Encourage client's participation in structured workshops. These offer training and ongoing supervision of workers who desire work but need training or support to maintain a position.

4. a. Offer supportive therapy to appropriate family members and friends.
   b. Encourage client's participation in supportive groups (e.g.; Alliance for Mental Illness, Emotions Anonymous).

5. Counsel and assess client for potential for sexual promiscuity, victimization, exposure to sexually transmitted disease, and pregnancy.
   a. Assess client regularly for violence potential, educate client's family and friends to recognize signs of impending violence.
   b. Provide sheltered environment when needed to prevent criminal behavior.

Chapter 33

1. psychotropic medications
   deinstitutionalization

2. ethnomethodologic

3. correctional

4. families or aggregates

5. H.M.O. (health maintenance organization)
   V.N.A. (visiting nurses association)

6. a. Primary prevention
      1. Health promotion
      2. Disease prevention
      3. Specific protection
   b. Secondary prevention
      1. Case finding
      2. Early diagnosis and treatment
      3. Prevention of complications
   c. Tertiary prevention
      1. Care and rehabilitation

7. a. Preplanning
   Acquire as much information as possible concerning the client, the client's diagnosis and history, and the plan of care. Contact client regarding visit.
   b. Entry of the home
      1. Nurse is both a professional and a guest.
      2. Nurse's clothing should be professional and official identification should be displayed.
      3. Establish a relaxed atmosphere for assessment.
   c. Intervention
      1. Provide structure and information about all treatments and length of visit.
      2. Establish goals.
      3. Monitor effect of medications.
      4. Monitor mental status.
      5. Organize complimentary multidisciplinary services.
   d. Documentation
      1. Communicate findings.
      2. Facilitate communication of treatment plan.
   e. Exit
      1. Leave client and supporting individuals with clear understanding of work to be accomplished at the next visit.

8. Values, beliefs, customs, social structure, health care practices, folk remedies, family customs, food preparation and preferences, the sick role, gender roles, experience of time, and attitude toward health care system.

Chapter 34

1. a. A search for the sacred; a need to have a conscious experience with the divine.
   b. A way of expressing one's spirituality; it may be formal or informal.
   c. The ability to draw on spiritual resources without having physical or empiric proof.

2. a. One who tends to do things in her/his own interest, is usually uninvolved in faith communities, and only has a casual acquaintance with faith community practices.
   b. A regular church attendee who adheres to institutional rules.
   c. One who has left a formal religious community and often challenges many of her/his beliefs and tenants.
   d. One who has internalized her/his faith; they fully accept the rules they obey and believe that they are just and right.

3. a. The 23rd Psalm, the poem "Footprints," the Serenity Prayer, the Lord's Prayer, or traditional hymns.
   b. Visits from the minister and members of their local spiritual community; formal use of prayer, anointing, and laying on of hands; use of prayer books and music specific to that demonination.
   c. Meditation, healing touch, devotional reading, communal prayer, and a variety of music.
   d. Traditional rituals, rites, and expressions of formal spirituality.

4-7. Students' responses will vary.

8. c

9. a

10. d

11. b

Test Bank

Chapter 1

Foundations of Psychiatric Mental Health Nursing

1. The nurse would evaluate which of the following characteristics as indicative of healthy boundaries?
    a. Giving as much as you can for the sake of giving
    b. Believing others can anticipate your needs
    c. Letting others define you
    d. Taking responsibility to meet one's own needs

2. The student nurse is planning to initiate a therapeutic relationship with a client, Paul. Which should she plan to incorporate in their interactions?
    a. Mutually sharing ideas and experiences
    b. Becoming subjectively involved
    c. Encouraging the client to choose a subject for discussion
    d. Giving and receiving friendship equally

3. A client frequently diverts the focus off himself by changing the topic or commenting on the nurse's appearance. The nurse recognizes this as an example of:
    a. Transference
    b. Resistance
    c. Countertransference
    d. A social relationship

4. An expected outcome of the nurse's attempts to maintain objectivity in a therapeutic relationship with a client is:
    a. Personally identifying with the client
    b. Processing information based on facts
    c. Subjectively determining the client's needs
    d. Using intellectualizing to remain separate from the client

5. The result of a nurse becoming subjectively involved in a therapeutic relationship is likely to be that the client will:
    a. Explore issues
    b. Expand on topics
    c. Feel accepted and understood
    d. Stop sharing information

6. An expected outcome of the preorientation phase of the therapeutic relationship is that the nurse will:
    a. Initiate a trusting relationship with the client
    b. Complete the required assessment process
    c. Examine his or her own feelings and perceptions about the client
    d. Recognize his or her own need for therapy

7. A client displays isolation, bizarre behaviors, unsafe actions, and poor hygiene. Which will be the first priority in the nursing care plan?
    a. Safety
    b. Hygiene
    c. Isolation
    d. Bizarre behaviors

8. Specific nursing interventions appropriate for the termination phase include:
    a. Exploring the client's past in depth
    b. Confronting changes not completed
    c. Helping client summarize accomplishments
    d. Identifying new problem areas

9. When diagnosing a client, the nurse incorporates an understanding of definitions of mental health and would describe an individual as healthy when:
    a. They do not conform to the nurse's beliefs
    b. Their behavior conforms to those specified in DSM-IV
    c. Based on presence or absence of precise physiological signs
    d. Measured by psychiatric and psychological standards

10. The student nurse is learning how to reduce the stigma associated with mental illness. Which of the following statements by the student nurse would reflect that learning has taken place?
    a. "A 34-year-old is being admitted for suicidal threats as a result of cocaine use."
    b. "We're admitting a cocaine addict who threatened to kill herself."
    c. "We're admitting an out-of-control, manic client."
    d. "They've added another psychotic to my caseload."

11. The nurse plans to teach the client conscious techniques to manage anxiety, which could include:
    a. Rationalizing problems
    b. Exercising
    c. Reaction formation
    d. Introjection

12. Which of the following would the nurse expect to observe in a client who uses projection?
    a. Engaging in lofty discourse of painful situations with little emotionality
    b. Viewing others as hostile
    c. Making excuses for shortcomings
    d. Attempting to atone for wrongdoings

13. A client on a medical unit is stable after treatment for pleurisy but repeatedly whines and asks the nurse to do things that she is very capable of performing for herself. The nurse interprets this as:
    a. Regression
    b. Sublimation
    c. Suppression
    d. Introjection

14. If a client was not included in a celebration but then spent her time imagining herself dressing and attending this event, the nurse would analyze this as an example of:
    a. Omnipotence
    b. Isolation of affect
    c. Fantasy
    d. Acting out

15. Which of the following would the nurse anticipate to observe in a client whose use of protective mechanisms is adaptive?
    a. Internal stressors that are greater than the capacity to defend against them
    b. The use of one defense exclusively
    c. The perception that he or she cannot overcome stress
    d. Maintenance of reality orientation

16. The community health nurse plans to implement primary prevention in her role. Which of the following activities should be incorporated in the plan?
    a. Teaching parenting skills
    b. Treating acutely ill clients
    c. Referring clients to mental health providers
    d. Providing family support to deal with a child's addiction

Chapter 2

Clinical Experiences: Rewards, Challenges, and Solutions

1. Mark, a student nurse, is very anxious about his clinical abilities. He plans to use positive affirmations to increase his confidence. He would include:
   a. "I should use therapeutic communication techniques."
   b. "I am relaxed and more capable each day."
   c. "I need to facilitate the healing process."
   d. "I can ask my instructor to tell me what to do."

2. Which of the following is an indicator that a nurse is functioning as a facilitator?
   a. The nurse taking care of the client
   b. The client waiting for the nurse to tell him what to do
   c. The nurse taking charge of the client
   d. The client working with the nurse towards goals

3. The student nurse evaluates that the client with low self-esteem has improved when the client:
   a. Stops crying every session
   b. Asks the student if she should leave her husband
   c. Asks the student if she is getting better
   d. Identifies her own strengths

4. John, a student nurse, seeks out his instructor and says he is worried he might become mentally ill. The instructor recommends that John:
   a. Put these thoughts aside
   b. Seek inpatient evaluation
   c. Obtain supervision or counseling
   d. Avoid focusing on these symptoms

5. Mary, a new psychiatric nurse, is concerned about maintaining appropriate boundaries in relationships with clients. An appropriate outcome for this concern is that Mary will:
   a. Set rigid boundaries with all clients
   b. Establish a close, friendly relationship with her clients
   c. Share her personal beliefs with her clients
   d. Establish a warm, caring relationship with clients

Chapter 3

Theoretic Perspectives

1. The nurse would evaluate that systematic desensitization has been effective with a client who has agoraphobia if the client:
   a. Understands why she has these fears
   b. Is able to go shopping
   c. Never experiences any further anxiety
   d. Identifies her irrational thoughts

2. A nurse has been using Beck's theory in working with a depressed client. Which of the following is an expected outcome of this approach?
   a. Decrease in automatic thoughts
   b. Development of insight
   c. Improved ability to speak about feelings
   d. Decreased feelings of depression

3. Mary, a student nurse, plans to use a strategic therapy approach with her client. Which of the following is an expected outcome of this therapy?
   a. Development of more balanced cognitions
   b. Modification of observable behaviors
   c. Awareness of aspects of self
   d. Reframing of the problem

4. George, a staff nurse, is developing a nursing care plan using a behavioral model. Prior to initiating fantasy desensitization, George will:
   a. Analyze the client's fantasies
   b. Teach relaxation techniques
   c. Challenge irrational ideas
   d. Use in vivo desensitization

5. Susan plans to use a gestalt approach with her withdrawn client. Which of the following techniques would be appropriate in this therapy?
   a. Alter ego playing
   b. Role playing
   c. Chair work
   d. Game analysis

6. If a client experienced a temporal lobe injury, the nurse would anticipate assessing problems with:
   a. Personality and intellectual function
   b. Attention selectivity and span
   c. Form and color recognition
   d. Visual recognition and memory

7. An alcoholic client exhibited staggering gait, clumsiness, and slurred speech while in an acute state of intoxication. The nurse evaluates these as indicative of a generalized malfunction of:
   a. Cerebral cortex
   b. Cerebellum
   c. Basal ganglia
   d. Brain stem

8. A client asks the nurse why he is depressed. He says, "My mother says it is chemical. What does she mean?" The nurse bases her or his response on the theory that depression involves:
   a. Decreased serotonin levels
   b. Decreased cortisol levels
   c. Decreased dopamine levels
   d. Decreased acetylcholine levels

9. When planning to use Freud's psychoanalytic approach with a client, the nurse will incorporate which of the following basic assumptions?
   a. The libido is always in control.
   b. Thought processes are always logical.
   c. The unconscious is in control.
   d. All behavior has meaning.

10. If a client repeatedly says she has nothing on her mind during her therapy sessions, the nurse may evaluate this as indicative of:
    a. Resistance
    b. Transference
    c. Counter transference
    d. Catharsis

11. When assessing a two-year-old boy using Freud's theory, the nurse would expect to focus on which stage?
    a. Oral
    b. Anal
    c. Phallic
    d. Latency

12. In determining the best approach, the nurse would recognize that which of the following populations would benefit from a behavioral therapy approach?
    a. Individuals with a bipolar disorder
    b. Individuals with phobic personalities
    c. Individuals with schizophrenia
    d. Suicidally depressed persons

13. Which of the following underlying assumptions would the nurse use in planning a behavioral therapy approach?
    a. All behavior is learned.
    b. Behavior is separate from the individual.
    c. Behavior results from the unconscious.
    d. All behavior is meaningful.

14. When assessing a depressed client according to Beck's Cognitive Triad, the nurse would expect that the client's thinking is:
    a. Slower because of brain chemical depletion
    b. Negative in view of self, ongoing events, and future possibilities
    c. Based on introjected anger
    d. Reflective of irrational thoughts, ideas, and cognitions

15. The client is an eight-year-old female with a fear of food poisoning. The client refuses to eat anything that has not been boiled or from a newly opened package. The parents have explained how they prepare foods to avoid food poisoning. They have taken her to a nutritionist to learn about food poisoning prevention, and they have read books to her on this topic. According to a strategic therapist, the parents activities represent:
    a. Reframing
    b. An indication of the client's position
    c. Attempted solutions
    d. Second order change

16. According to Berne's Transactional Analysis theory, healthy effective and functional interactions can be identified as those which:
    a. Occur between role-appropriate ego states
    b. Occur when the message sent is the message received
    c. Have no ulterior motive
    d. Originate from the adult ego state

17. Using Beck's theory, which of the following would be the most appropriate nursing diagnosis for a client who is depressed after losing his job?
    a. Alteration in thought processes related to automatic thoughts
    b. Alteration in self-esteem related to lost job
    c. Ineffective individual coping related to job loss
    d. Anxiety related to fears as a result of job loss

18. Sally is a 40-year-old client with chronic depression and alcoholism. Using a behavioral approach, which of the following would be an appropriate nursing diagnosis for Sally?
    a. Ineffective individual coping related to a poor self-concept
    b. Impaired self-esteem related to relapse of drinking
    c. Risk for self-directed violence related to negative thoughts
    d. Anger related to introjected feelings

19. If her nurse uses a psychoanalytic approach in Sally's therapy sessions, which of the following would be an expected outcome? Sally will:
    a. Bring aspects of herself into awareness and acceptance
    b. Develop skills to scientifically address irrational thoughts
    c. Decrease her pain and change her view of the situation
    d. Uncover unconscious conflicts

20. John, an advanced practice nurse, plans to use a strategic therapy approach with a client who is a perfectionist. A technique that John will incorporate in the nursing care plan is:
    a. Symptom prescription
    b. Dream analysis
    c. Use of a feeling log
    d. Relaxation training

21. If a nurse decides to use a Rogerian approach with her client, which of the following will be included in the nursing care plan?
    a. Reframing the symptoms
    b. Allowing the client to lead the therapy
    c. Structural analysis
    d. Homework assignments

22. Steve is a 34-year-old male being evaluated by the nurse. Steve describes himself as a failure and not worthwhile because he is not always competent and achieving in all respects. The nurse evaluates this as being:
    a. An automatic thought
    b. Faulty information introjection
    c. A basic irrational idea
    d. An example of top dog/underdog

23. In an attempt to learn more about transactional analysis, a student nurse decides to analyze her friends' interactions. Friend A says, "Let's go see Pocahantas tonight." Friend B replies, "You always get to choose what we do." The student interprets this as an example of:
    a. Adult to adult; child to parent
    b. Adult to child; child to adult
    c. Parent to child; child to parent
    d. Parent to child; child to adult

24. Sue is using a psychoanalytic approach with Doug, a client with depression. Which would be an appropriate response by Sue when Doug repeatedly 'forgets' to pay for the sessions?
    a. "We will continue only if you pay what you owe me."
    b. "I still care for you even though you are behind in the payments."
    c. "Let's look at what's going on in this relationship."
    d. "I feel you are devaluing my role as a therapist."

25. The idea that at the core of every human being is an organized and effective self whose basic energy is moving towards the integration of experiences would be incorporated to a nursing care plan using which of the following approaches?
    a. Gestalt therapy
    b. Cognitive therapy
    c. Client-centered therapy
    d. Strategic therapy

26. Which of the following types of brain-imaging techniques is based on the use of glucose in the brain?
    a. CT scans
    b. EEG
    c. PET scans
    d. MRI images

27. Neurotransmitters are best described as:
    a. Neurons
    b. Chemicals
    c. Synapses
    d. Gyri

28. The therapeutic action of psychotropic drugs is most often caused by their effect on the activity of:
    a. The cerebellum
    b. Dendrites
    c. Neurotransmitters
    d. The peripheral nervous system

29. Psychobiological treatments would include all the following *except*:
    a. ECT
    b. Reserpine
    c. Thorazine
    d. Psychoanalysis

30. The system responsible for the "fight-or-flight" response is the:
    a. Sympathetic system
    b. Endocrine system
    c. Parasympathetic system
    d. Extrapyramidal system

Chapter 4

Psychobiology

1. During a client admission it is important for the nurse to obtain the family history for mental disorders because:
    a. A positive history of mental disorders signifies the client will have those disorders
    b. Family history may assist in decisions about diagnosis and treatment
    c. Clients may be embarrassed about family history and withhold information
    d. Discussing family history will help prevent client from getting the disorder

2. The theory of biological basis for mental disorders:
    a. Is a relatively new approach for brain based etiology
    b. Was discovered in the "decade of the brain"
    c. Has a history dating back to ancient Greece
    d. First appeared in the United States

3. Understanding the normal function of the human brain is:
    a. Not necessary for psychiatric nurses who focus primarily on behavioral intervention
    b. A complex undertaking that nurses seldom use in their practice
    c. Important for nursing assessment, but not relevant during treatment
    d. Necessary for nurses in all aspects of psychiatric care

Chapter 5

Legal-Ethical Issues

1. Mr. H. is an advanced-practice nurse in a state where the nurse can sign the first certification for an emergency commitment. Ms. S. is being evaluated for emergency commitment because of the likelihood of serious harm to others. Ms. S. threatened to kill her mother, who she thinks is against her. In assessing the need for commitment, what would be the most important nursing response?
   a. "I understand you have had some difficulty today."
   b. "You have threatened your mother. Tell me why."
   c. "Because you threatened your mother, you are going to have to go to the hospital."
   d. "Tell me about your delusions."

2. Mr. W. is an inpatient with the diagnosis of bipolar disorder, manic type. Yesterday he became agitated and pushed another client. The staff responded by wrestling him to the floor and then placing him in seclusion. The charge nurse called a meeting to discuss the incident. The most appropriate approach for her to use is:
   a. "How did this situation get so out of control?"
   b. "Mr. W is very angry and might file a lawsuit. How can we protect ourselves?"
   c. "Why didn't you try a less restrictive intervention with Mr. W yesterday?"
   d. "Let's review what happened yesterday."

3. Karen is a nurse in a state where nurses have privileged communication. She has been subpoenaed to testify in court in the divorce trial of her client Sally—against Sally's wishes. When asked to describe Sally's diagnosis and treatment for the court, Karen respectfully tells the court:
   a. "I am refusing to testify based on the fifth amendment."
   b. "I am claiming an exemption under the privileged communication statute."
   c. "I have been treating Sally for chronic depression using cognitive therapy."
   d. "Sally does not want me to testify about what she has told me."

4. Sam has been treated on the inpatient unit for paranoia. Although he continues to have fixed delusions about his wife being unfaithful and has discussed his plan to 'get her for this,' the team has decided to discharge him now that he is stable on antipsychotic medications. Dawn, his primary therapist, should include which of the following in his discharge plan?
   a. Informing Sam of the consequences if he acts out at home
   b. Informing Sam's wife of his threats
   c. Requiring mandatory day hospital attendance
   d. Informing Sam when he can alter his medication dose

5. Paul has been on the inpatient unit for 5 days with a schizoaffective disorder and is being treated with lithium carbonate. He repeatedly states he is a prisoner and is being poisoned by the staff. He states his hand tremors are proof of the poisoning. The nurse analyzes this data as an indication that Paul:
   a. Needs information about his medication's side effects
   b. Needs to have his medication increased because of continued delusions
   c. Is experiencing symptoms of withdrawal
   d. Is manipulative

6. Patricia is an involuntary inpatient being treated for chronic depression with suicidal ideation. After one week, she demands to be released. The nurse plans to:
   a. Allow her to leave the unit
   b. Inform her that she can appeal her commitment
   c. Restrict her to her room
   d. Inform her she lost her right to leave the hospital

7. Sean, an involuntary inpatient, is being treated for an acute exacerbation of paranoid schizophrenia. He refuses his morning dose of prolixin. The most appropriate initial nursing response is:
   a. "If you do not take your medication, you will be placed in seclusion."
   b. "You have no right to refuse your medication; you are an involuntary client."
   c. "Can we discuss why you do not want to take your medication, Sean?"
   d. "I will give you an injection if you do not take this pill."

8. Sean, a paranoid client, has refused his morning dose of prolixin. Charley, another client on the unit, says, "You better take your medicine, or else they will throw you into the seclusion room and take away all your clothes." The nurse decides the clients need some information on their rights and treatment. Which of the following should the nurse plan to include?
   a. Advice on how to get discharged from the hospital
   b. Purposes of seclusion
   c. Commitment procedures
   d. Restraint procedures

9. Debby is a 15-year-old female brought by her mother to see a nurse. Debby's mother demands that her daughter be admitted for treatment of "behavior problems." Her mother says she stays out until 4 A.M. and is hanging out with "bad" kids. The CNS will recommend:
   a. Involuntary commitment
   b. That she work with Debby and her mom on an outclient basis
   c. That the mother start therapy
   d. That the mother take her daughter for emergency admission

10. Sandra Smith is a 42-year-old female who has had 12 previous hospitalizations for chronic undifferentiated schizophrenia. Since being discharged 9 days ago, she appears poorly motivated and sits around her house most of the day. Her sister asked the CNS to arrange for her to be committed because she thinks she needs more treatment. The CNS evaluates the data and informs Sandra's sister that she cannot be committed because:
    a. It is less than two weeks since her discharge
    b. There is no evidence she is a danger to herself or others
    c. She has used up her hospital coverage
    d. She has not voluntarily requested hospitalization

11. Mr. D. is a 34-year-old male charged with assault with intent to commit murder. He has been hallucinating, and his lawyer has requested a competency hearing. Select the question that is most appropriate to assess his competency to stand trial:
    a. "Mr. D., can you describe your hallucinations?"
    b. "Mr. D., were you ever abused as a child?"
    c. "Mr. D., can you describe for me the charges against you?"
    d. "Mr. D., can you explain to me why you would want to assault your brother?"

12. Steve is a 30-year-old male admitted for substance abuse detoxification. Nurse Rogers receives a call from a person who says he is Steve's coworker and is inquiring about Steve's condition. Nurse Rogers should respond:
    a. Without acknowledging that Steve is a client on the unit
    b. That the coworker should contact the physician about Steve's condition
    c. That Steve's condition is stable
    d. That the coworker should call Steve directly on the client's phone

13. Sue is agitated, is using profanity, and is physically threatening the other clients. Based on these symptoms, the nurse initially plans to:
    a. Speak to the physician about reevaluating Sue's medications
    b. Secure staff to seclude Sue
    c. Talk with Sue about better ways to manage stress
    d. Speak with the other clients about their feelings

14. A priority nursing diagnosis for Sue is:
    a. Impaired verbal communication as evidenced by cursing
    b. Ineffective individual coping
    c. High risk for violence to others
    d. Powerlessness

Chapter 6

Cultural Issues

1. When planning care for clients using a cultural focus, the nurse will incorporate which of the following beliefs regarding health?
   a. It is a belief of body and mind.
   b. It is equilibrium with mankind.
   c. It is harmony of the body, mind, and spirit.
   d. It is harmony with man.

2. A client refuses to participate in a group because of the presence of a person who 'can put spells on him.' The nurse recognizes that this client may believe in the superstition that illness can be caused by:
   a. Evil eye
   b. Biological factors
   c. Environment
   d. Unhealthy habits

3. Which would be the most appropriate nursing response to a client who refuses to join a group because another client may put a spell on him?
   a. Discuss this belief with the client later
   b. Inform the client that this is ridiculous
   c. Ask the group what they think
   d. Avoid focusing on this delusion

4. When assessing a client's cultural beliefs, which of the following might indicate an attempt by the client to ward off the evil eye?
   a. Avoiding the topic
   b. Displaying religiosity
   c. Wearing amulets
   d. Wearing black

5. When planning nursing care, the nurse should be aware that a belief that health depends on "the balance of hot and cold" is commonly found among people of:
   a. Asian-American culture
   b. African-American culture
   c. Hispanic-American culture
   d. Native American culture

6. When planning to use a 'person' orientation in providing nursing care, the nurse will incorporate principles of:
   a. Chiropractic medicine
   b. Osteopathic medicine
   c. Allopathic medicine
   d. Homeopathic medicine

7. When assessing a client for heritage inconsistency, the nurse would expect to observe:
   a. Evidence of knowledge about one's culture and customs
   b. Regular contact with the extended family
   c. Residence in a neighborhood predominantly of one's ethnic group
   d. An admitted change of last name

8. When working with a xenophobe, anticipate that the individual will:
   a. Welcome strangers to her or his home
   b. Admire foreign customs
   c. Be wary of alternative ideas
   d. Join diverse groups

9. The nurse plans to teach a newly immigrated engineer from Vietnam about his diabetes mellitus using pamphlets. Before initiating this education, the nurse should determine the client's:
   a. Willingness to participate and follow instructions
   b. Ability to read and understand English
   c. Readiness to learn this material
   d. Previous knowledge on the subject

10. When planning nursing care for an African-American client, the nurse will use an orientation which focuses on:
    a. The present
    b. The past
    c. The future
    d. No specific time

11. The nurse is working with a Native American client and observes that the person is future oriented with no boundaries. The nurse analyzes that this indicates:
    a. Psychopathology
    b. Abnormal behavior for a Native American
    c. Nontraditional Native American behavior
    d. Expected Native American behavior

12. When assessing a Hispanic client using a cultural focus, the nurse would anticipate that this person would be:
    a. Future oriented
    b. Embracing
    c. Adverse to physical contact
    d. Without boundaries

13. When interacting with a client from a culture about which the nurse is unfamiliar, the preferred action is to:
    a. Seek information about the specific cultural group
    b. Interact based on the predominant cultural group
    c. Interact based on the nurse's culture
    d. Interact in a way which combines several cultures

14. When implementing nursing care for a client from a different culture, the nurse observes the client take a pill from a container with a label in a foreign language. The nurse's best initial action would be to:
    a. Remove all medicines from the client's room
    b. Call security to seize this medicine
    c. Insist that the client only take medicine administered by the nurse
    d. Attempt to determine the medication type and purpose

15. Which of these cultural factors may affect a nursing assessment?
    a. Race
    b. Age
    c. Gender
    d. Education

16. Which of the following is useful advice for the nurse communicating with a client who speaks a different language?
    a. Use first names only to minimize confusion.
    b. Do not assume a client is angry if they speak loudly.
    c. Try to use an ethnic dialect so that the client feels accepted.
    d. Inform the client of friends you might know of the same ethnic background.

17. A student nurse is planning to incorporate a culturally sensitive focus in her nursing care. Which of the following should she include as an underlying principle explaining culture?
    a. Culture is the classification of human beings into groups based on particular physical characteristics.
    b. Culture is a condition of belonging to a group whose members share a unique heritage.
    c. Culture is learned patterns of behavior and thinking shared by a particular group and transmitted over time to other members.
    d. Culture is a group from which one's ancestors originated.

Chapter 7

The Nursing Process

1. Which of the following would be an appropriate question by the nurse in assessing a client's judgment?
    a. "Why did you run away?"
    b. "When did you first start hearing voices?"
    c. "Do you really believe that you hear voices, or do you think it is in your mind?"
    d. "What would you do if you smelled smoke in your home?"

2. When planning to determine if a client has memory problems, which would be the most appropriate approach?
    a. "Where are you?"
    b. "Do you know what day this is?"
    c. "Do you know who I am?"
    d. "What has happened to you?"

3. If a nurse said to a client, "Listen to me carefully. I am going to give you an address that I want you to remember. Later, I will ask you to repeat it to me." The nurse is assessing:
    a. Recent memory
    b. Remote memory
    c. Comprehension
    d. Abstraction

4. Which of the following would be a nursing diagnosis statement in relation to the sociocultural life process?
    a. Altered nutrition
    b. Impaired social interaction
    c. Sexuality pattern disturbance
    d. Self-esteem disturbance

5. If a client had a nursing diagnosis of ineffective individual coping related to ineffective problem solving which of the following comments would the nurse expect?
    a. "I can't stand my psychiatrist."
    b. "I can't decide if I should get my own apartment or not."
    c. "I'm not sure if I want any ice cream right now."
    d. "I don't think I will be able to manage that."

6. An expected outcome for a client with a nursing diagnosis of ineffective individual coping related to ineffective problem solving is that the client will:
    a. Decide if he wants dessert
    b. Develop a more positive self-esteem
    c. Identify pros and cons of getting own apartment
    d. Recognize the positive qualities of this psychiatrist

7. Which of the following would indicate improvement in a client who has a nursing diagnosis of ineffective individual coping related to impaired problem-solving skills?
    a. The client quit therapy with his psychiatrist.
    b. The client chose to remain living with his parents.
    c. The client joined an assertiveness training group.
    d. The client's appearance improved.

8. An appropriate nursing diagnosis for a client who frequently expresses guilt or shame, states he is unable to deal with situations, and is hesitant to try new things would be:
    a. Chronic low self-esteem
    b. Powerlessness
    c. Hopelessness
    d. Ineffective individual coping

9. Outcome criteria for a client with a nursing diagnosis of risk for loneliness related to social isolation would include which of the following?
    a. The client will no longer experience loneliness.
    b. The client will sit in group.
    c. The nurse will interact with the client.
    d. The client will interact with a peer.

10. The student nurse is learning to use the nursing process and attempts to develop appropriate measurable outcome criteria for a client with a nursing diagnosis of ineffective individual coping. Which of the following goals would indicate that learning has occurred? The client will:
    a. Exhibit less hopelessness
    b. Demonstrate effective coping skills
    c. Verbalize reasons to get well
    d. Verbalize feeling calm and relaxed

11. The process of planning includes which of the following?
    a. Determining needs and problems
    b. Analyzing effectiveness of care
    c. Establishing realistic outcome criteria
    d. Identifying priorities of care

12. Nursing interventions needed to help a client with mania accomplish a key outcome of achieving a stable lithium level would include teaching the client:
    a. When to stop using this drug
    b. When to increase the dosage
    c. How to recognize symptoms of toxicity
    d. How to inject this drug

13. Which of the following would be an example of a descriptive nursing intervention?
    a. Assisting the client to interact with others to decrease a sense of loneliness.
    b. Gradually engaging the client in interactions beginning with individual contacts
    c. Teaching the client and family about the prescribed medications
    d. Praising the client for socializing

14. The student nurse is learning to write meaningful nursing interventions rather than medically focused activities. Which of the following would be an example?
    a. Administering antipsychotic medications as prescribed
    b. Observing for extrapyramidal effects
    c. Teaching the client how to manage medication side effects
    d. Initiating Cogentin therapy as ordered

15. The evaluation step of the nursing process is based on:
    a. Attainment of expected client outcomes
    b. Nursing actions
    c. Diagnostic statement
    d. Client's feelings

16. Which of the following is an important nursing behavior to be incorporated in the plan of care when working with a client with severe anxiety?
    a. Giving detailed explanations of the plan
    b. Maintaining a calm, nonthreatening demeanor when interacting with the client
    c. Using open-ended questions during the client's initial hospital phase
    d. Maintaining a stimulating and challenging environment for this client

17. Which of the following are part of the nursing diagnosis step of the nursing process?
    a. Goal statements
    b. Problem statements
    c. Nursing actions
    d. Assessment tools

Chapter 8

Principles of Communication

1. The student nurse plans to reinforce healthy behaviors in her client. Which of the following statements should the student include?
    a. "How can that stress reduction plan help you at home?"
    b. "It sounds like you have made a healthy choice."
    c. "When you tried to do that, how well did it work?"
    d. "It sounds like this is very important to you."

2. When working with clients who exhibit aggressive behaviors, appropriate nursing interventions include:
    a. Setting firm limits
    b. Ignoring these outbursts
    c. Medicating the client
    d. Mimicking the client's behaviors

3. Jack has been labeled a "problem client" on the unit. Which of the following would the nurse expect to observe?
    a. He claims he is not ill.
    b. He produces feelings of sympathy in the staff.
    c. He isolates himself in room most of the time.
    d. He has problems brought on by self (e.g., substance abuse).

4. The student nurse is learning about specific responding techniques. Which should the student plan to use with her client?
   a. Giving advice
   b. Giving reassurance
   c. Giving information
   d. Giving approval

5. When analyzing communication, how would the nurse interpret the following interaction? Verbal—"I have been waiting a long time and was worried about you"
   Nonverbal—concerned facial expression
   a. Incongruent
   b. Congruent
   c. Contradictory
   d. Unclear

6. The student nurse plans on evaluating the client's paralinguistic communication. Which of the following should be included?
   a. Body posture
   b. Mannerisms
   c. Eye contact
   d. Audible sounds

7. Sally, the staff nurse, has been working with Paul, who is mute and has psychosis. After four weeks, Paul has suddenly encroached on Sally's personal space by smiling and touching her hair. The most therapeutic response by Sally would be to:
   a. Ignore this, since Paul is finally showing some response
   b. Firmly communicate acceptable boundaries to Paul
   c. Touch Paul's head and observe his reaction
   d. Smile at Paul and tell him you don't like his touching you

8. The student nurse is learning about principles of communication. Which of the following descriptions of the purpose of therapeutic communication would indicate learning has taken place? The purpose of therapeutic communication is to:
   a. Maintain relationships
   b. Mutually share information
   c. Promote growth and change in clients
   d. Offer advice, suggestions, and spontaneous messages

9. The expected outcome of conducting a periodic self-evaluation of responses to the client by a nurse is:
   a. Maintaining distance from the client's problems
   b. Recognizing the nurse's need for therapy
   c. Recognizing the nurse's responses to the client
   d. Maintaining a professional boundary

10. Which of the following nursing responses would indicate an empathetic approach to a client who is depressed over recent losses in her life?
    a. "I lost my job and family all in one month and continued working."
    b. "I lost my parents last year and still feel sad."
    c. "Tell me more about what you are feeling."
    d. "Let's not focus on sad topics today."

11. The CNS is holding an assertiveness training session for staff nurses. Which of the following should the CNS plan to include in her presentation?
    a. Avoiding eye contact
    b. Targeting behaviors to be changed
    c. Learning to be the 'nice' person at work
    d. Insisting on your rights at work

12. An individual has been labeled as aggressive. Which would you expect to observe?
    a. The person stands up for own rights and respects those of others.
    b. The person stands up for own rights and abuses those of others.
    c. The person does not stand up for own rights.
    d. The person allows domination and feels victimized.

13. Open-ended questions and statements result in fuller, more revealing responses by the client and typically stimulate discussion. Which of the following is an example of this technique by the nurse?
    a. "Where is your family?"
    b. "Tell me about your family."
    c. "Do you have a family?"
    d. "Would you like to talk about your family?"

14. When a client is struggling to explore and solve a problem, the nurse may offer alternatives. Which of the following should the nurse incorporate in the care plan to achieve this objective?
    a. "Have you thought of . . ."
    b. "You should . . ."
    c. "Why don't you . . ."
    d. "I think you need to . . ."

15. The expected outcome of the use of self-disclosure by the nurse is to:
    a. Inform client of expected behaviors
    b. Validate reality
    c. Foster the client's dependence
    d. Allow the nurse to ventilate

16. The student nurse is learning about the appropriate use of procedural touch. Which of the following should the student plan to incorporate?
    a. Holding an elderly client's hand while she speaks of husband's death
    b. Hugging an adolescent client on his discharge
    c. Positioning a client's arm for BP measurement
    d. Shaking the hand of a new client during an introduction

17. The nurse is working on the inclusion of therapeutic humor in interactions with clients. An expected outcome of this technique is:
    a. Elimination of negative emotions
    b. Decrease in alertness
    c. Willingness of client to allow others to laugh at him
    d. Decrease of fears and anxiety

18. Therapeutic techniques that the nurse can use to deal with both transference and resistance include:
    a. Listening to a client's highly charged and irrational responses
    b. Setting limits on what the client can verbalize
    c. Allowing the transference and resistance to remain in place
    d. Terminating with the client because they are unwilling to work

19. Which of the following would be interpreted as therapeutic communication on the part of the nurse?
    a. "Things will get better; you will see."
    b. "I'm sorry. What did you say?"
    c. "That's nothing compared to that other client's problems."
    d. "That's a difficult problem for you."

20. Joyce, 37 years old, is being interviewed by the CNS. Joyce was released from the hospital after a suicide attempt and has told the CNS she is planning to divorce her husband even though she is four months pregnant. Which of the following would be a therapeutic response by the CNS?
    a. "Why are you considering such a drastic move?"
    b. "You will really have problems if you attempt to raise this child yourself."
    c. "This is not the Christian thing to do."
    d. "Let's discuss this option further."

21. A chronic psychotic client tells the nurse that her arm is missing and therefore she cannot participate in the group activities. The arm is intact. Which of the following techniques should the nurse plan to use with this client?
    a. "If your arm is missing, how come you feed yourself?"
    b. "I see your arm right there."
    c. "Let's not focus on that right now."
    d. "It feels like you are missing an arm? Is that what you mean?"

22. Which of the following nursing responses is an example of the therapeutic technique of empathizing?
    a. "I know how difficult that is for you."
    b. "I see you are quite anxious."
    c. "Help me to understand how this is affecting you."
    d. "It sounds as if this is important to you."

Chapter 9

Children and Adolescents

1. Using Freud's developmental theory as a basis, the nurse would analyze that an individual whose major defense is projection is fixed at which stage?
   a. Phallic
   b. Anal
   c. Oral
   d. Genital

2. The nurse is leading parent education classes. The nurse instructs the parents that a helpful strategy to foster a child's initiative (based on Erikson's stages) would be to:
   a. Offer options for dressing
   b. Allow the child to simultaneously wash unbreakable dishes
   c. Place the child in enrichment learning programs at age 2
   d. Promote experimentation in playthings

3. When using Coles' theory as a basis for fostering moral development in a child, which of the following would the nurse incorporate in the nursing care plan?
   a. Healthy role models
   b. Exposure to controls
   c. The utilitarian principle
   d. The golden rule

4. The school nurse is discussing development issues with parents. Which of the following strategies would foster moral development according to Kohlberg?
   a. A laissez-faire approach by the parents
   b. A focus on justice in encounters with the child
   c. Affiliation with an established religion
   d. Enforcement of strict rules by the parents

5. The school nurse is involved with monitoring development and health markers of the students. When using Freud as the basis, the nurse recognizes that the expected outcome of the genital stage is:
   a. A sense of fidelity
   b. An ability to love and work
   c. A healthy relationship with same-sex peers
   d. A sense of competence

6. A nursing diagnosis for an individual who had inconsistent, unpredictable, and discontinuous care as an infant would be:
   a. Anxiety
   b. Ineffective individual coping
   c. Hopelessness
   d. Role confusion

7. Which of the following would the nurse expect to assess in a child who has not developed a sense of competence, based on Erikson's theory?
   a. Shame
   b. Guilt
   c. Alienation
   d. Inferiority

8. A parent is concerned with the interpersonal skills of her 12-year-old son. She asks the community health nurse what would be the expected behaviors of this age group according to interpersonal theorists. The nurse states that the child:
   a. Is able to work with peers towards a common goal
   b. Has developed a conscience
   c. Is able to be genuinely intimate with others
   d. Has developed a self-system with sublimation

9. The school nurse is discussing the importance of emotional and behavioral self-regulation in the development of competence in school-age children with a previous history of maltreatment. One foster parent asks the nurse how she can specifically work toward this with her child. The nurse suggests that the parents plan to:
   a. Avoid any constrictions on their children's behavior
   b. Target self-regulation of emotions
   c. Set up hard and fast rules for the child to follow
   d. Establish a daily schedule of chores

10. According to Piaget, the nurse would expect to assess which of the following in a three-year-old?
    a. Intuitive guesses about cause and effect
    b. The ability to conserve
    c. The ability to reverse operations
    d. Thinking in hypothetical terms

11. The nurse would analyze that a child who can think of future events and develop strategies for solving complex problems is functioning at what level (according to Piaget)?
    a. Preoperational level
    b. Concrete operations level
    c. Formal operations level
    d. Postconventional level

12. When assessing a five-year-old according to Kohlberg's developmental theory, the nurse would expect to observe a:
    a. Good boy/girl orientation
    b. Punishment-obedience orientation
    c. Law-and-order orientation
    d. Hierarchy of principles

13. Which of the following parental responses to a toilet training accident by a three-year-old child is likely to result in the development of a "not me" self-system as described by Sullivan?
    a. Ignoring this as inevitable
    b. Displaying mild parental frustration
    c. Giving punitive responses
    d. Showing acceptance of mistakes

14. If a child is able to focus and coordinate and imagine a series of events, the nurse would analyze that his cognitive developmental level is:
    a. Preoperational
    b. Concrete operational
    c. Formal operational
    d. Postoperational

15. When planning to use operant conditioning with a six-year-old child, the nurse will include which of the following strategies in the plan of care?
    a. Varied outcomes
    b. Reinforcement
    c. Self-efficacy
    d. Conditioned response

16. If a child stated, "people would think you are bad and did not come from a good family," the nurse would analyze that the level of moral development is:
    a. Conventional
    b. Preconventional
    c. Social contract
    d. Postconventional

17. The nurse would evaluate that a child is in which of Piaget's stages of moral development if she observed the ability to consider consequences and intentions when making moral judgments?
    a. Moral realism
    b. Autonomous morality
    c. Universal ethical principles
    d. Social contract

18. A nurse who is using an information-processing theory foundation will assess which of the following?
    a. Specific performance at a given time
    b. Competence
    c. Moral reasoning
    d. Emotional markers of independence

19. Sharon is an 11-year-old who is being treated by the CNS for ineffective individual coping related to school failure as evidenced by suicidal ideation. An appropriate expected outcome for this diagnosis is that Sharon:
    a. Will sign a 'no suicide' contract with the CNS
    b. Will initiate an activity with a peer
    c. And her family will discuss what behaviors are acceptable
    d. Will not focus on school performance

20. In order to assess the developmental history of a child, the community health nurse would ask a parent:
    a. "Did you experience any prenatal problems?"
    b. "What concerns you about your child?"
    c. "How old was your child when he first walked?"
    d. "What have you tried in the past for this problem?"

Chapter 10

The Adult

1. A nurse who is using Jung's theory as a basis for working with adults will incorporate which of the following principles when planning approaches for a 33-year-old male with depression?
    a. Adults continue to work on separation/individuation in their twenties and thirties.
    b. Adult development is fixed by mid-twenties.
    c. Adults feel the need to reevaluate their life in five-year increments.
    d. Adults continue to work on developmental issues until their late fifties.

2. The nurse would evaluate that an individual who displays stagnation, boredom, and interpersonal impoverishment has not successfully completed Erikson's stage of:
    a. Generativity
    b. Ego integrity
    c. Intimacy
    d. Identity

3. When assessing a client in Erikson's seventh stage of development, which of the following would indicate problems with this task?
    a. Mistrust
    b. Feelings of failure
    c. Pseudointimacy
    d. Isolation

4. The nurse would evaluate that an adult who displays satisfaction in a life well lived is adapting to the need for:
    a. Intimacy vs. isolation
    b. Integrity vs. despair
    c. Generativity vs. stagnation
    d. Identity vs. role confusion

5. The nurse who is working with a client with a defensive personality trait will focus on:
    a. Ways to eradicate this pathology
    b. Ways to convert this into an asset
    c. The need to develop insight
    d. The client's childhood experiences

6. The nurse who is working with clients experiencing life transitions will view the positive and negative aspects of social rituals as necessary for:
    a. Helping individuals achieve their potential
    b. Avoiding the fear of separation
    c. Helping troubled individuals mature
    d. Avoiding a focus on change

7. When analyzing the typical responses of both men and women in their thirties, researchers have identified that:
    a. Women tend to struggle between the need to start a family and a career
    b. Women tend to remain less concerned about career issues
    c. Men tend to struggle between family and career goals
    d. Men are less able to postpone the need to start a family

8. A nurse has assessed a 30-year-old female who has symptoms of depression related to her inability to conceive. The client repeatedly speaks of her feelings that she is not 'a real woman' and her fears that her husband will want a divorce. A potential nursing diagnosis would be:
   a. Alteration in body image
   b. Impaired self-esteem
   c. Fear
   d. Ineffective individual coping

9. When assessing a female client for depression, the nurse would focus on:
   a. Loss of an ideal
   b. Loss related to an achievement goal
   c. Loss involving a close relationship
   d. Loss related to a performance issue

10. Using Maslow's hierarchy as a foundation in planning care for an adult, initial priority needs are related to:
    a. Safety
    b. Psychological issues
    c. Physiological issues
    d. Self-esteem

11. When assessing a client based on Maslow's fourth level, the nurse would consider the individual's:
    a. Competence
    b. Intimate relationships
    c. Freedom from fear
    d. Vocation

12. Based on Erikson's theory, an expected outcome for an adult in the eighth stage is the development of:
    a. Fidelity
    b. Wisdom
    c. Care
    d. Love

13. Nursing interventions to assist the adult in achieving Erikson's eighth stage include:
    a. Encouraging a life review of triumphs and disappointments
    b. Aiding in the fusion of one's identity with another
    c. Focusing on embracing the future
    d. Assisting in the use of creativity

14. The nurse is assessing a 53-year-old female for symptoms related to a mid-life crisis. Which of the following typical mid-life biological changes would the nurse expect to assess?
    a. Increased reaction time
    b. Alterations in strength and endurance
    c. Enhanced muscle tone
    d. More acute hearing

15. In planning care for a 53-year-old client experiencing a mid-life crisis, the nurse would include:
    a. Group therapy
    b. Systematic desensitization to stress
    c. Family involvement in her care
    d. The client's previously used coping mechanisms

16. Nursing strategies to assist Miriam, a 53-year-old female experiencing a mid-life crisis, would include:
    a. Encouraging the development of insight
    b. Focusing on behavioral changes
    c. Exploring childhood traumas
    d. Promoting mourning of losses

Chapter 11

The Elderly

1. When caring for geriatric clients, the nurse would incorporate the biologic theory of aging, which states that aging:
   a. Is explained solely by internal factors
   b. Combines genetic and environmental factors that explain why persons age differently
   c. Hypothesizes that autoimmune responses attack normal cells and cause mutations
   d. Is explained by the accumulation of waste products and free radicals

2. The nurse would evaluate that an elderly person who seems to draw on past experiences in coping with losses in the present would be an example to support the theory of:
   a. continuity
   b. activity
   c. adaptation
   d. disengagement

3. A nurse working in a geriatric center would include which of the following principles when planning care for this population? Responses to loss by the elderly differ from responses by younger-aged cohorts in that:
   a. The elderly are less able to cope with losses because of ineffective coping mechanisms
   b. Losses are more intense for the elderly because of their increased vulnerability
   c. Loss has less meaning for the elderly because of their memory impairments
   d. Losses are usually multiple in nature, and past coping mechanisms may not be effective

4. The nurse assesses her client for the presence of presbycusis, which is the:
   a. Loss of the eye's ability to accommodate to distance
   b. Changes in the sense of touch due to dermal alterations
   c. Diminished ability in hearing acuity
   d. Changes in sense of balance

5. The community health nurse is asked by the elderly adults in a senior center to discuss how age affects sexuality. The nurse should inform these persons that:
   a. Sex can be an important part of their lives
   b. Aging affects the reproductive system and sexuality
   c. Production of sperm decreases with aging
   d. Production of androgen hormones increase with aging

6. A priority nursing assessment for Jennie, a 70-year-old female, would be:
   a. Joint mobility
   b. Muscle mass strength
   c. Flexibility
   d. Loss of bone mass

7. The nurse working in the geriatric OPD is aware that common cardiovascular changes in the elderly can include:
   a. Lowered blood pressure
   b. Increased heart rate
   c. Atrial arrhythmias
   d. Increased cardiac output

8. The nurse who uses a psychoanalytic approach as a basis for practice would assist the elderly client to:
   a. Deal with transitions
   b. Balance feelings of despair and integrity
   c. Continue recreational and creative activities
   d. Accept the life that one has lived

9. A nurse who is using Erikson's theory as the basis for practice with her elderly clients would focus on which of the following in the nursing care plan?
   a. Balance between wisdom and senility
   b. Balance between syntonic and dystonic
   c. Need for a mentor
   d. Current physiologic status

10. According to the life structure theory of Lowenthal, the expected outcome for the elderly client would be:
    a. Acquisition of wisdom
    b. Coping with transitions
    c. Higher-level needs
    d. Balancing wisdom with senility

11. A community health nurse working with elderly clients is using a sociologic model in planning care. Which of the following would be included?
    a. Current illnesses
    b. Family history
    c. Economic status
    d. Individual personality traits

12. While working in a senior center, the nurse assesses the clients for expected role transitions such as:
    a. Loss of sexuality
    b. Immobility
    c. Retirement
    d. Caregiver support

13. Nursing strategies to assist in meeting the needs of the elderly client for Maslow's fourth level include:
    a. Supporting needs for intimacy
    b. Assisting with obtaining financial help
    c. Identifying contributions of the person
    d. Promoting physical appearance

14. When developing a nursing diagnosis for Jessie, 76 years old, the nurse assessed she has an external locus of control. Which of the following would be an appropriate nursing diagnosis?
    a. Social isolation
    b. Powerlessness
    c. Hopelessness
    d. Personal identity disturbance

15. Sal is a 70-year-old male who has been diagnosed with disturbance in self-esteem related to forced retirement based on Maslow's hierarchy of human needs. Expected outcomes for Sal include feelings of:
    a. Security
    b. Self-fulfillment
    c. Acceptance
    d. Worth

16. Nursing interventions which would assist Sal would include:
    a. Encouraging of significant relationships
    b. Assisting client to establish appropriate roles
    c. Encouraging a nonrestrictive environment
    d. Providing a structured daily routine

Chapter 12

Anxiety and Related Disorders

1. The nurse would analyze the symptoms of urinary frequency, rigid muscles, and decreased hearing as indicative of which stage of anxiety?
   a. Mild
   b. Moderate
   c. Severe
   d. Panic

2. Jane has been under treatment for recurrent severe levels of anxiety. An appropriate nursing diagnosis would be:
   a. Sensory perceptual alteration related to narrowed perceptual field
   b. Risk for injury related to closed perception
   c. Hopelessness related to total loss of control
   d. Risk for violence related to combative behavior

3. Steve was an awkward child who was ridiculed by his father for his inability to catch a ball. As an adult, Steve developed panic attacks. Steve has pinpointed these attacks as occurring since his company established after-work team sporting activities. The CNS analyzes that Steve's anxiety occurs in relation to:
   a. A signal that predicts a feared event
   b. His physiological responses to sports
   c. A genetic deficiency of neurotransmitters
   d. An unresolved desire to be a baseball player

4. A client was admitted with a diagnosis of agoraphobia with panic attacks. Which of the following symptoms would the nurse expect to observe?
   a. Parasthesias
   b. Constipation
   c. Feigned fears
   d. Hypotension

5. The nurse is working with the family of a client with obsessive compulsive disorder. Which of the following should the nurse incorporate in the teaching plan?
   a. The thoughts, images, and impulses are voluntary.
   b. The family should pay immediate attention to symptoms.
   c. The thoughts, images, and impulses worsen with stress.
   d. OCD is a chronic disorder not responsive to treatment.

6. If a client is admitted with a diagnosis of somatoform disorder, the nurse would expect to observe that:
   a. The complaints begin after age 30
   b. The complaints are explained by general medical disorders
   c. There are structural abnormalities
   d. There is involvement of multiple organ systems

7. A client presents with a history of pain related to at least four different sites which cannot be explained by a known general medical condition. The nurse analyzes this as indicative of:
   a. Somatoform disorder
   b. Pain syndrome
   c. Generalized anxiety disorder
   d. Obsessive compulsive disorder

8. When differentiating between somatoform and conversion disorders, the nurse is aware that the critical defining factor in conversion disorder is that:
   a. The symptom cannot be fully accounted for by a medical condition
   b. The symptom is limited to pain or sexual function
   c. The symptom is intentionally feigned
   d. Symptoms are precipitated by psychological factors

9. Appropriate discharge criteria for a client with chronic anxiety disorder is that the client will:
   a. Experience no more anxiety
   b. Suppress his anxiety symptoms and focus on the future
   c. Identify situations and events which trigger anxiety
   d. Recognize his need to take medications for the rest of his life to control anxiety

10. The nurse is planning to determine whether the client has been experiencing anxiety. Which of the following questions should the nurse include?
    a. "Have you had more difficulty concentrating lately?"
    b. "Have you been feeling sad and lonely?"
    c. "Do you have a history of nerves?"
    d. "Do you frequently feel angry and upset?"

11. Sue is working with a CNS for her obsessive compulsive disorder. The CNS has identified a nursing diagnosis of impaired social interaction for Sue. An appropriate outcome for this problem would be:
    a. Sue will ask her peers to join her in her rituals.
    b. Sue will speak of the baselessness of her obsessions in group.
    c. Sue will avoid obsessing while interacting with the CNS.
    d. Sue will describe an increasing sense of control over intrusive thoughts.

12. Jill, an evening staff nurse, was raped six months ago while walking to the train station. She immediately returned to work and did not focus on this incident. Recently Jill has been having nightmares and problems communicating with her boyfriend. An appropriate outcome for Jill's problem would be that she will:
    a. Develop improved coping skills
    b. Participate in a rape support group
    c. Verbalize her anger towards her boyfriend
    d. Learn how to protect herself from rape

13. The nurse has been working with a client with chronic anxiety. The goal is that the client will identify early warning symptoms of anxiety. Which of the following would the nurse analyze as indicative that the client is moving towards accomplishing this goal?
    a. The client begins to connect her panic symptoms with thoughts about her marital separation.
    b. The client reports no symptoms of anxiety for one week.
    c. The client practices the relaxation techniques daily and when anxiety increases.
    d. The client recognizes that others also experience anxiety in varying situations.

14. Which of the following strategies should the nurse incorporate in the nursing care plan for a client with generalized anxiety disorder?
    a. Tell the client to calm down when anxious.
    b. Have client discuss childhood issues.
    c. Inform client of importance of limiting caffeine, nicotine and other CNS stimulants.
    d. Inform client that they will need to be calm if they wish to attend group therapy.

15. Steve is being treated on the unit for somatoform disorder. Steve approaches the nurse and says he feels dizzy and weak. The initial nursing intervention is to:
    a. Tell Steve to sit and breathe deeply
    b. Give Steve the Xanax
    c. Measure Steve's vital signs
    d. Instruct Steve in imagery exercise

16. The CNS is planning to use systematic desensitization with Margaret, a client with agoraphobia. The initial step the CNS will plan is to:
    a. Define the phobic stimulus
    b. Define a hierarchy of symptoms
    c. Expose the client to the stimulus
    d. Incorporate relaxation teaching

17. The nurse is working with Mike, who has symptoms of PTSD since returning from the Gulf War. An appropriate outcome for Mike is that he will:
    a. Verbalize his feelings about the war experience
    b. Put this experience behind him
    c. Recognize the symptoms are masking his fear
    d. Leave the military because symptoms are war related

18. Cognitive behavioral therapy is widely used in the treatment of anxiety disorders. The nurse interprets that the success of this approach centers on the client's understanding that:
    a. The antecedents of the anxiety are from childhood traumas
    b. Symptoms are related to delusional thoughts
    c. The problem is all in his or her mind
    d. Symptoms are a learned response to thoughts

19. The nurse is teaching a client with chronic anxiety in anxiety-reduction strategies such as:
    a. Focusing on the anxiety situation
    b. Using visual imagery
    c. Focusing on the whole room
    d. Interacting in a group

20. The nurse has identified a diagnosis of personal identity disturbance for Dwayne: inability to distinguish between self and non-self. A goal related to this diagnosis is that Dwayne will:
    a. Suppress feelings of dissatisfaction
    b. Refer to himself as 'the client'
    c. Use aggressive behaviors to meet needs
    d. Identify periods of increasing anxiety

Chapter 13

Mood Disorders: Depression and Mania

1. Which of the following is a priority assessment for the client with a major depression?
   a. Nutritional status
   b. Fluid and electrolyte balance
   c. Suicidal ideation
   d. Mood and affect

2. Which of the following statements would the nurse expect a newly admitted client with mania to make?
   a. "I can't do anything anymore."
   b. "I can manage our finances much better than my wife."
   c. "I can understand why my wife is so upset that I spend so much money."
   d. "I can't understand where all our money goes."

3. Ronald has been admitted with a diagnosis of major depression. The nurse would expect to assess which of the following personality types?
   a. Egocentric
   b. Eccentric
   c. Narcissistic
   d. Dependent

4. The nurse who is interviewing a new client understands that dysthymia differs from a major depression episode in that dysthymia:
   a. Typically has an acute onset
   b. Involves delusional thinking
   c. Is a chronic low-level depression
   d. Does not include suicidal ideation

5. Sally is a 42-year-old female admitted with a diagnosis of acute mania. Her husband states she has not slept, eaten, or drunk for three days. In addition, he says she is very agitated and has been fighting with the neighbors. He also states that she stopped her lithium last week. The priority nursing diagnosis for Sally would be:
   a. High risk for injury
   b. Self-esteem disturbance
   c. Noncompliance
   d. Sleep pattern disturbance

6. Steve has been admitted with a diagnosis of atypical depression. The nurse would expect to observe which of the following in Steve?
   a. Depression beginning around October or November and lasting until March or April
   b. Leaden paralysis
   c. Psychomotor agitation
   d. Increased depression in the morning

7. A priority nursing intervention for Sam, who underwent his first ECT treatment a half hour ago, would be:
   a. Monitoring vital-signs
   b. Offering oral fluids
   c. Encouraging group participation
   d. Evaluating ECT effectiveness

8. Mrs. Lopez is a 38-year-old married mother of two admitted to the psychiatric unit. Recently she has spent $10,000 on new furniture, made excessive long distance phone calls, and has not slept for three days. She is dressed in a green bathing suit. The nurse would initially plan to focus on:
   a. Assessing her needs for food, liquids, and rest
   b. Setting strict limits on her dress and actions
   c. Obtaining a complete and thorough psychosocial assessment
   d. Conducting an in-depth suicide assessment

9. Two weeks after admission, Mrs. Lopez and the nurse have had several sessions discussing medications. Which of the following statements by Mrs. Lopez would indicate the need for additional client education regarding her lithium treatment?
   a. "I will drink 8 to 12 glasses of liquids daily."
   b. "I will restrict my salt intake."
   c. "I will take my medications with food."
   d. "I will have my blood drawn as the physician orders."

10. The nurse would evaluate that client education regarding lithium therapy is effective if the client states:
    a. "I can stop my lithium when I feel better."
    b. "I will probably need to take the lithium for the rest of my life."
    c. "I will taper my lithium when a therapeutic serum level is achieved."
    d. "I can continue with my diuretic and cardiac medications."

11. Mary is the nurse in the OPD working with Fran, who has been taking lithium carbonate 300 mgm t.i.d. Which of the following medications, if also prescribed for Fran, would require reevaluation of the lithium dosage?
    a. Hydrodiuril
    b. Navane
    c. Ativan
    d. Cefobid

12. A.J. is a 60-year-old man who comes to the health clinic for his annual flu shot. As the nurse prepares him for this, A.J. says he feels tired all the time, finds little pleasure in things anymore, and has difficulty sleeping. The best nursing action is to:
    a. Have him remain in the clinic until evaluated by a mental health professional
    b. Instruct A.J. in how to manage these typical signs of aging
    c. Explore his past psychiatric history and further assess his current mental status
    d. Explain that this is not a psychiatric clinic and provide a list of referrals for follow-up

13. Which of the following client outcomes would be appropriate to determine response to antidepressant medication? The client will:
    a. Describe signs and symptoms of major depression
    b. Make plans to attend one community social activity a week
    c. Demonstrate assertive communication skills
    d. Complete own self-care activities

14. Prior to initiating medication therapy with Nardil, the nurse plans to determine the client's:
    a. Mood and affect
    b. Cognitive ability to understand information about the medication
    c. Support network and their willingness to participate in treatment
    d. Activity level

15. In planning care for a client with severe major depressive disorder, the nurse:
    a. Is careful not to create a stressful situation by asking for the client's participation in the plan
    b. Includes teaching about mania as a priority intervention
    c. Advises the client that electroconvulsive therapy may be indicated
    d. Assesses the client's cognitive functioning and ability to participate in planning care

16. M.B. recently underwent orthopedic surgery and has a history of bipolar disorder. When visited by the home care nurse, M.B. is speaking more slowly, crying, refusing to perform ADLs, and reporting feeling depressed. Which of the following nursing diagnosis would be appropriate at this time?
    a. Alteration in thought processes related to bipolar disorder
    b. Knowledge deficit related to depression and surgery
    c. Self-care deficit related to orthopedic surgery and possible depression
    d. Alteration in self-esteem related to immobility

17. As the nurse for Jane, an extremely withdrawn client with depression, you are trying to assist her to become more active. The best approach would be:
    a. "I know you'll feel better if you come out. Everyone does."
    b. "You look so gloomy. Do you need to be left alone?"
    c. "I need a partner for this card game. Come be my partner."
    d. "Let's explore how it feels to sit alone here all day and feel sad."

18. The physician prescribes amitriptyline (Elavil) 50 mgm t.i.d. for Jill. She has been in the hospital and on medication for 16 days. Which of the following nursing diagnosis would the nurse focus on?
    a. Altered self-esteem
    b. Risk for self harm
    c. Noncompliance
    d. Anxiety

19. The expected outcome of medication therapy for Jack, who has been placed on amitriptyline (Elavil) 50 mgm t.i.d., is:
    a. Cure of his depression
    b. Neurotransmitter balance
    c. Limited with such a small dose
    d. Related to his affect

20. Grace is a 40-year-old married female admitted for depression. She has been refusing to get out of bed. As the primary nurse, you use a behavioral approach. Which of the following statements would be appropriate for this approach?
    a. "Tell me more about your relationship with your mother. What is your earliest memory of her?"
    b. "You may need medication. I will call the psychiatrist to do a medication evaluation."
    c. "Come and spend time with me. We can discuss this TV show."
    d. "When you are able to be up and dressed, we will be able to increase your unit privileges."

21. Which of the following principles should the nurse consider when planning nursing care for Dave, who was admitted after a suicide attempt?
    a. Clients who attempt suicide and fail will not try again.
    b. The more specific the plan, the greater the risk of suicide.
    c. People who talk about suicide are less likely to attempt it.
    d. People who attempt suicide and fail did not really want to die.

22. Appropriate nursing strategies to assist Dave, who was admitted after a suicide attempt, include:
    a. Encouraging Dave to express his feelings rather than to suppress them
    b. Encouraging Dave to focus on peers rather than his self-absorption
    c. Discussing with Dave the impact of his suicidal thoughts on his family
    d. Avoiding any focus on the topic of suicide

23. Pat is a 33-year-old female admitted with bipolar disorder, manic phase. Pat is loud, garishly dressed, hyperverbal, and hyperactive. Which of the following principles should the nurse consider when planning care for Pat?
    a. Manic clients respond well to peer pressure.
    b. Decreasing stimulation tends to diminish symptoms.
    c. Increasing stimulation tends to focus the client.
    d. Detailed activities will help the client limit behavior.

24. Pat, from question 23, has been on the unit for two days. The clients are planning their weekend activity when Pat interrupts and insists they change their plans to a disco party. Pat curses and becomes louder when her suggestions are rebuffed. The best nursing intervention at this point is to:
    a. Ask the group to reconsider Pat's suggestion
    b. Tell Pat to quiet down or else
    c. Escort Pat to a quieter place
    d. Ignore her outbursts because it is related to her mania

Chapter 14

The Schizophrenias

1. Martin has been admitted with a diagnosis of catatonic schizophrenia. The nurse would expect to assess:
    a. Echopraxia
    b. Paranoia
    c. Regression
    d. Clanging

2. The nurse would evaluate that a client who has auditory hallucinations has improved when the client can:
    a. Tell the nurse what the voices say
    b. Tell the voices to be quiet
    c. Validate what is real
    d. Follow what the voices say

3. John is a 34-year-old client with chronic schizophrena who frequently displays ambivalence. A realistic short-term goal for the nurse to work towards in term of this problem is John will:
    a. Decide his own daily schedule
    b. Refuse to attend activities he doesn't like
    c. Choose which staff member he will work with
    d. Choose between two outfits to wear today

4. Larry, a 32-year-old with catatonic schizophrenia, has been mute and motionless for 2 days. The priority nursing diagnosis is:
    a. High risk for fluid and electrolyte imbalance
    b. Impaired mobility
    c. Impaired verbal communication
    d. Ineffective individual coping

...3-year-old female who was admitted 3
... she ran nude through the streets
... she was the "Queen of Hearts."
... n, Susan remains delusional, shouts
... is loosely associated. Based on this
... develops a nursing diagnosis of:
   a. ... for violence
   b. Defensive coping
   c. Alteration in thought processes
   d. Impaired verbal communication

6. Susan's nurse from question 9 plans to work with her on the diagnosis of alteration in thought processes as evidenced by delusions. An appropriate expected outcome would be that Susan will:
   a. Allow the nurse to dispute her delusions
   b. Distinguish her boundaries
   c. Speak in reality with the nurse
   d. Explain why she thinks she is the "Queen of Hearts"

7. Which of the following interventions by the nurse would be appropriate to use with Susan?
   a. Confronting the delusion
   b. Asking Susan why she would like to be the queen of hearts
   c. Explaining to Susan that she is not the queen of hearts
   d. Presenting reality

8. Which of the following would the nurse interpret as an indicator of improvement for Susan?
   a. Susan participates in unit activities.
   b. Susan discusses her delusion with her peers.
   c. Susan recognizes herself and staff for who they are.
   d. Susan avoids any mention of royalty.

9. If a client exhibited a sudden scream and self-mutilation and was responding to command hallucinations, the nurse would analyze these as indicators of:
   a. Poor impulse control
   b. Inability to manage anger
   c. Derealization
   d. Inappropriate affect

10. If a nurse has identified a nursing diagnosis of impaired self-esteem for her client, which would be an appropriate intervention to use?
    a. Encouraging verbalization of feelings in a safe environment
    b. Helping the client verbalize feelings
    c. Engaging the client in activities designed to promote success
    d. Providing large muscle activities to relieve stress

11. 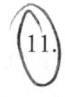 If a client developed extrapyramidal symptoms, the nurse would interpret this as an indication of symptoms:
    a. That occur from an overabundance of dopamine in the extrapyramidal system
    b. That are most likely to occur with the use of a low-potency, high-dosage antipsychotic
    c. Related to dopamine depletion occurring in response to antipsychotic medication administration
    d. Primarily related to high doses of antidepressant medications

12. Donna, 19 years old, is admitted for the second time in nine months, acutely psychotic with a DSM-IV diagnosis of undifferentiated schizophrenia. Donna sits alone rubbing her arms and smiling. She tells the nurse her thoughts cause earthquakes and the world is burning. The nurse understands that which of the following best characterizes the primary deficit in Donna's condition?
    a. Altered mood states
    b. Disordered thinking
    c. Withdrawal
    d. Increased impulse control

13. Bill has been admitted with disorganized type schizophrenia, and the nurse observes that his affect is blunted, he isolates himself, and he sits rocking in the corner. He occasionally will curse or call another client a "jerk" without provocation. The nurse asks Bill how he is feeling, and he responds "everybody picks on me. They frobitz me." The nurse's best response would be:
    a. "That's too bad."
    b. "Who is everybody?"
    c. "What difference does it make?"
    d. "Why do they frobitz?"

14. In making a nursing care plan for a client, the nurse recognizes the need to include:
    a. A significant symptom of the disorder
    b. A list of potential diagnoses
    c. Specific criteria for measuring goals
    d. An evaluative statement

15. Marc is a new nurse on the day hospital unit and he has been assigned to work with Maria, a 48-year-old woman with a diagnosis of residual schizophrenia. Marc would expect to assess which of the following in Maria?
    a. Somatic delusions
    b. Disorganized speech pattern
    c. Catatonic posturing
    d. Emotional blunting

16. An expected outcome for Sam, who hears voices telling him he is evil, would be that he will:
    a. Recognize why the voices say he is evil
    b. Respond verbally to these voices
    c. Identify events of increased anxiety that promote hallucinations
    d. Integrate these voices into his personality in a positive manner

17. Selena is a 22-year-old client with paranoid schizophrenia who has said she feels like throwing a chair in the dayroom. Mary, her nurse, attempts to encourage verbalization in order to deescalate Selena. Which would be appropriate?
    a. "Selena, tell me what's going on."
    b. "Selena if you throw something you will be restrained."
    c. "Selena, why are you so upset?"
    d. "Selena, it's time for group therapy. You can talk there."

18. Laura is a 34-year-old female admitted with catatonic schizophrenia, and she is mute and motionless. Which of the following nursing interventions would be a priority?
    a. Orienting Laura to the unit
    b. Assessing Laura for symptoms of physical problems
    c. Establishing a nonthreatening therapeutic relationship with Laura
    d. Reinforcing reality with Laura

19. Sean is a 35-year-old male with paranoid schizophrenia who has demonstrated a loss of control by punching the door and throwing his coffee down the hallway. When planning his approach, Marc the nurse, will:
    a. Speak loudly and clearly
    b. Stand within three feet of Sean
    c. Keep his hands at his side
    d. Give a detailed explanation of the rules

Chapter 15

Personality Disorders

1. When analyzing Mike, a 23-year-old who meets the criteria for antisocial personality disorder, the nurse recognizes that the following nursing diagnosis would be pertinent to his care:
    a. Risk for self-mutilation
    b. Personal identity disturbance
    c. Impaired social interaction
    d. Ineffective individual coping

2. Wanda is a 43-year-old woman diagnosed narcissistic personality disorder. Wanda would expect to observe which of the behaviors?
    a. Attention seeking
    b. Empathy towards others
    c. Lack of trust in others
    d. Labile affect

3. Sarah is a 35-year-old who is being interviewed by the CNS. Sarah's history indicates that she has few friends, fears criticism from others, and withholds information about her thoughts and feelings because she anticipates a negative reaction. Based on this data, the CNS suspects that Sarah may have a(n):
    a. Borderline personality disorder
    b. Histrionic personality disorder
    c. Avoidant personality disorder
    d. Schizoid personality disorder

4. When planning nursing care for a client with a dependent personality disorder, the nurse recognizes that this individual:
    a. Perceives his or her behavior to be embarrassing
    b. Believes he or she cannot function without help of others
    c. Exaggerates the potential dangers of ordinary situations
    d. Demands excessive attention from others

5. Josh is a 22-year-old man diagnosed with antisocial personality disorder. Which of the following should the nurse consider when planning care for Josh? Clients with antisocial personality disorder:
    a. Demand constant attention
    b. Tolerate frustration well
    c. Have well-developed super egos
    d. Can be charming initially

6. An expected outcome when the team implements a behavior modification approach is that Josh will:
    a. Learn how to avoid punishment
    b. Explain why he breaks rules
    c. Comply with behaviors specified in the contract
    d. Develop appropriate behavioral interaction skills

7. Karen is a 27-year-old woman diagnosed with borderline personality disorder. Karen displays a labile affect, impulsivity, frequent angry outbursts, and difficulty tolerating her angry feelings without self-injury. A priority nursing diagnosis for Karen is:
    a. Anxiety
    b. Risk for self-mutilation
    c. Risk for violence towards others
    d. Ineffective individual coping

8. Which of the following would the nurse expect to observe in a client diagnosed with schizotypal personality disorder?
    a. Brief psychotic episodes in response to stressful events
    b. Intense stormy relationships
    c. Incorrect interpretation of external events
    d. Lack of tender feelings towards others

9. Priority nursing interventions for a client with borderline personality disorder who has a history of self-mutilation and is currently angry, irritable, and impulsive would be:
    a. Establishing a contract for safety with the client
    b. Teaching the client ways to manage anger
    c. Helping the client tolerate feelings
    d. Implementing behavioral modification

10. Which of the following would the nurse analyze as indicating that a client with a diagnosis of high risk for self-mutilation related to feelings of abandonment and impulsivity has improved?
    a. Client verbalizes feelings of abandonment in a realistic way
    b. Client vows never to get involved in a relationship again
    c. Client expresses deep rage at the ending of this relationship
    d. Client suppresses feelings of abandonment

11. Garrett, currently imprisoned for embezzlement, has a history of blaming others for his problems and becoming defensive and angry when criticized. Garrett has expressed no remorse for his actions, nor any response to his conviction, and he continues to claim his actions were justified since his company did not pay him what he is worth. The nurse would diagnose Garrett with:
    a. Avoidant personality disorder
    b. Schizotypal personality disorder
    c. Antisocial personality disorder
    d. Borderline personality disorder

12. Sandra, who is diagnosed with schizoid personality disorder, is isolative, does not speak to her peers, and sits through the community meeting without speaking. Her mother describes her as shy with few friends. Which would be an appropriate nursing diagnosis for Sandra?
    a. Anxiety related to a new environment as evidenced by isolation and not talking to peers
    b. Impaired social interaction related to unfamiliar environs as evidenced by isolation and not talking with peers
    c. Ineffective individual coping related to new environs as evidenced by isolation and minimal interaction with others
    d. Altered thought processes related to a new environment as evidenced by isolation and minimal interactions with others

13. Ellen would do anything to "act out" a suicidal gesture, including grabbing the coffee jar to smash it and attempting to hang herself with her bra. The nurse would analyze Ellen's behaviors as indicative of which personality disorder?
    a. Narcissistic
    b. Histrionic
    c. Borderline
    d. Antisocial

14. Which should the nurse include when teaching a client with a personality disorder?
    a. "Journal writing will help you recognize feeling states."
    b. "Try to problem-solve on your own to help with your difficulty relating with others."
    c. "Identify people/circumstances which create conflict and avoid them."
    d. "Try to alleviate the behaviors that indicate problems relating with others."

15. Jim was threatening another client in group when the client spoke of drug use. The nurse determined that Jim is at risk to act violently against others as evidenced by his aggressive behavior, verbal threats, and a history of impulsivity. Which is the best response?
    a. Secluding Jim to protect the nurse and other clients
    b. Putting Jim in restraints to protect the milieu
    c. Exploring alternative ways to handle frustrating topics in the group
    d. Telling Jim to leave the group until he can speak appropriately

16. Janet is having difficulty with memories of sexual abuse and has a history of suicidal gestures, self-mutilation, sexual addiction, and substance addiction. She complains of back pain, menstrual problems, and headaches. Janet came to the partial hospital program to prevent another suicide gesture or self-mutilation. What type of collaborative therapy would be useful for Janet?
    a. Working with the occupational therapist, Janet and the nurse explore ways to reduce stress.
    b. Working with the physical therapist, Janet and the nurse explore ways to reduce back pain.
    c. Working with an acupuncturist, the nurse and Janet explore ways to reduce her pain.
    d. Working with a sexologist, the nurse and Janet explore healthy sexuality and safe sex.

17. Ralph is seeking treatment for depression after the recent breakup of a relationship. Ralph constantly procrastinated in terms of marriage and said his girlfriend complained that he did not show her affection and was too controlling. He described his inability to sleep and concentrate and a loss of energy since the breakup. When evaluating outcomes, which is a priority for Ralph?
    a. He will demonstrate assertive behavior and express his needs.
    b. He will express hope in terms of developing a future relationship.
    c. He will identify feelings of sadness related to the loss of the relationship.
    d. He will list three new ways to reduce stress.

Chapter 16

Substance-Related Disorders

1. Determinants of success for a substance abuser completing a rehabilitation program is based on:
    a. Willingness to recognize denial
    b. Number of drug-free days
    c. Ability to maintain employment
    d. Lack of symptoms of complications

2. The most effective nursing approach to deal with denial in a person with substance abuse is:
    a. Discussing the addictive personality
    b. Confronting client regarding his or her hopeless situation
    c. Having client identify the effects of alcohol on his or her life
    d. Describing the physiologic effects of alcohol on the body

3. A client presents with a 10-year dependence on alcohol and nicotine. [He is] separated from his wife and has problems [in] his everyday life. An appropriate diagnosis for this client is:
    a. Ineffective denial
    b. Risk for loneliness
    c. Ineffective individual coping
    d. Powerlessness

4. Mr. Jones has been admitted for the third time for alcoholism. He has relapsed immediately upon discharge previously and minimizes his problems with alcohol. An initial outcome during the hospital stay would be that Mr. Jones will:
    a. Remain compliant with the protocol for alcohol detoxification
    b. Verbalize that he is powerless over alcohol
    c. Remain abstinent
    d. Develop more effective coping skills

5. Mr. Brown has been admitted in delirium tremens. He is dehydrated with illusions and auditory hallucinations. He has a badly bruised, swollen tongue and is confused. In developing a care plan for Mr. Brown, what measures should the nurse include to ensure that he is physiologically stable?
    a. Applying ice to his tongue
    b. Encouraging oral fluids
    c. Keeping the room dark
    d. Monitoring his vital signs

6. The CNS is working with Jay, a 40 year old with chronic alcoholism, and his wife Sharon. Sharon describes how she has cut off all outside relationships over the past 20 years while focusing her life on trying to help Jay remain sober. Based on this, the CNS evaluates Sharon's behavior as an indication of:
    a. Enmeshment
    b. Concern
    c. Martyrdom
    d. Introversion

7. Which of the following characteristics would the nurse expect to observe in a substance abuser?
    a. Success-oriented personality
    b. Depressive personality organization
    c. Aggressive personality orientation
    d. Codependent personality

[...]n has consulted the school nurse because she is concerned about her 16-year-old son Robby and the possibility of drug abuse. What should the nurse plan to teach Jean about the signs of substance use/abuse in adolescents?
   a. Night sweats
   b. Increased thirst
   c. Daytime drowsiness
   d. Headaches

9. A client exhibited tremulousness, anorexia, hypertension, and confusion. The client, admitted for pneumonia, has a history of drug abuse. The nurse analyzes these symptoms as indicative of:
   a. Wernicke's encephalopathy
   b. Delirium tremens
   c. Alcoholic hallucinosis
   d. Korsakoff's syndrome

10. If an individual is admitted with a diagnosis of Wernicke's syndrome, the nurse would expect to assess:
    a. Confabulation
    b. Ataxia
    c. Peripheral neuropathy
    d. Auditory hallucinations

11. Which of the following should the nurse incorporate in the care plan of a client undergoing delirium tremens?
    a. Encouraging group participation
    b. Confronting his denial of substance abuse
    c. Forcing oral fluids
    d. Creating a quiet, nonstimulating environment

12. An appropriate outcome for Sheila, who has been admitted for detoxification from alcohol after a 20-year history of drinking and enablement by her family, would be that Sheila will:
    a. Maintain vital signs within normal range
    b. Identify the effect alcohol has had on her life
    c. Join a 12-step support group
    d. Commit to remaining alcohol free

13. Another client, Pete, has been on the unit for two weeks. He relates a 15-year history of polysubstance abuse with several detoxs followed by relapses when he "gets on with his life and tries to put this other stuff behind him." The nurse identifies an appropriate outcome for Pete. He will:
    a. Verbalize that recovery is a lifelong process which occurs one day at a time
    b. Identify reasons for his noncompliance
    c. Discuss childhood causes that impact on his drug use
    d. Recognize his need for methadone maintenance

14. Sal is a 25-year-old admitted to a drug rehabilitation program four days ago for chronic cocaine abuse. A priority nursing diagnosis for Sal is:
    a. Risk for self-violence related to suicidal depression
    b. Risk for noncompliance related to chronic drug use
    c. Sensory perceptual alteration related to stimulant drug use
    d. Risk for self-violence related to hyperactivity

15. Sandra, 19 years old, has been admitted to the ER after snorting heroin with her boyfriend. She is unconscious, with pinpoint pupils. The priority nursing diagnosis for Sandra is:
    a. Ineffective breathing patterns
    b. Fluid and electrolyte imbalance
    c. Impaired physical mobility
    d. Sensory perceptual alterations

16. When assessing a client for potential alcohol abuse problems, the nurse is aware that the laboratory test which is most sensitive for detecting the effects of chronic alcohol abuse is:
    a. Elevated erythrocyte mean corpuscular volume (EMCV)
    b. Serum glutamic-pyruvic transanimase (SGPT)
    c. Lactic dehydrogenase (LDH)
    d. Serum gamma-glutamyl transferase (GGT)

17. When medicating a client who is withdrawing from alcohol, which of the following principles should be followed? Medication should be:
    a. Administered based on the presence of withdrawal symptoms
    b. Administered at prescribed intervals for at least one month
    c. Used for twenty-four hours only
    d. Administered even if the client is asleep

18. When evaluating a client's drug use, the nurse analyzes the presence of tolerance as indicating the client's:
    a. Ability to adapt to side effects
    b. Consumption of drugs or alcohol on a regular basis
    c. Need for higher doses to produce desired effects
    d. Physiologic and psychologic dependence on a substance

19. When attempting to elicit an accurate substance abuse history, the nurse should:
    a. Progress from the most prohibited chemical of abuse to the most accepted
    b. Avoid the drug history and question the spouse later
    c. Progress from the most acceptable chemical of abuse to the most prohibited
    d. Wait for the client to disclose use

20. The probable occurrence of withdrawal symptoms in a person with a history of chronic alcoholism is most accurately assessed by determining:
    a. The blood alcohol level
    b. Drinking history, quantity consumed and time of last drink
    c. Experiences following previous cessation of drinking
    d. The kind of alcoholic beverage last consumed

21. Steve's physician has prescribed methadone 40 mg qd orally. The nurse recognizes that methadone maintenance can be used as an effective drug replacement for individuals addicted to:
    a. Opiates
    b. Amphetamines
    c. Barbiturates
    d. Hallucinogenic

22. The CNS is conducting a community health education series on substance abuse. Which of the following descriptions of abuse or addiction should the CNS plan to include?
    a. Abuse and addiction are interchangeable terms.
    b. Abuse is characterized by physical dependence, whereas addiction is characterized by psychological dependence.
    c. Both abuse and addiction indicate disease entities with severe withdrawal symptoms.
    d. Addiction is characterized by both psychologic and physiologic withdrawal symptoms.

23. Hedy's husband has chronic alcoholism, and she is concerned about the possibility that their children may develop this disease. She asks the CNS what causes alcoholism. The CNS's best response is:
    a. "The risk for developing alcoholism is increased if there is a family history of alcoholism."
    b. "Studies have confirmed that individuals with dependent personality traits are at high risk for this disease."
    c. "Cultures that include alcohol as part of the ritualized behavior have a higher rate of alcoholism."
    d. "Twin studies have indicated that the environment of a person is more important than the biological influences of parents."

24. A client is admitted to your unit with delirium tremens. Symptoms you are most likely to observe include:
    a. Depression, isolation, and fearfulness
    b. Tachycardia, tremors, and confusion
    c. Lethargy, depression, bradycardia
    d. Rhinorrhea, nausea, diaphoreses

Chapter 17

Delirium, Dementia, and Amnestic and Other Cognitive Disorders

1. Mr. Peters repeatedly says he has just finished an important business meeting, when in fact he has been napping. How should the nurse plan to deal with this problem?
   a. Ignore this confabulation
   b. Confront this delusion
   c. Present reality
   d. Change the topic

2. The nurse is to assess Mrs. Jones in her home using the Mini Mental Status examination. When the nurse arrives, Mrs. Jones is seated at the table with her husband, the TV is on, and several grandchildren are visiting. Mr. Jones says, "Let's get on with this business." Mrs. Jones is quiet, but her hands are gripped tightly, and she is staring at the ceiling. The nurse's best action would be to:
   a. Explain to Mr. Jones that you want accurate data and ask him to take the grandchildren out
   b. Explain the importance of the testing process and make an appointment for another day when the environment can be better controlled
   c. Delete the test from the assessment (because it will not be valid) and rely on observations and reports from her family
   d. Ask Mr. Jones to make an appointment to bring his wife to the clinic for testing

3. Shelly Howe has been admitted to the hospital for cholecystitis. She is accompanied by her sister Jane, who provides all of the assessment data while Shelly sits and nods. You determine that Shelly is 63 years old, single, lives alone, and lost her job as a secretary last year when a new computer system was installed that she was unable to learn. Jane says she is older but has recently had to manage Shelly's shopping, meal preparation, and finances. Which of the following are appropriate nursing diagnoses at this time?
   a. Pain, self-care deficits, situational low self-esteem
   b. Anxiety, self-care deficits, altered thought processes
   c. Impaired home maintenance management, altered thought process, impaired verbal communication
   d. Body image disturbance, anxiety, pain

4. Which of the following should the nurse consider when analyzing the etiology of Alzheimer's disease?
   a. A secondary dementia indicated by loss of recent memory and disorientation to time and place
   b. A primary dementia which is incurable, irreversible, and fatal, caused by the presence of a beta-amyloid protein in the neurons resulting in senile plaques
   c. A secondary dementia which is treatable with analysis of the diet and removal of toxic substances from the diet and environment
   d. A primary dementia characterized by stepwise decreases in cognitive abilities which is irreversible but treatable with antihypertensive medications

5. Which of the following indicates realistic outcome identification for a client with Alzheimer's disease?
   a. Appropriate long-term placement will be obtained to maintain caregiver's health and well-being.
   b. The client will maintain the highest possible functional level.
   c. All decision making will be taken over by a caregiver.
   d. The client's physical status will remain fully functional, since Alzheimer's affects the brain.

6. The home care nurse has assessed Mr. Paul, who is status post herniorrophy, with a history of senile dementia. Mr. Paul has short-term memory loss, disorientation of time and place and dysphasia and lives in a senior retirement community with no close family. Appropriate goals for Mr. Paul include:
   a. Participating in a geriatric assessment program; regaining speech; managing public transportation
   b. Attending English class to improve speech; transferring finances to a conservator; remembering his meds
   c. Discontinuing meal prep; attending speech therapy; relocating to a skilled nursing facility
   d. Eating a balanced diet; having a safe environment; participating in a dementia program

7. Bess, diagnosed with Alzheimer's disease, has a catastrophic reaction during an activity involving simultaneous music playing and a craft project. Bess starts shouting "no, no, no" and leaves the room. The nurse should plan which approach?
   a. Isolate Bess until she is calm, and then direct her back to the activity.
   b. Follow Bess, reassure her, and redirect her to a quieter activity.
   c. Discontinue the activity program since it upsets the clients.
   d. Give Bess a prn antianxiety medication and restrict her activity participation.

8. Which of the following indicators measure the success of a therapeutic activity program for a client with Alzheimer's disease?
   a. Accurate recent memory, positive emotional response, increased verbal expression
   b. Increased attention span, verbal expression of remote memory, positive emotional response
   c. Positive use of preservation, reduction in use of habitual skills, improved abstract reasoning
   d. Positive emotional response, ability to remember multiple steps, accurate recent memory

9. Which of the following nursing techniques are appropriate for successful interaction with a client who has been diagnosed with Alzheimer's disease?
   a. Using multiple memory cues and giving all directions at one time to increase understanding
   b. Correcting errors by the client, and speaking in a loud, clear voice
   c. Encouraging verbal and nonverbal communication, and maintaining a calm demeanor
   d. Setting strict time limits and rephrasing misunderstood questions

10. Jim Poll is a 45-year-old male admitted with a diagnosis of acute onset delirium. The nurse would expect to assess:
    a. Fluctuating levels of consciousness
    b. Gradual onset of symptoms
    c. Apathetic affect
    d. Negative thought content

11. A client has been diagnosed with a dementia secondary to a toxic cause. Which of the following would the nurse expect in the history?
    a. Vitamin B_{12} deficiency
    b. Alcoholism
    c. Hepatic disease
    d. Tuberculosis

12. Sean told the CNS that he is concerned about his mother, who lives alone, seems more forgetful, and is 75 years old. Which of the following, if also mentioned by Sean, would be indicative of Alzheimer's disease?
    a. "Mom continues to participate in senior center activities each week."
    b. "Mom insists on cooking and cleaning herself."
    c. "Mom forgot to pay her bills last month."
    d. "Mom refuses to stop driving even though she is very slow."

13. Susan is an 84-year-old woman with dementia who lives with her daughter and son-in-law. Her daughter tearfully tells the CNS that she doesn't know what's wrong with mom, who has begun accusing them of stealing her lingerie and keeping her a prisoner. Based on the above, the CNS identifies the following nursing diagnosis for Susan:
    a. Altered thought processes
    b. Powerlessness
    c. Ineffective individual coping
    d. Defensive coping

14. An expected outcome for a client experiencing delirium is:
    a. Managing symptoms
    b. Irradicating the cause
    c. Maintaining present level of functioning
    d. Managing regressive symptoms

15. If a client has been diagnosed with Alzheimer's disease, stage I, the CNS would interpret which of the following as expected in this stage?
    a. Recent memory loss
    b. Catastrophic reactions
    c. Progressive gait disturbances
    d. Perseveration

16. Gail is an 85-year-old client with dementia who has a nursing diagnosis of impaired ADL. She lives at home and has not bathed for a month. What is an appropriate outcome for this problem?
    a. Gail will bathe daily.
    b. Gail will bathe three times a week.
    c. The nurse will totally manage Gail's hygiene.
    d. Gail will remain free of skin diseases.

17. Which of the following is an appropriate nursing intervention for a client with dementia who develops a catastrophic reaction?
    a. Employing neutral behavioral interactions
    b. Using touch to communicate
    c. Eliminating or reducing all outside stimulation
    d. Maintaining close personal boundaries

18. Success of a plan incorporating activities for a client with dementia can be measured by which question?
    a. Is the client less involved in ADL activities?
    b. Do caregivers feel more of the stress instead of the client?
    c. Have incidents of sundowning increased?
    d. Has client's aimless pacing decreased?

19. Which of the following should the nurse incorporate in the nursing care plan of a client with dementia to aid in memory retention?
    a. Daily activity schedule
    b. Large motor activities
    c. Simple word games
    d. Discussion groups

Chapter 18

Disorders of Childhood and Adolescence

1. Which of these statements is true concerning mental disorders in children and adolescents?
    a. Mental disorders diagnosed during childhood may continue into adulthood.
    b. In childhood, mental disorders are relatively easy to diagnose.
    c. Medications are not prescribed for the treatment of mental disorders prior to puberty.
    d. The younger the child when a diagnosis of a mental disorder is made, the more positive the outcome will be.

2. The following children are diagnosed as being mentally retarded. Which one of the children meets the DSM-IV criteria for moderate mental retardation?
   a. Joe, who requires constant supervision
   b. Steve, who works every day and supports himself
   c. Ann, who will not likely advance beyond the second grade in school
   d. Beth, who attends the local junior college

3. Which of these behaviors is a classic manifestation of pervasive developmental disorders?
   a. Repetitive and stereotypical use of language
   b. Imagination and creative play
   c. Interest in developing peer relationships
   d. Flexibility in adapting to environmental change

4. Tommy, age 8, was diagnosed with attention deficit hyperactive disorder. From the data collected about Tommy, which statement best supports this diagnosis?
   a. Crying when separated from his mother or father
   b. Refusing to pick up his toys as instructed by his parents
   c. Fascination with spinning and moving toys and objects
   d. Inability to concentrate long enough to complete his school work

5. Brad, age 6, is a new client on the children's unit and has started to act out and break the unit rules. The health care team developed a treatment plan which included setting limits on his behavior. What is the rationale for limit setting in this situation?
   a. Brad's behavior indicates a lack of internal control.
   b. The health care team needs to maintain the position of authority.
   c. Brad will benefit from the extra attention from the staff.
   d. Brad will not be responsible for the outcome of his behavior.

6. Which of these theories supports the view that symptoms are learned behaviors and change occurs only through relearning and environmental change?
   a. Structural theory
   b. Family theory
   c. Reactive theory
   d. Genetic theory

7. Joy, age 9, is being evaluated in the emergency room at the hospital, having fallen down the steps in her home. Her mother is with her and describes her as a "clumsy kid." The nurse practitioner suspects child abuse. Which of these findings indicate that physical abuse may be a chronic problem for Joy?
   a. Bloody nose and blackened eyes
   b. Unhealed fractures revealed on x-ray
   c. Clinging to her mother as she attempted to leave
   d. Struggling with the staff who attempt to obtain a blood specimen

8. Which of these nursing actions is best to assist an adolescent client who was admitted to the unit because of impulsivity and acting-out behavior at school?
   a. Isolating him from the other clients on the unit
   b. Explaining the unit rules and the consequences of breaking the rules to him
   c. Placing him on close watch to insure his safety
   d. Administering an antianxiety medication to him

9. Roy, age 17, was admitted to the adolescent unit after cutting his wrist with a knife. The wound was treated and bandaged by the emergency room staff. Which of these basic needs should be given highest priority by the unit admissions nurse?
   a. Food
   b. Comfort
   c. Love and belonging
   d. Safety

10. Asperger's disorder differs from autism in that Asperger's disorder is characterized by:
    a. Repetitive patterns of behavior
    b. Age-appropriate language development
    c. Stereotypic movements and speech patterns
    d. Obsession with moving objects

11. Which of these children is displaying characteristics of oppositional-defiant disorder?
    a. Jimmy, who blames others for causing his symptoms
    b. Tommie, who is mildly retarded and attends a special school program
    c. Judy, who is consistently able to follow directions but has difficulty completing her work
    d. Robbie, who successfully completes his work after being reminded by his parents

12. The nurse from the adolescent unit was participating in the orientation program for new nurses on the unit and was reviewing adolescent development. Which of these tasks is considered major for the adolescent?
    a. Developing a trusting relationship with older siblings
    b. Individuation from one's parents
    c. Mastering a competitive sport
    d. Completing career goals

13. Torrie, age 5, was admitted to the children's unit, having been sexually abused by an acquaintance of her family. Torrie refuses to talk and participate in unit activities, choosing to stay in her room with her stuffed animals. Which one of these therapeutic interventions will likely be best to help Torrie release pent-up feelings about the abuse?
    a. Individual communication with the nurse
    b. Play therapy
    c. Family therapy
    d. Role play with other children on the unit

14. Which of these statements best demonstrates acceptance of the adolescent's expression of painful feelings?
    a. "After you share your feelings with others, you will feel better."
    b. "You will feel better soon. Time will heal your wounds."
    c. "It must be difficult feeling the way you do."
    d. "Telling me those horrible stories makes me feel bad."

15. Brad, age 9, is a client on the children's unit. He was referred to a therapist, having been involved in several altercations at the school and having been suspended. On the unit Brad avoided talking to staff about his feelings. The staff would expect that Brad, in an effort to mask his true feelings, will probably:
    a. Select solitary games and activities
    b. Display acting out behaviors on the unit
    c. Refuse to participate in family visits
    d. Fail to complete homework assignments

16. Sue, age 17, was physically and sexually abused by her uncle when she was a child. Which of these remarks indicates that Sue has effectively dealt with the abuse she suffered?
    a. "I volunteer one day a week after school at a woman's shelter."
    b. "I spend time with my uncle whenever I can."
    c. "I do not watch television programs that involve abuse issues."
    d. "I do not date even though I am asked out frequently."

17. Patty, age 10, is on the children's unit, having been diagnosed with conduct disorder. She frequently throws eating utensils, books, and toys at the other clients. The staff developed a treatment plan for Patty. Which of these client outcomes would be appropriate in this situation?
    a. Patty will eat her meals in her room until she can refrain from throwing utensils.
    b. Patty will not throw any objects while in the hospital.
    c. Patty will be given time out in her room for one hour each time she throws an object.
    d. Patty will be discharged after her acting-out behaviors decrease.

18. The nurses on the adolescent unit are planning group activities for the weekend. Which of these group activities would encourage the development of interpersonal skills and learning how to function in an adult world?
    a. Watching a video and eating popcorn in the community room
    b. Taking a day trip to tour a local landmark
    c. Preparing a picnic for the clients and staff
    d. Playing basketball in the hospital gymnasium

19. Which of these nursing interventions would enhance the development of a therapeutic relationship with a child or adolescent?
    a. Using terminology and slang words the client can understand
    b. Offering personal opinions to assist the client with decision making
    c. Remaining nonjudgmental when the client shares sensitive feelings
    d. Refraining from responding empathetically to the client

20. Bucky, age 16, is being discharged to a group home as a continuing treatment option rather than returning to his own home. Bucky's father stated to the nurse, "I really wish my son was well enough to go home with us. I feel awful about this." Bucky's father is expressing to the nurse his feelings of:
    a. Guilt
    b. Anger
    c. Denial
    d. Relief

21. Jane, age 6, has been on the children's unit for three weeks and is getting ready for discharge. Her acting-out behavior has decreased, and she has been attending school and completing her work on time. She has begun to trust the staff and to develop a trusting relationship with them. What is the likely reason for her to start to act out again as discharge approaches?
    a. Her compliance in the hospital was a way to obtain positive attention.
    b. The treatment was not as effective as the staff had thought.
    c. She was having difficulty terminating positive relationships.
    d. She is trying to get her hospital stay lengthened.

22. Adam, age 15, has been diagnosed with major depression and admitted to the adolescent unit. Which of these behaviors would you expect to observe in Adam?
    a. Discussing repeated offenses with the law enforcement authorities
    b. Crying and refusing to get out of bed
    c. Blaming others for causing him to be admitted to the unit
    d. Reporting a decrease of enjoyment in school related activities

23. The nurse is leading a discussion group with parents of adolescents. One of the parents asked about the increase in the number of suicides in recent years. The nurse was accurate in reporting that the most common method used in adolescent suicide is:
    a. Drug overdose
    b. Use of firearms
    c. Carbon monoxide poisoning
    d. Hanging

24. Which of these activities would be appropriate to use for a child who has difficulty expressing angry feelings in an acceptable manner?
    a. Kicking a football across the day room to another client
    b. Painting a picture in the activities room
    c. Working on an intricate project with a peer
    d. Pounding on a woodworking project in the activities room

25. Elizabeth, age 16, has been on the adolescent unit for seven days, having been admitted for attempted suicide by overdosing on an undetermined number and mixture of over-the-counter medications. Which of these statements by Elizabeth would warrant additional information before she is released from the unit?
    a. "I have learned about myself since I have been here and realize how foolish I was to try to hurt myself."
    b. "Sometimes I wonder whether my friends would have attended my funeral had I died."
    c. "I feel secure now that I know who to call should I become desperate again."
    d. "What a beautiful day! I'm glad I can enjoy it."

Chapter 19

Eating Disorders

1. Which of these events have contributed to the increased number of eating disorders in recent years?
    a. Abundance of nutritious foods available
    b. Trend toward thinness in the fashion industry
    c. Competition in the work place
    d. Increase number of divorced and blended families

2. Which of these personality traits are common in a person with an eating disorder?
    a. Excellent coping skills
    b. Security in social relationships
    c. Noncompliance
    d. Interceptive deficits

3. Cognitive therapy literature describes distortions in the thinking patterns in the person with an eating disorder. Which statement exemplifies dichotomous thinking?
    a. Viewing a situation as all good or all bad
    b. Feeling responsible for another person's unhappiness and failure
    c. Comparing oneself with others in most situations
    d. Believing the behavior of others is a direct reaction to oneself

4. A group of teenagers were discussing their individual problems associated with having an eating disorder. Which of these findings is probably a result of purging?
   a. Excessive facial hair
   b. Elevated blood pressure
   c. Polyuria
   d. Dental enamel erosion

5. Beth, age 18, believes she is overweight, yet her weight is 120 pounds on a 5 ft. 10 in. frame. Her desired weight is 100 pounds. On the days that Beth is scheduled for a weight check, the nurse should be aware of which of these possible responses from Beth?
   a. Eagerness to determine her present weight
   b. Dressing in several layers of clothing
   c. Suggesting that the scale numbers be hidden from her view
   d. Reminding the nurse that she is ready to be weighed

6. Doris, who has anorexia nervosa, states she believes she will have fewer problems in college and gaining popularity if she continues to lose weight. What nursing intervention would be useful at this time?
   a. Assisting Doris to identify what problems are causing her concern
   b. Determining what she hopes to gain from this behavior
   c. Explaining that her chances for getting ill from losing weight are likely
   d. Having a physical report indicating her condition sent to college officials

7. Many clients with eating disorders have difficulty translating their pain into words. Which of these possible approaches may be used to allow greater self-disclosure?
   a. Personality inventory testing
   b. Dance and movement therapy
   c. Letter writing
   d. Cooking and meal planning classes

8. During the nursing assessment on a newly admitted client to the eating disorders unit, the nurse stated to the client, "How do you feel about being here today?" The purpose of this question is to:
   a. Reduce the client's anxiety
   b. Encourage the client to talk
   c. Determine the client's willingness to engage in treatment
   d. Assess the client's level of guilt and shame

9. Virginia, age 16, is hospitalized with b vosa having lost fifty pounds during th months. She has dry skin with poor tu breakage, and brittle nails. When prov mation concerning her menstrual histo of these findings is likely to be reported?
   a. Heavy menstrual flow
   b. Amenorrhea
   c. Premenstrual syndrome
   d. Dysmenorrhea

10. A 14-year-old client on the eating disorders unit refused to eat her meals and said to the nurse on the unit, "There is nothing wrong with me, and you cannot make me eat." Which one of these defense mechanisms was the client using?
    a. Repression
    b. Rationalization
    c. Sublimation
    d. Denial

11. A group of nurses were discussing how food is used in their families and the effect this might have on their ability to work with clients who have eating disorders. Which one of these nurses will probably be most effective?
    a. John, who requires that his children eat everything on their plate each meal
    b. Sam, who permits his children to have dessert only after cleaning their plate
    c. Mary, who refuses to engage in power struggles related to food consumption
    d. Ruth, who grew up poor and frequently did not have enough food to eat

12. What is the primary reason that the medication bubroprion (Wellbutrin) is contraindicated for the treatment of bulimia nervosa?
    a. Increase in appetite and intake of food
    b. Adverse interaction with other medications
    c. High incidence of seizure disorders
    d. Risk of hypertensive crisis

13. Which of these axis 1 disorders is most commonly seen in the client with bulimia and anorexia nervosa?
    a. Anxiety disorders
    b. Depressive disorders
    c. Dissociative disorders
    d. Somatoform disorders

14. Which of these medications would the nurse expect to see prescribed for the client who is being treated for comorbid eating/affective disorder?
    a. Sertraline (Zoloft)
    b. Diazepam (Valium)
    c. Lorazepam (Ativan)
    d. Lithium

15. Which of these measures should be initiated first for a new client admitted with malnutrition, extreme weight loss, weakness, and fatigue?
    a. Determining electrolyte levels
    b. Placing on suicide precautions
    c. Providing a nutritious meal
    d. Placing on bed rest with bathroom privileges

16. Jane, who is hospitalized with anorexia nervosa, stated during a one-to-one session with the nurse, "I'm freaking out. I'm losing it." Which of these nurse responses would be most therapeutic at this time?
    a. "Perhaps this is a good time to call your parents."
    b. "You need to relax and maintain control."
    c. "Let me sit with you for a while."
    d. "Tell me what thoughts are going through your head at this time."

17. Which of these expectations should be considered prior to discharging a client with anorexia nervosa from the eating disorders unit?
    a. Absence of weight loss for at least 2 days
    b. Demonstration of the use of adequate coping abilities to deal with stress
    c. Knowledge of caloric and nutritional value of foods required for a balanced diet
    d. Reduction of periods of active exercise to three times daily

18. During a counseling session the mother of one of the clients with an eating disorder stated to the nurse, "I feel like such a failure. How can I be sure my daughter has no more problems like this?" Which of these responses is the most therapeutic?
    a. "You are not responsible for your daughter's behavior."
    b. "Avoid giving advice and engaging in power struggles with your daughter."
    c. "It sounds like you are blaming yourself for your daughter's problems."
    d. "Try to ignore any problems your daughter has related to her eating disorder."

19. Ms. Smith, the charge nurse on the eating disorders unit, in discussing boundaries in the family, referred to Salvador Minuchin, a family therapist, who described an enmeshed family as a unit in which:
    a. Individuality is encouraged
    b. Boundaries are poorly defined
    c. Conflict is effectively resolved
    d. Social acceptance is deemed unimportant

20. In an art therapy session, Linda, a client with anorexia nervosa, was asked to draw a picture of herself. Which of these drawings would likely depict the view that Linda has of herself?
    a. A tall, slim girl with obvious muscle definition
    b. A malnourished teenager with thin, lanky extremities
    c. A grossly obese figure lacking feminine characteristics
    d. A shapely figure of a model whom she admires

21. Susie, a high school cheerleader, was admitted to the eating disorders unit, having developed the electrolyte imbalance, hypokalemia. Which of these medications will probably be prescribed for Susie?
    a. Potassium supplements
    b. Calcium gluconate
    c. Metoclopramide (Reglan)
    d. Ferrous sulfate

22. The nurse working with Clemmie, whose diagnosis is bulimia, asked her to recall a time in her life when eating was a positive experience and she could enjoy small amounts of food without purging. What is the purpose of this intervention?
    a. To gain additional information about Clemmie's bulimic condition
    b. To emphasize the fact that Clemmie is capable of engaging in episodes of successful eating
    c. To incorporate specific foods into Clemmie's meal plan that reflect pleasant memories for her
    d. To assist Clemmie to become more compliant with the eating disorders treatment plan for her

23. Three clients on the eating disorders unit were involved in group therapy and planned to continue attending an outpatient group after discharge. What is the rationale for using group therapy for the treatment of eating disorders?
    a. Spending time in a group setting helps the client focus on things other than food-related issues.
    b. Interacting with clients with similar problems helps prevent secondary gains related to being different.

c. Focusing on problems experienced by other group members helps the client avoid having to deal with personal concerns.
d. Many insurance companies are more willing to pay for group rather than individual therapy.

24. The nurse who works with clients who have eating disorders is involved in teaching the family members about the disorder, the symptoms, and management. What is the rationale for including the family in this manner?
    a. Eating disorders are usually caused by dysfunctional family interaction.
    b. Knowledge promotes power and reduces fear and anxiety.
    c. Family members need to learn to monitor the eating pattern of the identified client.
    d. Having an understanding of the disorder will prevent other family members from developing a similar problem.

25. Tracy, who was treated for anorexia nervosa, was seen by the therapist for a follow-up visit one month after discharge from the hospital. Which of these statements indicates that Tracy has met the goal, "demonstrate improvement in body image with more realistic view of body shape and size?"
    a. "When I go shopping, I always select clothes that are several sizes too large for me."
    b. "My boyfriend says I really look good now that I'm out of the hospital."
    c. "I had my class picture taken, and I think it looks really good."
    d. "My mother bought me a whole new wardrobe since I've been home."

Chapter 20

Sexual Disorders

1. Which of these individuals is experiencing a symptom of the DSM-IV diagnosis, sexual aversion disorder?
    a. Client A, who has delayed orgasm following sexual excitement
    b. Client B, who has absence of desire to engage in sexual activity
    c. Client C, who has an avoidance of genital sexual contact with a partner
    d. Client D, who has genital pain associated with intercourse

2. A group of nurses were attending a lecture on sexual disorders. Which statement best describes the evolution of research on sexuality?
    a. Kaplan was instrumental in identifying the need for psychoanalysis in treating sexual dysfunction.
    b. Sigmund Freud, a sexologist, based his work on scientific data from studying human sexual behavior.
    c. Masters and Johnson were the first persons to explore the area of sexual dysfunction.
    d. Increased knowledge about sexual dysfunction has been available since the late 1960s.

3. A special unit was getting ready to open which would only admit clients who were experiencing sexual dysfunction and seeking treatment. The nurse manager was interviewing nurses to staff the unit. Which of these qualifications would be most important for a nurse working with this specific group?
    a. Previous experience working with individuals with sexual dysfunction
    b. A keen awareness of personal feelings about sexuality
    c. The belief that all types of sexual dysfunction can be corrected
    d. Knowledge of having worked through personal issues of dealing with sexuality

4. The nurse was collecting data from a client who is to be treated for sexual dysfunction. Which of these questions is best to determine the presence of cognitive distortions?
    a. "Is there a family history of sexual dysfunction?"
    b. "Were you sexually abused as a child or adolescent?"
    c. "What makes you think you have a sexual dysfunction?"
    d. "Why did you come for treatment at this time?"

5. Ms. Smith was seeking help at the community health clinic, complaining of lack of sexual desire and the problems this was causing in her marriage. Which of the following data is likely related to her sexual dysfunction?
    a. Being an adopted only child
    b. Taking an antidepressant medication
    c. Growing up in a dysfunctional family
    d. Living in an isolated area in the country

6. A group of nurses were discussing types of sexual dysfunctions. Which of these behaviors is characteristic of fetishism?
   a. Standing on the street corner exposing genitals to others
   b. Achieving sexual pleasure from rubbing against a stranger in an elevator
   c. Feeling sexually attracted to a 10-year-old child who lives next door
   d. Utilizing various objects for sexual arousal

7. Mr. Darris was being treated on the sexual disorders unit, having been arrested for molesting two neighborhood children. At the team meeting to evaluate his progress, the staff reported his continued use of denial. Which comment by Mr. Darris supports this belief?
   a. "My parents abused me when I was a child."
   b. "I only acted inappropriately because I was stressed."
   c. "I am sorry for what I have done."
   d. "There is nothing wrong with the way I behave."

8. The nurse documented in the chart that Mr. Luther, who has a paraphilic disorder, was noncompliant in helping develop his plan of care. What is the likely reason for his noncompliance?
   a. Anger at being hospitalized
   b. Embarrassment about what he had done
   c. Fear of failing in treatment
   d. Failure to recognize that he has a problem

9. The nurse would evaluate the plan of care for a paraphilic client as having been effective if the client displayed which of these behaviors?
   a. Willfully withdrawing from the program
   b. Asking to include his wife in the treatment program
   c. Acknowledging that he has a sexual disorder
   d. Requesting an antianxiety medication to help him cope

10. The sex therapist was explaining to the client that the nocturnal penile tumescence test (NET) is a means of:
    a. Comparing daytime and nocturnal erectile potential
    b. Determining erectile responses during the sleep cycle
    c. Incorporating visual erotic stimuli
    d. Measuring penile and brachial blood pressures

11. A client being interviewed at the community health clinic stated to the nurse, "I have a sexual problem." Which of these comments led the nurse to suspect the problem to be dyspareunia?
    a. "I cannot maintain adequate lubrication during intercourse."
    b. "I do not enjoy sexual intercourse and try to avoid it."
    c. "I experience genital pain during intercourse."
    d. "My perineal muscles contract at the wrong times during intercourse."

12. Which of these interventions is required prior to administering the medication Depo-Provera to a client?
    a. Assessing height and weight
    b. Determining approximate intake of alcoholic beverages
    c. Obtaining informed consent
    d. Providing printed material explaining desired and undesired effects of the drug

13. The clients on the sexual disorders unit are required to attend group psychotherapy as part of their treatment plan. The purpose of group psychotherapy is to deal with cognitive distortions and to:
    a. Assist the clients to identify triggers that may affect their behavior
    b. Teach the clients how to therapeutically interact with others
    c. Explain legal implications involved with certain sexual behaviors
    d. Explore methods to structure time to assist in relapse prevention

14. Which of these client behaviors indicates a potential relapse of treatment in the paraphilic?
    a. Requesting a visit from family members
    b. Refusing to take the prescribed medications
    c. Sitting alone in the day room writing poetry
    d. Attempting to develop a social relationship with the staff

15. A group of individuals were discussing types of sexual disorders. Which statement best expresses the feelings of an ego-syntonic pedophile?
    a. "I know what I do is wrong, but I am comfortable the way I am."
    b. "Being this way makes me so miserable that I want to get help."
    c. "If parents supervised their children more closely, molestation may stop."
    d. "I decided on my own that I needed help. No one sent me here."

16. Fred, who was seen in outpatient therapy, described symptoms indicative of scatoalgia. He acknowledges that he has a problem and asked for help in avoiding a repeat of these behaviors. Which of this information should be included in Fred's teaching plan?
    a. Triggers must be identified that provoke the inappropriate behavior.
    b. Making obscene phone calls relates to his hatred of women.
    c. The obscene message is generally not a problem to the receiver of the call.
    d. The etiology of this disorder is usually related to dysfunctional parenting.

17. Uncle Ted loves to babysit his three- and five-year-old nieces. Frequently he fondles them while they sit on his lap and touches them inappropriately. After the girls were observed touching their dolls the same way, they confessed that Uncle Ted had done this to them. Which of these statements indicates Uncle Ted's use of rationalization?
    a. "The children always want me to hold them in my lap."
    b. "There is absolutely nothing wrong with me."
    c. "It's your fault for expecting me to babysit for you."
    d. "My babysitter used to do the same things to me."

18. Mr. Larson has been diagnosed with Klinefelter's syndrome? Which of these findings would be expected in this disorder?
    a. Elevated sperm count
    b. Decreased secretion of FSH
    c. Female characteristic present at birth
    d. Gynecomastia in the teenage male

19. Mr. and Mrs. Moses are in marriage counseling for the initial visit because of Mr. Moses's decreased interest in an intimate relationship with his wife. He admitted that his job is a constant source of worry and that he feels "tied in knots all the time." They admit that any mention of sex results in a verbal battle. Which of these client outcomes is realistic at this time?
    a. Mr. Moses will be able to focus on body feeling during intimacy rather than anxiety.
    b. Mr. and Mrs. Moses will express their perception of the problem in the presence of the therapist.
    c. Mr. and Mrs. Moses will discuss job concerns creating stress in their lives and strategies for change.
    d. Mrs. Moses will talk openly about her feelings of inadequacy.

20. The physician ordered that the medication Depo-Provera (500 mg) be administered to a client being treated for a paraphilic disorder. Which of these findings are related to this medication?
    a. Increased testosterone levels
    b. Potential for elevated blood pressure
    c. Loss of appetite and weight loss
    d. Increased motor activity

Chapter 21

Adjustment Disorders

1. According to the DSM-IV, adjustment disorders is a classification for a group of disorders that:
    a. Involve psychotic thinking in adolescents
    b. Include behaviors that are seen primarily in the child and adolescent population
    c. Address issues of anxiety and depression
    d. Manifest as transient episodes of dysfunction in response to specific stressors

2. Mr. Light, age 45, was diagnosed with an adjustment disorder, chronic type. The nurse who was obtaining admission data would expect to learn that Mr. Light's symptoms had existed for a period longer than:
    a. 2 months
    b. 4 months
    c. 6 months
    d. 8 months

3. During a group session, Ruth stated that she could not get a job because everyone thought she was so stupid. The group leader stated, "Would other members think Ruth was stupid if you interviewed her for a job?" What is the purpose of this intervention?
    a. To offer members of the group a chance to state their opinion of Ruth
    b. To cause Ruth to look at herself more closely
    c. To encourage Ruth to compare her perception with others' perceptions of her
    d. To discourage Ruth from making negative remarks about herself

4. The nurse manager is teaching a class to new staff members about working with clients with adjustment disorders. Which of these interventions will be most helpful in working with clients with this diagnosis?
   a. Including family members in the treatment plan
   b. Reducing the client's level of anxiety to prevent escalation of behaviors
   c. Identifying the stressful event and current problems
   d. Including pertinent data in the client's record

5. Mr. and Mrs. Long accompanied their daughter, Amy, to the hospital. When discussing the client's diagnosis, Mr. Long stated, "I don't understand what the doctor means by saying my daughter has an adjustment disorder." The nurse explained that this disorder often results from:
   a. Failure of existing coping skills
   b. Lack of emotional support
   c. Denial that a problem exists
   d. Overcompensation to present a controlled appearance

6. Mr. Storms visited his wife, who was a client on the psychiatric unit. The nurse heard them arguing about their financial situation and lack of resources to pay bills. After her husband left, Mrs. Storms complained of a severe headache. The nurse was likely correct in stating the headache was a result of:
   a. Feeling unloved
   b. The argument
   c. Lack of control
   d. Having to be hospitalized

7. Mr. Burns is celebrating his 65th birthday and planning to retire from the job he has held for 35 years. His place of employment is providing information on how to adjust to the change in lifestyle. The industrial nurse leading the workshop is aware that should Mr. Burns experience an adjustment disorder it will likely be related to:
   a. Loss of identity and purpose
   b. Concern about finances
   c. Boredom from having no interests
   d. Loneliness from having to spend time alone

8. Which of these actions by inexperienced health care professionals may prohibit grief resolution when a client experiences a loss?
   a. Attempting to obtain detailed information about the loss
   b. Feeling intense sadness for the client
   c. Failing to recognize cultural customs
   d. Seeking assistance from the pastoral care department

9. The nurse was presenting a seminar on Erikson's developmental theory. She was correct in stating that his theory supports the belief that adjustment disorders usually occur:
   a. When family dysfunctional behavior causes chronic stress
   b. After the individual experienced a sudden loss
   c. When failure to complete closure appropriately exists
   d. When age-appropriate behaviors are not completed

10. Amber, age 24, lives at home and has provided care for her two younger siblings since her mother died two years ago. When she is asked to participate in activities after work, she always declines, making up an excuse to avoid explaining her situation. She rarely gets phone calls and spends free time reading and sewing. Which of these nursing diagnoses would be appropriate for Amber?
    a. Potential for self-harm
    b. Disturbance in self-esteem
    c. Impaired social interaction
    d. Dysfunctional grieving

11. The nurse was admitting a client with an adjustment disorder to the unit. In assisting the client to identify what may have preceded her difficulty, which of these questions is best?
    a. "Tell me about your support system?"
    b. "Have you been in therapy before?"
    c. "What has happened in your recent past?"
    d. "How do you handle problems in your life?"

12. Mrs. Santos, age 56, was admitted to the mental health facility stating she felt blue and lonely and had no reason to live. Her husband had been killed in an airplane crash two years ago while on a business trip, and she had been continuing to grieve. Which of this information gained from the nursing history should be considered first when assisting Mrs. Santos to deal with the death of her husband?
    a. Length of time they had been married
    b. Support system available to her
    c. Names of family members who can assist with her care
    d. Culturally and socially accepted manners for expressing grief

13. The mental health team had written a client outcome to assist an elderly client deal with the loss of his wife: "Client will verbalize loss as a process." Which of these statements by the client indicates the goal was met?
    a. "I no longer feel lonely and sad."
    b. "My favorite day of the week is Friday, when I bowl with my friends."
    c. "I know that loss is a natural process and will resolve in time."
    d. "I have reached the stage of anger in dealing with my grief."

14. Sue, age 15, was admitted to the adolescent unit with the diagnosis, adjustment disorder. Which of this data collected from the assessment interview will be given highest priority when planning Sue's care?
    a. Recently being picked up by the police for breaking curfew
    b. Parents being divorced eight years ago
    c. Stating she finds no pleasure in living
    d. Failing most of her high school classes

15. Which of these questions asked by the nurse would be effective in gaining data about the client's ability to identify a stressor preceding an adjustment disorder?
    a. "Can you tell me about your family and available support system?"
    b. "What has happened in your life recently?"
    c. "Have you been in counseling before?"
    d. "How have you handled events like this in the past?"

16. The nurse manager was admitting to the unit a client who had a mastectomy four months ago and had been experiencing insomnia, depression, and anxiety. The client stated, "I don't think I will ever be the same again." Which response by the nurse is most appropriate?
    a. "I understand. Healing can be a slow process."
    b. "Your incision is healed nicely. The scars are almost invisible."
    c. "Could you tell me more about your feelings?"
    d. "I'm glad you came for help before you become more depressed."

17. Jane, age 23, is a client in the mental health treatment facility, having had emotional problems since relocating far away from family and friends because of her job. Which of these approaches will best assist Jane in identifying patterns of thoughts and identifying feelings?
    a. Listing past experiences when she was lonely
    b. Writing entries in a journal when she is upset
    c. Identifying her expectations from being in treatment
    d. Asking group members to validate her concerns

18. The nurse working with a client with adjustment disorder with depressed mood would accurately evaluate that the crisis had been resolved based on which of these findings?
    a. Absence of presenting symptoms
    b. Decreased need for medications
    c. Increased socialization with peers
    d. Significant weight gain

19. Which of these statements is accurate when teaching a family the usual outcome of an adjustment disorder?
    a. The symptoms will likely resolve completely.
    b. The client may continue to be in danger of self harm.
    c. Medications are frequently used to mask the symptoms.
    d. Relaxation is an effective tool to decrease stress.

20. Which of these activities may be prescribed for a client with adjustment disorder with anxious mood as a constructive outlet for tension and anxiety while enhancing self-esteem?
    a. Knitting scarves for a homeless shelter
    b. Painting a "paint-by-number" picture
    c. Working on a large picture puzzle
    d. Engaging in physical exercise

21. Which of these observations suggests an improvement in a client who was diagnosed with adjustment disorder with depressed mood?
    a. Asking to participate in preparing a meal as a group activity on the unit
    b. Walking to the medicine room to get her p.r.n. meds
    c. Visiting with her minister during visiting hours
    d. Attending group therapy

22. Mark, age 25, has been diagnosed with adjustment disorder, unspecified. His wife requested a divorce two months ago, and his work has been adversely affected with the possibility of losing his job. Which of these statements indicates that Mark needs assistance in structuring his daily activities?
    a. "My work hours are 9 am to 5 pm, which is not that bad."
    b. "All I want to do is get the job done, come home, and sleep."
    c. "I guess I should include exercise in my daily schedule."
    d. "Going out to eat with friends might be an enjoyable activity for me."

23. Which of these modalities will best assist the nurse to assess the decrease or continuation of symptomatology displayed by a client?
    a. Psychological testing
    b. Group therapy
    c. Laboratory studies
    d. Written documentation

24. Which of these client outcomes would best address a nursing diagnosis of risk for self-directed violence?
    a. Client will notify nurse if he feels more depressed.
    b. Client will verbalize no suicidal ideations while hospitalized.
    c. Client will keep a journal describing any self-destructive thoughts.
    d. Client will not harm self while in the hospital.

25. Mr. Todd, age 54, was getting ready for discharge, having been diagnosed with adjustment disorder with anxious mood and admitted to the mental health facility. One nursing diagnosis was Sleep pattern disturbance. Which of these statements indicates that Mr. Todd has a better understanding of dealing with this problem?
    a. "I know I must take a sleeping medication in order to sleep."
    b. "Listening to relaxation tapes helps me get to sleep."
    c. "I sleep better after I drink a small glass of wine."
    d. "When I can't sleep, I will call my friend, who is always willing to listen to me."

Chapter 22

Interactive Therapies and Methods of Implementation

1. Which of these interventions will be most valuable for the nurse in developing a therapeutic nurse-client relationship?
    a. Administering the prescribed medications accurately
    b. Interacting with members of the health care team
    c. Being aware of therapeutic modalities
    d. Possessing self-awareness and understanding

2. A therapeutic relationship differs from a social relationship in that in a therapeutic relationship:
    a. The focus is shared equally between the participants.
    b. Absence of boundaries is generally accepted.
    c. Time constraints do not apply.
    d. A specific goal is established that implies the reason for the relationship's existence.

3. Paplau identified four roles of the psychiatric nurse. What role has the nurse assumed as she listens to the client and assists to clarify feelings?
    a. Counselor
    b. Surrogate
    c. Resource person
    d. Technical expert

4. Which of these statements best describes the goal of a therapeutic relationship?
    a. To accomplish tasks in a timely manner
    b. To provide a support system for the client
    c. To assist the client in becoming a healthy responsible individual
    d. To plan the necessary care for the client

5. The nurse was working with the client in the hospital when the client stated, "I don't like to have you as my nurse. You're just like my mother." Which of these possible responses would be most appropriate by the nurse?
    a. "Perhaps I remind you of her because we are about the same age."
    b. "I sense that you are uncomfortable with me, so you will be assigned another nurse."
    c. "I'm sorry. I had no idea I was acting like your mother."
    d. "Even though I remind you of your mother, I care about you in a different way."

6. The psychiatric nurse should continually be involved in the act of autodiagnosis, which is the process of:
   a. Individual therapy
   b. Self-examination
   c. Determining the mechanics of communication
   d. Gaining supervision in practice

7. Which of these behaviors displayed by the nurse is considered effective attending behavior?
   a. Maintaining continuous eye contact with the client
   b. Sitting behind the desk during the initial client interview
   c. Leaning slightly forward in the chair during the interaction
   d. Determining the content of the interaction

8. The nurse working with a client in the outpatient department stated, "Even though I can see the situation from your point of view, I must follow the hospital rules." The nurse is demonstrating:
   a. Respect
   b. Genuineness
   c. Sympathy
   d. Empathy

9. The maintenance of boundaries is necessary in the nurse-client relationship. Which of these statements describes the purpose of boundaries?
   a. To define responsibilities and duties to one's self in relation to others
   b. To determine objectives of the working stage of the relationship
   c. To differentiate the roles of the nurse and the client
   d. To prevent the possibility for undesired material to emerge during the interaction

10. John, the psychiatric nurse, asked the client for his perception of his problem and the reason for hospitalization. At which phase of the therapeutic relationship should this be done?
    a. Orientation phase
    b. Working phase
    c. Termination phase
    d. Prior to discharge

11. During a nurse-client interaction, the nurse attentively listens for themes which are described as:
    a. Definite repetition of words voiced by someone else
    b. Recurring patterns reflective of the client experiences
    c. Unhealthy human responses
    d. Effective methods of dealing with problems

12. The nursing student is concerned that a client not be able to trust her enough to establish a therapeutic relationship. Which of these actions will likely facilitate the development of trust?
    a. Responding positively to the client's demands
    b. Following through with what was promised
    c. Clarifying with the client when in doubt
    d. Staying with the client for the entire shift

13. Jane, the nurse on the unit, is meeting with her client, Mr. Doss, for the first time. After introducing herself, which of these possible statements best define Jane's role as the client's ally and helper?
    a. "Mr. Doss, I will work with your doctor to help you get better."
    b. "Mr. Doss, I'm glad to see you. I'm here to help you."
    c. "Your medications will help you feel better soon."
    d. "You will be expected to attend group activities while you are here."

14. The nurses on the unit were planning care for a group of clients and determining whether they could best meet their needs in a task or a process group. Their decision was based on their understanding that a task group focuses on:
    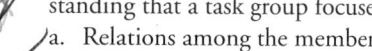
    a. Relations among the members
    b. Communication styles
    c. Content issues
    d. The "here and now"

15. The treatment team was planning how group therapy could be included as a part of the structured daily activities of the unit. A new team member asked, "Why is group therapy a useful treatment modality for the clients?" The most accurate response would be based on the assumption that:
    a. Disordered relationships can create psychopathy
    b. Some persons do not relate well on an individual basis
    c. Hidden agendas frequently surface in group sessions
    d. Group therapy is far more cost-effective for the clients

leader and co-leader were discussing
... and the way it was meeting the needs
... ts. Which of these clients is demon-
... havior indicating Yalom's therapeutic
... ned universality?
a. ... who realizes he is not the only person
   who has a particular problem
b. Larry, who continues to display dysfunctional interaction patterns learned in his family of origin
c. Bill, who states he finally feels a strong sense of belonging
d. Joe, who expresses his anger openly about his work

17. A group of nursing students were attending a lecture tracing the history of psychiatric treatment. The lecturer was correct in stating that the concept of "therapeutic community" is attributed to:
    a. Sigmund Freud
    b. Maxwell Jones
    c. Florence Nightingale
    d. Irvin Yalom

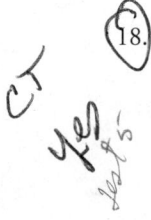

18. Jan, the nurse, was leading an inpatient group dealing with women's issues. Which of these behaviors demonstrated by a member characterizes the role of aggressor in the group?
    a. Seeking a position between contending sides
    b. Mediating conflicts and disagreements
    c. Attempting to manipulate others
    d. Criticizing the contributions of others

19. The nurse manager was gathering information as to the possibility of starting an inpatient group for women on the unit. Which of these factors would cause the nurse manager to reconsider?
    a. Two clients reported sexual abuse in childhood.
    b. Several clients were divorced and raising their children alone.
    c. Sixteen clients expressed interest in joining the group.
    d. One of the clients was recently widowed.

20. The nurse was reviewing notes she had written following a family session with the Diggs family who had begun therapy in hopes of becoming a more unified family. Because of their schedules, they were feeling alienated and estranged from each other. Which statement by the 16-year-old son was considered by the therapist as positive in problem resolution?
    a. "I have stopped playing football since practice required me to be away from home so often."
    b. "Eating dinner with my parents on Sunday nights has helped us be more aware of each other's needs."
    c. "Since my mother quit her job, she is more available to keep the home running smoothly."
    d. "My Dad has stopped giving me advice on how to live my life."

21. The nurse and client were interacting during a one-to-one session on the psychiatric unit. In response to the nurse's statement, "Tell me about your family," the client became silent and displayed nonverbally that he was uncomfortable. Which of these statements reflects the nurse's sensitivity to the client?
    a. "I'm so sorry. I didn't realize your family was a problem for you."
    b. "Learning to express negative feelings will assist you in getting well."
    c. "Perhaps you can talk about your feelings to the physician later."
    d. "That seems to be a difficult statement for you. We can discuss it later if you prefer."

22. After attending a group session for six weeks, Ms. Dean was terminating from the group. She believed she had successfully met her established objectives and could manage without the group support. When sharing her feelings about separating, Ms. Dean stated, "I feel a bit sad and empty that I won't be seeing you folks again." What is the most accurate evaluation of Ms. Dean's statement?
    a. It indicates regression and her lack of readiness to terminate.
    b. Unconsciously, Ms. Dean is hoping she will be permitted to continue the group.
    c. Ms. Dean is demonstrating normal terminating behaviors, and the nurse should explain this to her.
    d. Ms. Dean needs further evaluation by her individual therapist to determine her readiness to terminate.

23. The nurse was evaluating team leadership styles from observing a variety of inpatient groups led by different leaders. Which of these group leaders was using the democratic style of leadership?
    a. Leader A, who asked for input from the group members in decision making
    b. Leader B, who stated the manner in which the group would run
    c. Leader C, who viewed his lack of structure as a positive force in goal attainment
    d. Leader D, who discouraged members from giving individual opinions related to the group

24. Mrs. Lee, a 60-year-old client on the psychiatric unit, was angry because of a remark another client had made to her. Mrs. Lee asked the nurse manager if she would talk to the client about her behavior. Which of these actions would best support Mrs. Lee in resolving this situation?
   a. Assisting Mrs. Lee as she confronts the client about the incident
   b. Intervening on Mrs. Lee's behalf in approaching the client about her behavior
   c. Suggesting that Mrs. Lee ignore the situation since the client likely was not aware of her behavior
   d. Encouraging Mrs. Lee to report the incident to the client's physician

Chapter 23

Psychopharmacology and Other Biologic Therapies

1. Jane, the nurse manager on the psychiatric unit, was explaining to the new staff the differences in typical and atypical antipsychotics. She correctly stated that atypical antipsychotics:
   a. Remain in the system longer
   b. Act more quickly in reducing psychotic behaviors
   c. Show reduced evidence of extrapyramidal effects
   d. Can be administered as depot injections

2. Tom, age 25, diagnosed with schizophrenia, paranoid type, was admitted to the hospital and prescribed haloperidol (Haldol). The nurse would investigate further for signs of neuroleptic malignant syndrome (NMS) if Tom had a:
   a. 30 mm Hg. decrease in blood pressure reading
   b. Respiratory rate of 24 per minute
   c. Temperature reading of 104° F
   d. Pulse rate of 70 beats per minute

3. Mr. Johnson is taking fluphenazine (Navane) and has been complaining of dry mouth and blurred vision. What is the likely cause of these symptoms?
   a. Decreased available dopamine at receptor sites
   b. Blockade of histamine
   c. Anticholinergic effects of cholinergic blockade
   d. Adrenergic-blocking

4. A group of clients were sitting in the day room of the psychiatric hospital. Which client is showing behaviors characteristic of tardive dyskinesia?
   a. Jane, who rocks from side to side and
   b. Clara, who falls asleep in her chair and refuses to eat lunch
   c. Sam, who is experiencing muscle rigidity and tremors
   d. Luther, who has excessive salivation and drooling

5. Mr. Raymund, age 45, a chronic schizophrenic, was admitted to the hospital one month after his last hospitalization, demonstrating psychotic behaviors. He lives alone and has not been taking the Haldol that was prescribed for him. Which of these interventions would best assist Mr. Raymund to get the medication he needs?
   a. Instructing him to have a friend monitor his medications
   b. Giving him Haldol Decanoate prior to discharge
   c. Writing instructions in detail for Mr. Raymund to follow
   d. Changing the Haldol to an atypical antipsychotic

6. During a medication management class for nurses, the pharmacist was discussing tricyclic antidepressants. How do these medications affect neurotransmitter activity?
   a. By decreasing available dopamine
   b. By increasing availability of norepinephrine and serotonin
   c. By making available increased amounts of monoamine oxidase
   d. By increasing the effects of gamma-aminobutyric acid

7. Mrs. Smallwood, a 56-year-old school teacher, was admitted to the adult psychiatric unit, having attempted to harm herself by taking an overdose of a prescribed medication. She had never been treated for depression and was prescribed clomipramine (Anafranil). The nurse would monitor Mrs. Smallwood for which of these side effects of the medication?
   a. Polyuria and extreme hand tremors
   b. Orthostatic hypotension and constipation
   c. Excess salivation and drooling
   d. Muscle rigidity and restlessness

8. The nurse was leading a medication management group for clients who were being discharged from the hospital. Which of these statements from John, who was taking isocarboxazid (Marplan), would warrant further instruction?
   a. "I sometimes forget to wear sunscreen when I go for a walk."
   b. "I need to restrict the amount of sodium in my diet."
   c. "I should not use over the counter cold medications."
   d. "I usually order liver and onions when my wife and I eat out."

9. The nurse was making rounds following the evening report to learn the current status of each client. Which of these client complaints should receive priority from a client who is taking tranylxypromine (Parnate)?
   a. "My legs get stiff when I sit in the chair for a while."
   b. "Will you take my temperature? I feel warm."
   c. "I have a splitting headache."
   d. "I haven't had a bowel movement today."

10. A client with symptoms of a major depression has been prescribed sertraline (Zoloft). What has contributed to the increase in the use of SSRIs in recent years?
    a. Mild side-effect profile
    b. Less expense for the client
    c. Increase in compliance
    d. Rapid rate of absorption from the GI tract

11. Mr. Rawles, age 50, was admitted to the hospital with a diagnosis of bipolar disorder. He was placed on lithium and will continue to take it after discharge. Which of these statements by Mr. Rawles requires further instruction?
    a. "I will not take my morning lithium until after I have my blood work done."
    b. "When I get home, I may go on a salt-free diet."
    c. "I have learned not to restrict my intake of water."
    d. "I understand some people gain weight on lithium."

12. What effect does a benzodiazepine have on the activity of gamma aminobutyric acid (GABA), the primary inhibitory neurotransmitter in the brain?
    a. Enhances the activity
    b. Reduces availability of GABA
    c. Interacts with serotonin to increase availability
    d. Creates less activity of GABA

13. Mrs. Johnson, age 45, was prescribed alprazolam (Xanax) for symptoms of anxiety she was experiencing since a recent divorce and relocation. She stated to the nurse, "I feel out of it and spacy after I take the Xanax." What is the likely cause of this feeling?
    a. The combination of the medication with an antidepressant
    b. Rapid penetration into the brain
    c. Sensitivity of the mesencephalic reticular activating system
    d. Long elimination half-life

14. Which of these client outcomes would be most applicable for the client who has been taking benzodiazepines?
    a. Client will list specific foods to avoid while on this medication.
    b. Client will state understanding of how to increase medication dosage.
    c. Client will list alcohol as substance to avoid while on the medication.
    d. Client will state understanding that he or she can not return to work while on this medication.

15. Which of these persons is the least likely candidate to receive the medication depakene (Valproate)?
    a. Jean, who is recovering from a hysterectomy
    b. Jane, who is displaying symptoms of postpartum depression
    c. Lois, who is three-months pregnant
    d. May, who is taking hormone replacement therapy

16. Tommy, age 6, has ADHD, and his mother was attending a class to learn about his prescribed medication, methylphenidate (Ritalin). What is the rationale for giving the medication at breakfast and again at midday?
    a. To prevent Tommy from experiencing the return of symptoms
    b. To decrease afternoon sleepiness
    c. To provide the opportunity to monitor Tommy's behavior closely
    d. To avoid possibility of toxicity

17. Jo Ryan has been diagnosed with seasonal affective disorder (SAD) and is planning to begin phototherapy treatment. Effective treatment with phototherapy is best achieved if the:
    a. Skin is exposed to direct light for at least four hours at a time
    b. Treatment is done early in the day
    c. Client is exposed to light at a distance of five to six feet
    d. Light strikes the eyes directly

18. The nurse was taking Ms. Ames' vital signs in preparation for her first electroconvulsive treatment (ECT). Which of these statements from Ms. Ames would result in cancellation of the treatment?
    a. "I'll be so glad when this treatment is over."
    b. "Will I remember having this treatment?"
    c. "I just had some crackers and milk since I'll miss breakfast."
    d. "I'm so tired of being depressed."

19. Three clients were talking in the day room in the psychiatric hospital. Beth, who has been experiencing extreme anxiety, demonstrated her understanding of Ativan, which she is prescribed p.r.n., when she stated:
    a. "I can talk with my therapist much better after my medication takes effect."
    b. "I wonder if I will have to take this medication for the rest of my life."
    c. "I don't want anyone to know I'm on this medication."
    d. "I'm going to ask for my p.r.n. so I can sleep this afternoon."

20. A client has been taking chlorpromazine (Thorazine) for the past two weeks. He is complaining of drooling and walking with a shuffling gait. The nurse would correctly attribute these behaviors to:
    a. Tardive dyskinesia
    b. Impending neuroleptic malignant syndrome
    c. Akinesia
    d. Pseudoparkinsonism

Chapter 24

Alternative Therapies

1. Gerald has an anxiety panic attacks when h teaches Gerald to do he feels anxious. The
    a. Is difficult to learn when doing techniques
    b. May result in a wide range of physiologic and psychologic effects
    c. Is beneficial only for individuals who have mild anxiety
    d. Often results in increased anxiety

2. A client complains of little change in her sleep pattern, and even though she has been doing the biofeedback exercises, "the machine has not been successful." The nurse tells her she will observe the next session. The nurse is aware that:
    a. Biofeedback assists the individual to gain own control of a problem or situation
    b. The machine is a critical component of biofeedback during all phases
    c. Client's muscle responses determine success of biofeedback
    d. The client's mood affects results of biofeedback

3. The nurse entered the room of a client who had been diagnosed with terminal cancer, and found client and her husband laughing loudly at old movies of The Three Stooges. The nurse left the room and postponed a planned treatment, knowing that humor
    a. has no place in serious hospital situations
    b. can affect positive changes on several physiologic systems and functions.
    c. only serves to prolong the client's denial of the real situation
    d. may help the very young who are unaware of serious situations

orhood clinic, the client listened as [...] neutrally told of traditional medicine [...] that were available to treat his health problems. The client thanked the nurse and said he was going to continue treatment with acupuncture and Ayurvedic medicine before doing any of the suggested treatments. The nurse told the client to carefully consider his choices, told him the staff was available if needed, and wished him good health. The nurse's response demonstrates:
   a. A superficial understanding of current accepted traditional treatment modalities
   b. Lack of concern for the client's well-being
   c. Inability to confront clients
   d. Respect for client's health care choices

Chapter 25

Crisis Intervention

1. Following the Coconut Grove fire in Boston in 1942, Eric Lindemann and his colleagues reported which of these findings?
   a. Persons should seek individual counseling after crisis events.
   b. Community caretakers can help the mourner work through the grief process.
   c. Delayed grief is a precursor to depression.
   d. Crisis is a natural phenomena and should be expected.

2. Which of these events has the potential for causing a situational crisis?
   a. A flood destroying a home
   b. Losing a job after 10 years
   c. Leaving home to attend college
   d. Retirement from teaching school

3. Peter, age 30, was experiencing marital problems with his wife of two years. After his wife walked out, Peter became angry, breaking china and destroying potted plants. A neighbor convinced him to seek help at the local crisis center. Which of these questions will the crisis nurse ask to determine Peter's immediate problem?
   a. "What did you do to cause your wife to leave?"
   b. "Do you feel in control at this time?"
   c. "Why did you come for help today?"
   d. "How would you handle this situation if you had a second chance?"

4. Tammy, age 16, was anxious because she had to change schools during the middle of the school year because of her father's job. Three of these coping methods would be acceptable for Tammy in relieving her anxiety. Which one is the exception?
   a. Talking to a friend or family member
   b. Crying
   c. Keeping a journal
   d. Screaming at her sister

5. Mrs. English was admitted to the hospital after an attempted suicide following the sudden death of her husband. She reported they were together most of the time and did not socialize with others. Now she is experiencing extreme loneliness and lack of companionship. Which of these nursing diagnoses will address this issue?
   a. Hopelessness related to death of husband
   b. Potential for self-harm related to loneliness
   c. Social isolation related to failure to establish outside relationships
   d. Delayed grief reaction related to sudden death of husband

6. The nurse manager of the unit was leading a discussion on crisis intervention and asked the question, "What is the usual length of time for crisis intervention?" Which of these group participants responded correctly?
   a. Lydia: "1 to 2 weeks"
   b. Dorothy: "2 to 4 weeks"
   c. Roger: "4 to 6 weeks"
   d. Mark: "6 to 8 weeks"

7. According to Caplan's developmental phases of crisis, what happens during a crisis if the problem continues and can be neither solved nor avoided?
   a. Tension rises, and more discomfort is felt.
   b. Tension increases, and major disorganization occurs.
   c. Internal and external resources are mobilized.
   d. Balancing factors can bring about a return to equilibrium.

8. A group of school-age children were brought to the emergency room having been injured in a school bus accident. Family members and friends paced back and forth in the waiting room. Members of the crisis team were called in to:
   a. Assist the medical team with the physical injuries
   b. Determine level of individual family coping
   c. Wait with the families and friends
   d. Provide immediate emotional support

9. The crisis nurse was interviewing a client who had come to the center in a state of panic. Which of these interventions would assist the nurse to help the client?
    a. Learning about the crisis-precipitating event
    b. Talking with a family friend about the client
    c. Requesting a copy of old health information
    d. Outlining a strategy to deal with the panic

10. Jake had recently been involved in assisting with the clean-up from a flood that washed away many homes in his area and caused loss of life. Which of these interventions would assist Jake in dealing with the traumatic experience?
    a. Providing him the opportunity to talk about the experience
    b. Encouraging him to leave the area in order to forget the experience
    c. Suggesting he be admitted to a mental health facility
    d. Arranging for his minister to meet with him

Chapter 26

Activity Therapies

1. What is the primary reason for the nurse to have an understanding of the various types of adjunct therapies?
    a. The nurse is expected to interpret the clients' involvement in the therapies.
    b. The nurse needs to be supportive of the treatment team members who direct these therapies.
    c. The nurse is responsible for placing the client in the appropriate group based on the diagnosis.
    d. The nurse chooses the most cost effective therapy group based on the client's ability to pay.

2. Which of the adjunctive therapies available would be best to assist a client to achieve increased awareness of her body?
    a. Psychodrama
    b. Music therapy
    c. Dance therapy
    d. Recreation

3. Adjunct therapies may be more useful in specific situations than verbal therapies because adjunct therapies:
    a. Allow the client to express feelings on multiple levels at the same time
    b. Do not require specific training or expertise to facilitate
    c. Provide the client the opportunity to use ego-protective mechanisms
    d. Are readily available in the treatment setting

4. Which of these statements reflects information a client would have learned in an independent living skills group?
    a. "I can now take care of all of my physical needs."
    b. "I know how to request reimbursement for services rendered."
    c. "I am sure I will have a more active social life."
    d. "I know some new methods to use to help me relax."

5. Mr. Smith, age 38, attended an occupational therapy group to work on the identified goal of "recognizing and using more effective coping techniques." How can the nurse continue to support Mr. Smith's attainment of this goal after he returns to the unit?
    a. By avoiding limit setting which might increase his level of anxiety
    b. By praising him for positive behavior changes
    c. By isolating him from more seriously ill clients
    d. By permitting him to make mistakes prior to intervening on his behalf

6. The nurse is assisting the recreational therapist with a dance activity for a mixed adult inpatient group of clients. How can the nurse encourage an extremely shy male client to participate?
    a. Offering to dance with the client
    b. Asking the client if this is the first dance he has attended
    c. Sitting with the client away from the group
    d. Encouraging another client to ask him to dance

7. Amy, age 12, was referred for art therapy. The therapist directing the activity assessed Amy's level of functioning prior to the selection of art materials to use. Which of these art materials has the potential to promote regression?
    a. Colored pens and pencils
    b. Magic markers and crayons
    c. Large unlined paper
    d. Finger paints and play dough

8. A group of nurses were attending a lecture on the effective use of adjunct therapies with psychiatric clients. The instructor was correct in identifying the Romanian psychiatrist who developed psychodrama as:
   a. Marian Chase
   b. Jacob L. Moreno
   c. Sigmund Freud
   d. Elinor Ulman

9. A nursing student participating in a group enactment was asked to serve as an alter ego. The function to the alter ego is to:
   a. Operate as the inner voice
   b. Portray significant others in a client's life
   c. Provide an opportunity for catharsis
   d. Direct the psychodrama

10. Jim, age 30, a schizophrenic client on the adult unit, was attending an art therapy session for the first time. Which of these art materials would be best for Jim to use?
    a. Marking pens and a defined space on which to draw
    b. A large blank sheet of paper and a pencil
    c. Small brushes and pencils
    d. Brightly colored finger paints

11. The nurse is collecting the paintings from the clients after the art session is over. A client hands the nurse his empty sheet of paper, which revealed he had not done the art project. Which of these statements indicates the nurse's knowledge of art therapy?
    a. "John, do you want to complete your painting?"
    b. "What happened, John, don't you like to paint?"
    c. "Can you tell me what happened, John?"
    d. "Thank you, John, I'll put this away for you."

12. What is the purpose of the "warm up" exercise associated with movement/dance therapy?
    a. Provides an opportunity to get to know other members in the activity group
    b. Increases comfort with movement and heightens awareness
    c. Decreases cardiovascular activity and intake of oxygen
    d. Prevents injuries as the activity progresses

13. Florence Nightingale, an early English nursing leader, first introduced recreational services to which of these groups?
    a. Nursing students
    b. Hospitalized soldiers
    c. Mentally ill clients
    d. Physically handicapped

14. The nurse is assisting with a psychodrama activity working on unresolved grief. During the closure the nurse observes two clients who are markedly upset and anxious. What would be an appropriate intervention at this time?
    a. Asking the activity for assistance
    b. Suggesting the clients leave the group to avoid embarrassment
    c. Encouraging the clients to process their reactions within the group
    d. Evaluating the activity as unsuccessful in grief resolution

15. The nurse is orienting to the activity department since he will be required to assist clients who will be involved in adjunct therapy. Which of these statements describes the function of music therapy?
    a. It allows for an immediate experience promoting self-organization and social connection.
    b. It enables clients to learn more about individual musical abilities.
    c. It provides the opportunity to reduce anxiety and stress.
    d. It affords the client a method of getting in touch with unresolved feelings and issues.

Chapter 27

Survivors of Family Violence

1. The nurse is leading a group for women who have experienced interpersonal violence. The nurse is aware that the perpetrator of interpersonal violence is:
   a. Usually under the influence of drugs and/or alcohol
   b. Most often someone the victim knows
   c. A stranger to the victim in most cases
   d. Often in a psychotic state during the act

2. Which of these nursing interventions will assist a client to disclose an experience of domestic violence?
   a. Interviewing her in the presence of another professional
   b. Speaking with the client in the absence of her husband
   c. Providing a safe, nonintimidating environment
   d. Allowing the client to initiate the topic of violence

3. A new client admits to having been battered by her live-in boyfriend several times over the past two years. She states to the nurse, "We plan to get married next June and I think things will be better then. He is always so sorry after the incident that I think I can trust him to change." Which of the following should be included in the client's teaching plan?
   a. Supporting her hope that the battering will end after they are married
   b. Assisting her to enroll in a class to learn self-defense
   c. Emphasizing that the battering pattern usually remains the same in frequency and severity over time
   d. Assisting her in developing an emergency plan since the pattern of violence is likely to continue

4. The nurse in the emergency room is taking a history from a family accompanying a child with suspicious traumatic injuries. The nurse should:
   a. Be covert in obtaining information
   b. Avoid responding to any hints that abuse is suspected
   c. Be open, concerned, and honest
   d. Separate the family from the child during the interview

5. Mrs. DeLong was brought into the emergency room with family members who reported a fall. During the assessment the nurse became suspicious that the client had suffered physical abuse. Mrs. DeLong denied that she had been abused. Her denial is most likely based on:
   a. A strong belief that nothing could be done to help her
   b. Her fear of the possibility of being removed from her family
   c. Her feeling that she deserved the abuse
   d. Her lack of trust that the situation could be changed

6. Steve, age 30, has been attending a group to help batterers learn more effective ways to cope. The group leader explained that the key component in wife battering is:
   a. The need for the batterer to control
   b. Alcohol abuse by the batterer
   c. History of psychotic behavior
   d. Failure of the woman to assert herself

7. The most common reason that a child may resist disclosing the experience of being sexually abused by a close family member is:
   a. Knowledge that he or she will be repeatedly questioned by others
   b. Fear of being blamed or disbelieved
   c. Fear of losing the love and affection of the abuser
   d. Embarrassment about facing family members

8. The nurse is planning to report a child abuse/neglect case to protective services in her city. Before making the report, the nurse needs to:
   a. Obtain her supervisor's permission to report it
   b. Have strong evidence that the abuse/neglect has occurred
   c. Notify the parents of the intent to report the suspicions of abuse/neglect
   d. Have suspicions that the abuse has occurred

9. A community health nurse is working with a family in which an elderly woman was neglected by her son and his wife. The elderly woman insists on remaining with the young couple despite the threat of future neglect. Which of these factors should be given highest priority at this time?
   a. Identifying community resources to decrease the caregiver's stress
   b. Establishing the probability of the elder's safety and potential for further abuse
   c. Educating the caregivers on the aging process and how to cope with it
   d. Providing stress management techniques for the caregivers

10. In order for the nurse to provide nursing care to abused children and their families, what must the nurse do first?
    a. Complete a comprehensive physical and mental assessment
    b. Recommend that the children be separated from their families until treatment is complete
    c. Refer each case to the appropriate social worker for follow up
    d. Examine personal feelings regarding the trauma of child abuse and neglect

11. According to statistical research data, which of these children is at the greatest risk for fatal abuse?
    a. Timmy, who is 2 years old
    b. Ben, who is 5 years old
    c. Daren, who is 8 years old
    d. Dean, who is 11 years old

12. The community health nurses are evaluating the success of interventions for working with the problem of family violence. Which of these nursing interventions is directed toward primary prevention?
    a. Assisting the victim to overcome abuse effects and prevent reoccurrences
    b. Identifying families at risk and attempting to avoid abuse from occurring
    c. Addressing the current abuse crisis and preventing future occurrences
    d. Enlisting the assistance of other community health officials for improved services

13. Tyler, age 18 months, was admitted to the hospital for treatment after his father hit him in the head with a piece of wood because he soiled his diaper. Which of these nursing diagnoses would be appropriate in this situation to include the parents?
    a. Maladaptive coping related to ineffective discipline methods
    b. Altered parenting related to unrealistic expectations
    c. Potential for abuse related to child's disobedience
    d. Anxiety related to removal of child from their home

14. Ms. Turner, age 34, has been physically abused by her husband five times during the past two years. During her last discussion with the nurse, Mrs. Turner stated, "I probably should not keep going back to my husband since he continues to abuse me." The nurse is aware that the final decision to leave a batterer:
    a. Often occurs after the victim suffers a serious injury
    b. Is usually a gradual process that occurs over time
    c. Is more likely if the client has approval from her church
    d. Is done with the batterer's permission

15. Mrs. Cone, age 42, has been battered by her husband since they were married eight years ago. Until this hospitalization for major depression, she had avoided dealing with the pain but now expresses a desire to deal with the situation. The attacks are occurring more often at this time. Which client outcome is realistic for Mrs. Cone?
    a. Citing possible ways she may have contributed to the abusive episodes
    b. Verbalizing an awareness of her increasingly dangerous situation
    c. Setting a goal date for divorcing her husband
    d. Employing methods of retaliating in order to get even with her husband

16. Which of these statements meets the criteria of the most recent American Medical Association Guidelines on the treatment of domestic violence with the victims informed consent?
    a. At least two photographs of each trauma area should be taken if battery is suspected.
    b. To avoid embarassing the victim, assessment for sexually transmitted disease is not done.
    c. Rape protocol is followed in abuse cases even when rape is not suspected.
    d. Protective services must be made aware of the abuse.

17. Recent studies dealing with the factors contributing to an increase in violence support the contention that exposure to violence in the media:
    a. Has no effect on the increase of violence in society
    b. Assists the client in distinguishing appropriate from inappropriate behaviors
    c. Desensitizes people to the violence around them
    d. Broadens the viewer's knowledge about happenings in the world

18. A group of children were discussing how their parents discipline them in their homes. Which of these children will likely exhibit physical aggression when dealing with his peers?
    a. Brian, who was placed in time-out for misbehaving
    b. Trudy, who lost certain privileges for inappropriate behaviors
    c. Anne, who was spanked when she was in trouble
    d. Katie, who had to miss a special television program as punishment

19. Which of these symptoms reported by Diane, age 35, who was sexually abused as a child, is reflective of the diagnosis, posttraumatic stress disorder (PTSD)?
    a. Reexperiencing the trauma via recurrent dreams
    b. Refusing to go to public places from which escape may be difficult
    c. Seeking advice and guidance prior to making any significant decision
    d. Ruminating over the abuse with friends and acquaintances

20. Play therapy is commonly used with young children who have been either physically or sexually abused. Play therapy is especially valuable in assisting the child to:
    a. Act out his aggression in an acceptable manner
    b. Express feelings that he cannot verbalize
    c. Interact with other children in his age group
    d. Learn adaptive behaviors through acting

Chapter 28

Suicide

1. Durkheim classified the social and cultural aspects of suicide. Which of these statements describes anomic suicide, one of the four subtypes?
    a. Deaths of individuals who were influenced by a group to turn against their own conscience
    b. Acts of self-destruction by individuals who have become estranged from important relationships in their groups
    c. Self-inflicted deaths based on obedience to a group's goals that override one's own best interests
    d. A death resulting from excessive regulation

2. Freud presented a psychoanalytic view of suicide. He stated that suicide results from:
    a. Feelings of failure from unresolved interpersonal conflicts
    b. Hostility directed inward toward the internalized love object
    c. The wish to kill, the wish to be killed, and the wish to die
    d. Unconsciously wishing for spiritual rebirth

3. Congress declared the 1990s as the decade of the brain, and research has been done to determine the structure and chemistry in relation to affective disorders. Which of these abnormalities have been found in relation to suicide?
    a. Irregularities in the serotonin system
    b. Abnormal electroencephalogram (EEG) readings
    c. Atrophy of the brain
    d. Enlarged lateral ventricles

4. A group of nurses were presenting a seminar on suicide prevention. A person in the audience asked the question, "Are there any medications that can prevent a person from committing suicide?" Which statement best answers the question?
    a. There are no medications available that affect suicidal behavior.
    b. Antipsychotic medications are used primarily for suicide prevention.
    c. Antidepressants are effective in the treatment of mood disorders that accompany suicidal ideations.
    d. If people want to harm themselves, they eventually will.

5. Research by Cummings (1993) correlated the dimensions of depression with alterations in specific brain areas. Which area of the brain seems to be associated with feelings of hopelessness and worthlessness?
    a. Thalamus
    b. Temporal lobe
    c. Frontal lobe
    d. Motor strip

6. Which one of these behavioral approaches for suicidal ideation is based on the learning theory?
    a. Intense psychotherapy to deal with the issues
    b. Group therapy with clients with similar problems
    c. Decreasing unpleasant events and increasing pleasant events
    d. Including significant others in the plan of care

7. The nurse manager was presenting a lecture at a community center on "Suicide Prevention." Which of the following correctly describes the problem of suicide in America today?
    a. The decreased rate of suicide is related to increased availability of antidepressants.
    b. Children are not considered a high-risk group for committing suicide.
    c. The highest suicide rate is among the white middle-aged population.
    d. Suicide is the eighth leading cause of death in America.

8. A group of adolescents were involved in group therapy, discussing their feelings about their progress. Which one of these statements should receive highest consideration when planning care?
    a. "I have a necktie in my room that I can use to hang myself."
    b. "If I fail another class, I'm going to kill myself."
    c. "When I leave home to live on my own, I'm buying myself a gun."
    d. "I took two bottles of Mom's pills and had to have my stomach pumped."

9. Of the four client problems listed, which one is most closely related to the development of suicidal thinking?
    a. Diabetes
    b. Mood disorder
    c. Thought disorder
    d. Hypertension

10. Mr. Reeves, age 58, was admitted to the hospital for severe depression. The nurse, gathering data about his past medical and psychiatric history learned of a suicide attempt four years ago after the death of his wife. Based on this information, it is likely that Mr. Reeves:
    a. Will avoid attempting suicide again after the past experience
    b. Try to minimize the seriousness of the suicide attempt
    c. May express suicide ideations and threats at this time
    d. Will report that he has recently written a will

11. Mr. Saul, age 46, was admitted to the hospital with major depression. The nurse asked, "Mr. Saul, do you feel like hurting yourself at this time?" What is the rationale for gaining this information since nothing in his referral note implied that he was suicidal?
    a. It is likely that he was hiding the desire to harm himself.
    b. This information must be reported to the physician.
    c. Additional safety measures must be implemented if he is in danger of self-harm.
    d. He would be placed on a locked unit if he is a threat to himself.

12. The nurse working at the crisis center received a call from a client who stated he was depressed and wanted to die. Further investigation revealed that the client had all of these items within reach that he could use "to get the job done." Which one of these items would cause the nurse the most concern?
    a. Two bottles of Prozac
    b. A loaded gun
    c. A garden hose
    d. A bottle of an alcoholic beverage

13. Mr. Leigh, a client with major depression was admitted to the hospital after attempting self-harm by over-dosing on a variety of medications and drinking alcohol. He was improving and interacting with peers and the staff. Which one of these statements would cause the nurse to observe his behavior more closely?
    a. "When I'm discharged, I guess I'll stay with my son until I feel better."
    b. "I do not enjoy shopping at the mall since my wife died."
    c. "It puzzles me that anyone would want to harm themselves like I did."
    d. "My wife and I would have been married 36 years tomorrow."

14. Roberta, age 15, was being interviewed by the psychiatric nurse to obtain information related to her admission earlier today. From the data listed, which finding is most significant in planning care?
    a. She ran away from home twice during the past month.
    b. Her mother died from suicide one year ago.
    c. Her father recently remarried.
    d. She has expressed a dislike for new stepmother.

15. The nurse was completing a plan of care for a client who was admitted to the hospital after threatening to harm himself, having been stopped by the police for speeding excessively in his automobile while intoxicated. He was depressed, anxious, and hostile. Which of these client outcomes is the priority?
    a. Client will not harm himself while in the hospital.
    b. Client will report feelings of self-harm to the physician.
    c. Client will accept referral to the substance abuse program.
    d. Client will recognize unconscious intentions to harm self.

16. Mrs. Ware was taking prescribed antidepressants having been experiencing severe depression with feelings of hopelessness, helplessness, and expressing suicide ideations. She was hospitalized because she was not improving, and her physician planned further evaluation. When would Mrs. Ware be at the greatest risk for suicide while she is hospitalized?
    a. Within the first 12 to 24 hours after admission
    b. At night after her visitors leave
    c. Within the first 24 hours after admission and as discharge approached
    d. When she realizes she must go home and be by herself

17. The nurse is preparing a client for discharge. He was hospitalized for 10 days, having attempted to kill himself by overdosing on medications. Which statement indicates that he meets the criteria for discharge?
    a. "The next time I get depressed, I'll be careful who I tell."
    b. "I enjoy living alone and don't need to socialize."
    c. "I have a person I can call if I should get depressed again."
    d. "I do not feel like harming myself."

18. The emergency room nurses were discussing James, a client who seeks help almost every holiday, having attempted suicide or expressing suicide ideations. One of the nurses stated, "I don't think James is serious about hurting himself. Maybe we should not see him the next time he comes." Which response from the charge nurse is accurate in dealing with James, who may be using suicidal behavior as a ploy to enter the hospital?
    a. "Telling James we cannot see him may be the answer to stop this behavior."
    b. "Each episode must be individually evaluated and all options explored."
    c. "He obviously needs the support he gets at the hospital."
    d. "We should avoid showing any emotion to James the next time he comes."

19. Mr. Troy, age 56, had been diagnosed with cancer of the prostate one month ago and underwent surgery. After returning home, he became more and more depressed and was negative about the future. His doctor admitted him to the hospital after Mrs. Troy reported he was trying to mix a lethal dose of medications and alcohol that he could drink. Which of these client outcomes are applicable to his situation?
    a. Mr. Troy will list five reasons to live.
    b. Mr. Troy will not direct harm to another client.
    c. Mr. Troy will learn ways to handle his unresolved anger.
    d. Mr. Troy will list reasons he does not want to live.

Chapter 29

Grief and Loss

1. Which of the following physical disturbances are common in acute grief?
    a. Increased appetite
    b. Tightness in the chest
    c. Cardiovascular problems
    d. Hypersomnia

2. Bereavement differs from depression in that in bereavement:
    a. Psychomotor retardation is obvious
    b. Suicide thoughts are common
    c. Symptoms are of shorter duration
    d. Guilt feelings are overwhelming

3. A Grief Support Group was held at the local community center to assist persons who were dealing with issues of loss. Which remark by one of the members indicates unresolved feelings of guilt?
    a. "I know that my husband had a good life."
    b. "It seems I miss my son more as time goes on."
    c. "I still wish I had gotten to him sooner."
    d. "Christmas is always a sad time for me."

4. A young woman had just learned of the death of her husband in an automobile accident. During a meeting to plan the funeral, she began to cry and stated, "It's not fair. How could he do this to me?" This remark could be correctly intermediated as:
    a. A plea for help
    b. An expression of anger
    c. An explosive episode
    d. Fear of making decisions alone

5. Mrs. Jamison was preparing a birthday dinner for her college son who was to return home for the celebration. On the way home he was killed in an automobile crash. Family and friends rushed to the home to offer support to Mrs. Jamison. Which of these persons, through their act of kindness, may contribute to prolonging Mrs. Jamison's grief?
   a. The physician who prescribed antianxiety agents to dull the pain
   b. The nurse who offered to spend the night at her home
   c. The next-door teenager who provided care for the two puppies
   d. The accountant who assisted with financial affairs

6. What are the most common initial responses to the sudden death of a loved one?
   a. Despair and protest
   b. Disorganization and confusion
   c. Anger and hostility
   d. Shock and disbelief

7. A grief counselor was discussing the concept of "grief work," a term coined by Lindermann. The counselor explains that "grief work" refers to:
   a. Actively seeking assistance to cope with the loss experiences
   b. Establishing new methods of coping with stress
   c. The means by which one moves through the grief process
   d. Evaluating progress made toward accepting the loss

8. Jamie, age 16, was grieving the loss of her pet dog who was killed by a car when he ran into the street. She stated to her mother, "I miss my dog so much but I know that if I start crying, I will never stop." The fear expressed by Jamie is:
   a. Loss of control over her emotions
   b. Embarrassment in front of her friends
   c. Behaving immaturely
   d. Lack of available support

9. During a grief processing group an elderly client stated, "For the first time since my husband died, I'm having more good days than bad." This statement suggests that the client has:
   a. Completed her "grief work" successfully
   b. Determined she is ready to terminate the support group
   c. Reached the phase of resolution
   d. Replaced old memories with new ones

10. Mr. Eades had returned from attending the service memorializing his wife who died after a sudden illness. Although those around him were visibly shaken, he smiled and remained in control. He refused support from friends stating, "I can handle anything that comes my way." Mr. Eades' behavior is an example of:
    a. Converted grief
    b. Inhibited grief
    c. Distorted grief
    d. An expected male response to loss

11. Which of these persons is most likely suffering from chronic sorrow, a form of grief recently described in the literature?
    a. The mother of a six-month-old baby who has frequent ear infections
    b. The father of a son who has schizophrenia
    c. The daughter whose father recently had a hip replacement
    d. The wife whose husband wants a divorce

12. A client, Mrs. Dean, was being seen by her family physician for symptoms of insomnia and significant weight loss over the past two months. The physician, aware that Mrs. Dean's husband had died recently, said, "Describe how it has been for you since your husband died." What is the purpose of this request?
    a. To determine the risk of pathologic grief and the need for grief therapy
    b. To learn whether Mrs. Dean has a significant support system
    c. To rule out psychological factors that may interfere with accurately diagnosing her illness
    d. To display an attitude of concern and sympathy to Mrs. Dean

13. Acute grief is different from anticipatory grief in that anticipatory grief:
    a. Is associated with an expected loss
    b. Requires a longer period to resolve
    c. Is associated with fewer expressions of guilt
    d. Prevents development of symptoms of depression

14. Ruth Ames was referred to a grief therapist having developed physical symptoms related to prolonged grief. Her husband, an alcoholic who regularly abused her, was killed in an automobile accident two years ago. Since his death, Ruth tends to idealize him and focus on their wonderful relationship. Which of these client outcomes is appropriate for Ruth?
    a. Keeping a daily journal recording pleasant memories of time spent with her husband
    b. Expressing both positive and negative feelings about her husband and their relationship
    c. Reading information on alcoholism and support groups available to her
    d. Enlisting emotional support from family and friends

15. During a bereavement group, one of the members stated, "I should have been the one to die. My husband had so much to offer." This statement is likely an indicator that the member was expressing:
    a. Intention to commit suicide
    b. Ambivalence and low self-esteem
    c. Need for attention from group members
    d. Unresolved anger toward her husband

16. The community health nurse was visiting a client diagnosed with dysfunctional grieving since the death of his wife and child in a head-on collision over a year ago. Which of these actions should the nurse take first?
    a. Facilitate expression of feelings related to the loss
    b. Determine the degree of ambivalence toward the loss
    c. Promote interaction with others
    d. Assess risk of violence toward himself and others

17. The nurse was teaching a group of nurses about the grief experience. One of the nurses commented, "When my mother died, I never saw my father show any emotion. He wanted to be strong for the children. What do you think will happen with those unexpressed feelings?" Which of these answers is most appropriate?
    a. "Pent-up emotions may be directed inward, leading to depression or other disorders."
    b. "Your father probably has worked through his grief by this time."
    c. "Maybe you can teach him how to express his feelings."
    d. "If feelings are not expressed openly, the person may develop self-destructive behaviors."

18. What is the rationale for including a physical exercise program in the treatment plan for a client dealing with unresolved grief?
    a. Provides a way for interacting with others
    b. Promotes expenditure of anxious energy, anger, and tension
    c. Affords an opportunity for thinking and processing information related to the loss
    d. Contributes to a feeling of well-being

19. Mr. and Mrs. Lawrence have lived in their same home for the past 50 years. Now that neither are able to drive and take care of the home, they have moved into an Adult Retirement Center in a nearby town. Changes in lifestyle such as the Lawrences are experiencing could result in which type of crisis?
    a. Situational
    b. Maturational
    c. Adventitious
    d. Unresolved grief

20. Donald, age 16, was deer hunting with his best friend who was accidentally killed by another hunter two weeks ago. Donald's parents consulted their physician because of his decreased appetite, insomnia, and inability to function at his previous level in school. He seemed obsessed with his friend's death, talking about the accident repeatedly. What is the best explanation for Donald's behavior?
    a. He is attempting to avoid dealing with his pain.
    b. He is feeling responsible for his friend's death.
    c. He is experiencing a normal grief reaction.
    d. He is at risk for self-harm in an attempt to be with his friend.

Chapter 30

Persons With HIV/AIDS

1. Matthew, age 27, who had received a diagnosis of HIV seropositivity, reported feeling jittery and distracted. His heart and respiratory rate increased, and he expressed feeling tense. Matthew's symptoms most likely indicate that he is experiencing:
    a. Suicidal ideations
    b. Acute anxiety
    c. Disappointment at lab results
    d. Guilt

2. Roy, age 30, was diagnosed with AIDS, having had numerous complaints of fatigue, night sweats, and fever. During his hospitalization he placed a "no visitors" sign on his door and refused phone calls. He stated to the nurse, "I know you don't want to be around me." Which of these nursing diagnoses is applicable to this situation?
   a. Fear of dying related to medical diagnosis
   b. Social isolation related to fear of rejection
   c. Lack of knowledge related to possible cause of his illness
   d. Anger related to having to face death at such a young age

3. Which of these factors should be considered when assessing the advisability of prescribing psychotropic medications for PWA's?
   a. Length of time since diagnosis was made
   b. Nutritional status of the client
   c. Characteristics of emotional distress
   d. Tolerance for oral medications

4. James, age 27, had been diagnosed with AIDS and was having more physical complaints. The nurse observed him reading a medical journal on the subject of lethal injections. As he attempted to hide the journal, which response by the nurse would be most appropriate?
   a. "I noticed what you are reading. Why are you trying to hide it?"
   b. "Let me have the journal. An article like that will only upset you."
   c. "Tell me what you think of the article. That way I won't have to read it."
   d. "I'd like to spend some time with you. Is that all right with you?"

5. Mark, age 37, an AIDS client, was talking to the nurse about his symptoms. Which of these statements indicates that Mark is exhibiting signs of acute psychotic-type dementia?
   a. "I move more slowly than I used to."
   b. "I don't enjoy being with others anymore."
   c. "Sometimes I hear voices."
   d. "I can't always remember where I put things."

6. Which one of these factors may contribute to the higher death rate in women with AIDS than in the male population?
   a. Delay in seeking treatment
   b. High rate of metabolism
   c. Presence of estrogen
   d. Increased fat cells

7. Which of these AIDS related complaints are common in the individual who is HIV positive and is symptomatic?
   a. Fever, night sweats, nausea
   b. Confusion, disorientation, and forgetfulness
   c. Elevated pulse, respirations, and blood pressure
   d. Increased appetite, specific food and drink cravings

8. Dinah, age 19, is concerned that she may have been exposed to the HIV virus. For months she thought about it and knew that she should be tested. What is the primary reason she would not have the HIV testing?
   a. She was waiting to develop symptoms.
   b. She was afraid her parents would hear about it.
   c. She feared she may test seropositive.
   d. She was concerned about losing her current boyfriend.

9. Tommy, a client with AIDS, was feeling threatened by his inability to work and take care of the yard and garden as he had always done. Which of these client outcomes is appropriate for Tommy at this time?
   a. Accepting the fact he will not be able to assume previous roles
   b. Realigning goals to achieve a positive emotional state
   c. Enlisting others to help him carry out his former tasks
   d. Explaining his declining state of health to the family

10. Mr. Teague, age 54, has been hospitalized with problems related to AIDS and is experiencing profound dementia. The nurse was talking with Mrs. Teague and her son about his condition. Which of these suggestions will be most helpful in assisting the family through this difficult experience?
    a. Providing information on support groups available to them
    b. Encouraging the placement of Mr. Teague in an adult home
    c. Explaining the importance of engaging in social activities with friends
    d. Focusing on present, rather than future problems

11. While being bathed, Ms. Taylor, a client with AIDS, asked the nurse, "Aren't you afraid of getting this disease from me?" Which of these answers best reflects the client's feelings?
    a. "You sound surprised that I want to spend time with you."
    b. "No, I always use universal precautions."
    c. "Statistics show that few nurses get AIDS from their clients."
    d. "I firmly believe that whatever will be, will be."

12. The nurse manager was interviewing staff to work on the AIDS unit in the hospital. Which of these applicants is the best candidate based on her answer to the question, "Tell me how you feel about working with AIDS clients."
    a. Nurse A: "I know I will have to be more careful on this unit especially with injections and IVs."
    b. Nurse B: "I firmly believe there will soon be a cure for AIDS."
    c. Nurse C: "I have done extensive research on AIDS and understand the disease."
    d. Nurse D: "I believe that everyone is worthy of the best care I can provide."

Chapter 31

Psychologic Aspects of Physiologic Illness

1. The nurse, in preparing a historical overview of the mind-body connection, learned that the belief that "an unexamined life was not worth living" can be attributed to which of these individuals?
    a. Thales
    b. Socrates
    c. Aristotle
    d. Hippocrates

2. The nurse was teaching a class on the health contributions of different cultures. She stated that Buddhism, founded in 500 B.C., supports the belief that individuals strive to reach Nirvana, which is:
    a. The attainment of spiritual enlightenment through meditation and self-discipline
    b. The integration of body, mind, and spirit
    c. The state of perfect peace
    d. Healing through finding one's center

3. The nurse was admitting a client to the unit and gathering information in order to plan his care. The client stated that his belief system reflected the philosophy that spiritual enlightenment is attained through meditation and self-discipline. The nurse is aware that this belief is attributed to:
    a. Confucianism
    b. The law of Karma
    c. Christian teachings
    d. The Zen philosophy

4. The nurse manager was discussing the concept of holistic health care with the nursing staff. He was correct in stating that holistic health care:
    a. Views man as a total being
    b. Supports separation of mind, body, and spirit
    c. Incorporates the belief that individuals are more alike than different
    d. Denies genetic factors as influencing individual responses to illness

5. The nurse is obtaining data about a client. Which of these behaviors might be an indicator that the client is experiencing spiritual distress?
    a. Attending worship services weekly in the hospital chapel
    b. Questioning as to the meaning of his suffering
    c. Expressing interest in learning about beliefs of other religions
    d. Reading a daily devotional from a magazine every morning

6. Transactional or process theories of stress are classified as irrelevant, benign-positive, or stressful. Which of these demands would be perceived as irrelevant?
    a. Harmful threats of losses
    b. Challenges and potential for growth
    c. Responding to a particular stimulus
    d. Requiring minimal attention

7. Three of the psychiatric nurses had attended a workshop on therapeutic touch and were reporting information they had learned. One of the nurses stated that therapeutic touch is derived from the "laying on of hands," which is based upon the theory that:
    a. Energy flow can cure most diseases if used correctly.
    b. Body contact signifies caring and concern for the individual experiencing illness.
    c. The release of excess energy from the healer assists the ill person in the healing process.
    d. The illness and pain experience enhance the flow of environmental energy.

8. During a group session the members were discussing the types of stressors that have an impact on their lives. Which one of these members is experiencing a psychologic stressor in her life?
   a. Mary, who was exposed to extreme cold while skiing
   b. Dot, who has just learned that her job is being eliminated
   c. Torrie, who has a history of hypertension now controlled
   d. Louise, who has been receiving radiation treatment

9. Timothy Brown, age 18, a college sophomore, was admitted to the hospital, having been injured in a football game. Timothy was an honor student. He was also involved in physical fitness, and he was popular with his peers. Which of these initial concerns will likely be most difficult for Timothy?
   a. Inability to take a scheduled test next week
   b. Distance from home and family
   c. Appearance of weakness and frailty
   d. Temporary loss of control over his life

10. A group of clients dealing with management of chronic pain had been meeting daily with the therapist and nurse. During the process session after the group dismissed, the nurse stated, "I think Mr. Lee is using his pain for 'secondary gains.'" Which of Mr. Lee's behaviors caused the nurse to make this remark?
    a. "I don't have to worry about my teenage son getting in trouble since he has to stay with me after school."
    b. "I still try to help around the house even if I don't feel like it."
    c. "My wife is still involved with her community and volunteer activities."
    d. "I think I will someday be able to feel normal again and feel better about life in general."

11. The nurse was presenting a seminar on "Stress Reduction" to a community group. In preparation, he reviewed Nuernberger's general inhibition syndrome which is based on:
    a. The fight-or-flight mechanism
    b. Positive reinforcement
    c. Primary appraisal stressors
    d. Self-protective mechanism

12. A nursing student who was studying the mind-body connection stated to the instructor. "I still don't understand how a placebo could help relieve a client's pain." The instructor based the answer on which of these factors?
    a. Increase in serotonin
    b. Decrease in dopamine
    c. Release of endorphins
    d. The catecholamine imbalance

13. Mrs. Laws, age 72, was admitted to the hospital to learn to deal more effectively with pain she is experiencing from a recent injury. Which of these sources of information will be most helpful to the nurse in planning her care?
    a. A written report from Mrs. Law's physician detailing the injury
    b. Mrs. Law's subjective report of what she is experiencing
    c. A family member who explains methods of pain control already implemented
    d. A detailed account of the medications Mrs. Laws' is currently taking

14. The use of a dilute solution containing poison ivy compound to treat a skin rash is an example of:
    a. Homeopathic medicine
    b. Witchcraft
    c. Ayurvedic medicine
    d. Herbal medicine

15. The group therapist asked the clients to visualize their tension as a rope tied in a knot, then relaxed like a limp rubber band as they tense and relax their muscles. This exercise is an example of:
    a. Yoga
    b. Mental imagery
    c. Biofeedback
    d. Thought stopping

16. Mrs. Miers, a 56-year-old client, was being treated for severe hypertension at the community health center. Several medications had been tried, but her blood pressure was unaffected. Although Mrs. Miers denied any significant problems, the nurse detected that she had been crying and was wringing her hands during the interview. On what basis did the nurse seek additional information?
    a. Physical and mental processes are directly related in maintaining equilibrium.
    b. It is possible that Mrs. Miers had been harmed enroute to the center.
    c. At her age, Mrs. Miers could have suffered multiple losses.
    d. It is likely that Mrs. Miers was not taking her medication.

17. During the community health rotation, nursing students were learning about the contribution epidemiologic studies have made in determining disease causing factors. Which of this information was gained through epidemiologic studies?
    a. The average age of community high school teachers is 38 years.
    b. More Baptist children attend church-related kindergarten than public kindergarten.
    c. Widowed persons had higher death rates than married persons of the same age.
    d. There is a greater risk of academic failure in the low socioeconomic class.

18. Mr. Ross, age 46, an avid golfer, suffered a myocardial infarction two weeks ago and had bypass surgery. When talking with the nurse, Mr. Ross refused to acknowledge that the recent illness will alter his lifestyle in any way. Which client outcome would be applicable in this situation?
    a. Client will discuss ways he can continue his former activities.
    b. Client will avoid isolating in his room during activity hours.
    c. Client will be able to express feelings about effects of heart problem on future lifestyle.
    d. Client will focus on issues he can handle at this time, rather than dwell on the future.

19. The nurse was leading a group for geriatric clients who were attending a day hospital program. When discussing stressors that affect their lives, which of these clients is likely having difficulty finding meaning in life at this time?
    a. Mr. Harris, who uses a wheel chair in order to accompany his wife to the mall
    b. Mr. Lewis, who reflects on the good times he had as a young man
    c. Mr. Scott, who states he sometimes wonders what life after death is like
    d. Mr. Brown, who recently was forced to move to an adult home, having lived alone for five years

20. Mr. Mao, a 20-year-old Chinese exchange student, is attending a local university studying medicine. While on spring break, he was injured in an automobile accident and admitted to the hospital. He had to undergo surgery and was in extreme pain. Which of these nursing diagnoses should receive priority when planning his care?
    a. Anxiety
    b. Impaired verbal communication
    c. Pain
    d. High risk for infection

21. The nursing instructor was teaching Hans Selye's theory of stress and asked the students to identify the stage when there is a total expenditure of energy. Which of these responses is correct?
    a. The stage of exhaustion
    b. The stage of alarm
    c. The stage of resistance
    d. The stage of acceptance

22. The nurses on the unit were responding to a lecture they had attended, including "the concept of hardiness" as a means for mastering or controlling stress. Which of these components is included in this concept?
    a. Viewing stress as a block to reaching a designated goal
    b. Perceiving stress to be a challenge
    c. Lacking internal sense of control
    d. Placing self-needs as unimportant

23. Mrs. Lin was admitted to the hospital for surgery, having been diagnosed with breast cancer. The nurse observed that she was tearful and avoided interaction with staff except to request a "nerve pill." The staff identified anxiety as a nursing diagnosis. Which is the best outcome criteria for measuring the success of goal accomplishment?
    a. Client asks the nurse if she will likely experience much pain.
    b. Client sleeps through the night.
    c. Client walked up the hall to the unit kitchen.
    d. Client waited for three hours before requesting a "nerve pill."

24. The nurse was interviewing Ms. James, a new client on the unit, and stated, "Tell me how you happened to come to the hospital today." What is the purpose of obtaining this information from the client?
    a. To identify client's level of stress related to the admission
    b. To be able to correctly report to the client's physician
    c. To determine the client's perception of her illness
    d. To accurately document the admission findings

25. The nurse working on the pain management unit was explaining to her client the use of biofeedback, one of the modalities available to them. The best explanation about biofeedback is that it is a technique that:
    a. Uses equipment to assist the client to gain voluntary control over striated muscles
    b. Decreases the release of endogenous morphines from the brain
    c. Involves manipulation to restore proper body placement
    d. Releases a controlled amount of analgesic on a continuous basis

Chapter 32

Persons With Chronic Mental Illness

1. The definition of chronic mental illness from the National Plan for the Chronically Mentally Ill in 1981 applies to individuals with mental disorders which:
    a. Are thought to be time limited
    b. Interfere with one's ability to perform ADLs
    c. Are often curable since the advent of improved psychotrophic medications
    d. Create stress for family members

2. Bert, age 28, who has minimal brain damage, has been employed part time as a bagger at a local store. Testing indicates that he is capable of learning additional skills which may lead to a more secure job. What is the most likely reason for Bert's hesitancy to make a change?
    a. Fear of failure
    b. Disinterest in learning
    c. Job satisfaction
    d. Lack of family support

3. Which of these clients is at the highest risk for committing suicide?
    a. An adult who developed chronic mental illness later in life after experiencing successes
    b. A middle-age man who has chronic schizophrenia without depression
    c. A child who has minimal brain damage and attends regular classes at school
    d. An individual who was diagnosed with chronic brain damage at age 3

4. Why do many chronic mentally ill individuals experience problematic behaviors after discharge from the inpatient setting?
    a. Lack of adequate supervision
    b. Involvement in a dysfunctional family
    c. Noncompliance with psychotrophic medications
    d. Impaired judgment

5. In which of these settings do the majority of the chronic mentally ill population live?
    a. Halfway houses
    b. Low-rent apartments
    c. Foster care
    d. Family homes

6. The nurse was visiting in the home of a family who care for an 18-year-old chronic schizophrenic. The parents remarked, "We never go anywhere alone and are thinking about taking a weekend trip. What do you think?" Which of these responses will be most helpful to them?
    a. "It has to be tough, but you surely do a good job with your son."
    b. "Maybe you should leave for a few hours first to see if your son objects."
    c. "It will be difficult to find someone willing to stay in your home."
    d. "You do need to have some time away together."

7. Ned, age 34, a chronic schizophrenic, lives in a half-way house which houses other chronically mentally ill adults. Recently he has been found on the streets, having ingested large amounts of alcohol. What is the most likely reason Ned is abusing alcohol?
    a. As a suicide attempt
    b. For symptom relief
    c. To decrease inhibitions
    d. To gain attention

8. The nurse is meeting with a group of parents of chronically mentally ill children. Which of these statements from Timmy's mother indicates feelings of guilt?
    a. "I wonder what I could have done differently to prevent this problem."
    b. "Timmy would be like other kids if my doctor had not been so careless."
    c. "If Timmy is permitted to attend regular classes, he'll be more like the other kids."
    d. "Even though Timmy has this illness, he is such a joy to me."

9. Jason, age 7, has pervasive developmental disorder and requires constant supervision from his parents. Which of these suggestions for recreational activities would be most helpful to Jason's parents?
   a. Planning a picnic that would include the entire family
   b. Arranging for someone else to stay with Jason so that both parents can get out
   c. Planning activities on different nights and take turns staying with Jason
   d. Getting involved in activities that provide childcare services

10. Ralph, a chronic paranoid schizophrenic, has been threatening to harm his neighbors, whom he claims talk about him on the telephone. He was admitted to the hospital for evaluation. What is an appropriate client outcome for Ralph?
    a. Client will demonstrate absence of verbal intentions to harm others.
    b. Client will apologize to his neighbors for his behavior toward them.
    c. Client will demonstrate socially acceptable behavior.
    d. Client will initiate conversation with the staff.

11. One of the problems associated with deinstitutionalization has been the process of transinstitutionalization, which refers to:
    a. Overusing private hospitals rather than public institutions
    b. Transferring clients from one institution to another
    c. Discharging clients from institutions before they are ready
    d. Placing clients in the least restrictive settings

12. A nursing student organization was planning to work at a homeless shelter and earn points for community service. While at the shelter, they would be responsible for serving lunch. The staff explained that the shelters do not provide services to individuals who are:
    a. Retarded
    b. Intoxicated
    c. Depressed
    d. Divorced

13. Which of these actions should the nurse place first when assessing a client who was just admitted to the hospital?
    a. Determine if the client has family support.
    b. Develop a sense of trust.
    c. Ask the client for his perception of the illness.
    d. Provide privacy during the interview.

14. The nurse was interviewing a client with chronic mental illness. During the nurse asked, "Have there been times life wasn't worth living?" What was purpose in asking this question?
    a. To determine the patterns of violence
    b. To determine the presence of hopelessness
    c. To determine the content of his hallucinations
    d. To determine the adequateness of his living arrangements

Chapter 33

Community Psychiatric Mental Health Nursing

1. A nursing student was beginning a clinical rotation with home health nurses. She asked the instructor, "How does home health nursing differ from community health nursing?" The instructor explained that home health nursing:
   a. Focuses on the care of the individual in the home setting
   b. Employs a transindividual perspective in providing care
   c. Is a service available to clients discharged from the community hospitals
   d. Is a "pay for service" type of assistance available to families who can afford it

2. Mrs. Day, age 67, was discharged from the hospital, having been diagnosed as an insulin dependent diabetic. Because of declining dexterity, Mrs. Day had difficulty in administering the insulin correctly. The discharge summary specified that a home health nurse would visit daily to teach and assess the situation until Mrs. Day was able to safely prepare and administer the insulin. Which level of care is described in this situation?
   a. Intermediate
   b. Maintenance
   c. Concentrated
   d. Primary prevention

3. Which of these factors differentiate the role of the home health nurse from the role of the nurse in the hospital setting?
   a. The home atmosphere is more relaxed.
   b. A larger number of family members are present.
   c. There are fewer supplies with which to work.
   d. The nurse is a guest in the client's home.

Jane, the home health nurse, arrived at her client's home at the expected time. A relative from out of town had gotten to the home just before the nurse, and the family has made a fresh pot of coffee. The client stated to Jane, "Come have some coffee with us and you can meet my cousin." Which of these nurse responses is most applicable to the situation?
  a. "Thanks, but I never eat or drink when I'm working."
  b. "Thank you so much. I'd like that."
  c. "I really need to get started. Could you drink the coffee after I leave."
  d. "I'm trying to limit my intake of caffeine. It makes me hyper."

5. Mr. Cone, a home health nurse, was planning to visit a Hispanic family the following day who needed help caring for their elderly grandfather. Mr. Cone had never worked with the Hispanic culture, and did not feel adequately prepared for this assignment. Of these available resources, which one would be most helpful to Mr. Cone at this time?
  a. Viewing a video dealing with health needs in the Hispanic culture
  b. Talking with a fellow nurse who is experienced in working with the Hispanic culture
  c. Reading literature on transcultural nursing
  d. Enrolling in a class on cultural health care practices

6. The home health nurse is visiting a client who has just been referred to the agency for services. During the initial visit, which of these interventions should be done first?
  a. Develop a plan of care and discuss it with the client.
  b. Explain the nurse's role in assisting the client.
  c. Determine the client's need for additional services.
  d. Complete a physical assessment.

7. Which of these precautionary measures should the nurse take if assigned to visit a client in a high-crime neighborhood?
  a. Consulting the client as to the best time to visit
  b. Notifying the nursing supervisor upon arriving at the client's home
  c. Obtaining a permit to carry a concealed weapon
  d. Scheduling the appointments in the daylight hours

8. Mrs. Miller was receiving home health care since being discharged from the hospital and was beginning to ambulate with assistance. The home health nurse was evaluating the client outcome. "Will walk from bedroom to kitchen with assistance twice a day for a week." Mr. Miller responded, "My wife didn't walk but once a day, and that was tough for her." How should the nurse handle this situation?
  a. Reemphasize the fact that Mrs. Miller has no choice if she wants to improve.
  b. Enlist the help of a more objective family member to assist Mrs. Miller.
  c. Praise Mrs. Miller for walking once a day and reset the goal for the following week.
  d. Examine Mrs. Miller's skin for possible breakdown related to inactivity.

9. Wirth, a chronic schizophrenic, recently moved to the area and was admitted to the hospital because of noncompliance in taking the prescribed medications. Which of these individuals in the community will be responsible for overseeing Wirth's treatment plan after he is discharged from the hospital?
  a. The physician
  b. The case manager
  c. The home health aide
  d. A legally appointed guardian

10. When planning community health care for the chronically mentally ill client, which of these factors is most significant?
  a. Care should be provided in the least restrictive environment possible.
  b. Clients with similar disturbances should be housed together.
  c. Instructions in accessing the crisis line must be understood by the clients.
  d. Family members should supervise the client's activity when possible.

11. The community health nurse, during a home visit to her client, observed that a family member was hearing voices and threatening to hurt himself. Identifying that the client was in need of care and was at risk fits which level of prevention?
  a. Primary prevention
  b. Secondary prevention
  c. Tertiary prevention
  d. Intermediate prevention

12. Which of these activities is an example of the nurse intervening at the primary level of prevention?
    a. Notifying a physician of change in the client's condition
    b. Enlisting the services of a social worker to assist with a specific client problem
    c. Screening individuals for hypertension at the local mall
    d. Teaching a client to administer her own insulin

13. Home Health Agencies are eligible for third-party reimbursement for services provided pertinent to the client's need for assistance. Which of these incidents may negatively affect third-party payment?
    a. Care was given by an unlicensed provider.
    b. There was failure to document availability of family support,
    c. Need for care was not described in nursing note.
    d. No signs of improvement were indicated in the record.

Chapter 34

Spirituality

1. Which of the following best describes the role of the chaplain in a mental health setting?
    a. Assists clients in practicing their religion while in a hospital environment
    b. Assures clients that there is a divine power that will help them overcome their illness
    c. Addresses the spiritual needs and goals of clients who request or require their services

2. A client confides in you that she is guilty about the poor relationship she had with her mother-in-law who is now deceased. She tells you that she is sure God will punish her for this and needs to confess her sins to someone. Your best response is:
    a. "I think you need to speak to the chaplain about this. He'll be here later today. I'll let him know you want to meet with him."
    b. "It sounds as if you need to talk about this. Let's sit down in a private area, I'd like to hear more about your relationship with your mother-in-law."
    c. "We all have trouble with our in-laws occasionally. God doesn't punish us for that. You can confess to the chaplain when he comes later today."

3. A client is spending a great deal of time praying, chanting, and reading religious doctrine. He is reluctant to attend therapeutic groups as a result of his religious preoccupation. Your best response is to:
    a. Allow the client a set amount of time each day to express his religion, with the understanding that he attend groups and adhere to the treatment program
    b. Inform the client that he can only express his religion with the chaplain and needs to follow the treatment program the rest of the time
    c. Tell the client he is inappropriate and disruptive to others, then notify the client's physician to increase the client's medication as soon as possible

4. A client tells you that she is possessed by the devil who is telling her to harm herself. Your best response is:
    a. "There is no such thing as a devil, but tell me more about what 'he' is telling you to do."
    b. "You seem troubled about this. I'm concerned about you. We will keep you safe and give you medication that may help you."
    c. "The chaplain will be here soon and can explain about the devil. In the meantime someone will stay with you."

Test Bank Answers with Rationales

Chapter 1

1. **d. This would signify healthy boundaries.**
   a, b, and c. These are all signs of unhealthy boundaries.
   Nursing Process: Evaluation
   Cognitive Level: Analysis

2. **c. This would be a component of a therapeutic relationship.**
   a, b, and d. These are components of a social, rather than a therapeutic, relationship.
   Nursing Process: Planning
   Cognitive Level: Application

3. **b. This indicates resistance on the part of the client, which commonly occurs in therapy.**
   a. Transference occurs when the client 'transfers' unresolved feelings onto the nurse.
   c. Countertransference occurs when the nurse 'transfers' unresolved feelings onto the client.
   d. This indicates more avoidance than characteristics of a social relationship.
   Nursing Process: Assessment
   Cognitive Level: Comprehension

4. **b. The goal is to process information about the client based on facts.**
   a. The goal is to remain free of this.
   c. The goal is to avoid this.
   d. This would indicate a barrier.
   Nursing Process: Outcome identification
   Cognitive Level: Comprehension

5. **d. This is a typical result of the nurse becoming subjectively involved with the client.**
   a. This is doubtful.
   b. This is unlikely.
   c. The client is more likely to feel misunderstood.
   Nursing Process: Outcome identification
   Cognitive Level: Comprehension

6. **c. During the preorientation phase, the nurse examines his or her own feelings, thoughts, perceptions, and attitudes about the client, which may have an impact on the relationship.**
   a. This occurs in the next stage, the orientation phase.
   b. This occurs in the next phase.
   d. This is not an expected outcome.
   Nursing Process: Outcome identification
   Cognitive Level: Comprehension

7. **a. Safety needs are met first.**
   b. Hygiene needs will follow.
   c. Isolative behaviors will also follow safety.
   d. Bizarre behaviors will be modified after the client's safety is assured.
   Nursing Process: Planning
   Cognitive Level: Comprehension

8. **c. Termination involves summarizing accomplishments and ending the relationship.**
   a. This would be appropriate for the working phase.
   b. Confrontation is a working-phase technique.
   d. Termination does not involve identifying new problems.
   Nursing Process: Implementation
   Cognitive Level: Application

9. **d. The individual's responses are considered healthy as measured by standards.**
   a. The nurse's beliefs are not the benchmark.
   b. The behaviors specified in DSM-IV define psychopathology.
   c. Mental health disorders are not easily measured on precise signs.
   Nursing Process: Nursing diagnosis
   Cognitive Level: Comprehension

10. a. **This reflects that the client is not the disorder, but a person with an illness.**
    b. This is labeling the client as an addict.
    c. This labels the client as the disorder.
    d. This also labels the client as the disorder.
    Nursing Process: Evaluation
    Cognitive Level: Analysis

11. b. **Exercising is a healthy way to manage anxiety.**
    a. This would avoid responsibility for managing problems.
    c. This involves assuming the opposite reaction than one feels.
    d. This would not consciously manage anxiety.
    Nursing Process: Implementation
    Cognitive Level: Application

12. b. **The person who uses projection views others as hostile and accuses them of having his or her own unacceptable feelings.**
    a. This would be intellectualization.
    c. This is rationalization.
    d. This would indicate undoing.
    Nursing Process: Assessment
    Cognitive Level: Comprehension

13. a. **Regression is returning to an earlier developmental level.**
    b. This is modification of an instinctual, but socially unacceptable, impulse.
    c. This is conscious inhibition of an impulse.
    d. This is treating something outside the self as if actually inside the self.
    Nursing Process: Evaluation
    Cognitive Level: Analysis

14. c. **Fantasy involves the gratification of frustrated desires by substituting them with daydreams and imagery.**
    a. This involves feeling or acting as if the person is superior to others.
    b. This is separation of feelings from thoughts and ideas originally associated with them.
    d. This is the use of actions to deal with stress.
    Nursing Process: Evaluation
    Cognitive Level: Analysis

15. d. **Healthy individuals employ defenses that help to maintain reality orientation.**
    a, b, and c. These are all examples that indicate problems with the use of defense mechanisms.
    Nursing Process: Assessment
    Cognitive Level: Comprehension

16. a. **Teaching basic skills that will prevent problems is primary prevention.**
    b. This is secondary prevention.
    c. This is secondary prevention.
    d. This is tertiary prevention.
    Nursing Process: Planning
    Cognitive Level: Application

Chapter 2

1. b. **This is a positive statement to increase his confidence.**
   a. This will increase his stress.
   c. This will increase his stress.
   d. This will decrease his self-confidence.
   Nursing Process: Planning
   Cognitive Level: Application

2. d. **This is an example of the nurse facilitating the client's growth.**
   a. This would decrease the client's growth.
   b. This implies the client is not capable.
   c. This would increase the client's dependency.
   Nursing Process: Evaluation
   Cognitive Level: Analysis

3. d. **This is an indicator of client improvement.**
   a. This does not indicate improved self-esteem.
   b. This indicates dependency.
   c. This indicates the need for approval.
   Nursing Process: Evaluation
   Cognitive Level: Analysis

4. c. **This will help John deal with stress of clinical rotation and personal issues.**
   a. This will not help this problem.
   b. This is not appropriate at this point.
   d. This will not help solve this problem.
   Nursing Process: Implementation
   Cognitive Level: Application

5. d. **The nurse-client relationship should be warm and caring.**
   a. This might preclude the development of trust and client sharing.
   b. Nurse-client relationships are not friendships.
   c. This is nontherapeutic.
   Nursing Process: Outcome identification
   Cognitive Level: Comprehension

Chapter 3

1. **b. Systematic desensitization is a behavioral modification, and a positive result with the client who has agoraphobia would be the ability to leave her house and shop.**
   a. Systematic desensitization does not work towards insight.
   c. This would be an unrealistic goal.
   d. This would be a goal of RET.
   Nursing Process: Evaluation
   Cognitive Level: Analysis

2. **a. One of the principles of Beck's theory is that people have automatic thoughts which label and interpret situations and which can lead to depression. A goal is that the client will reduce these automatic thoughts.**
   b. Insight development is associated with psychoanalytic approaches.
   c. This is associated with gestalt therapy.
   d. This is not an outcome of cognitive therapy, although it will hopefully result as the client reduces automatic thoughts.
   Nursing Process: Outcome identification
   Cognitive Level: Application

3. **d. Strategic therapy is solution-oriented and begins with reframing the problem.**
   a. This is a goal of cognitive therapy.
   b. This is goal of behavioral approach.
   c. This is goal of client-centered approach.
   Nursing Process: Outcome identification
   Cognitive Level: Application

4. **b. Prior to initiating fantasy desensitization, the nurse teaches the client specific relaxation techniques, which the client uses during this process.**
   a. This is not part of desensitization.
   c. This is related to RET.
   d. This would be implemented after fantasy desensitization.
   Nursing Process: Planning
   Cognitive Level: Application

5. **c. Chair work is frequently used in gestalt therapy. It allows the client to interact with an imaginary, or nonavailable, provocateur.**
   a. This is part of client-centered approach.
   b. Role playing is used in rational emotive therapy.
   d. Game analysis is a part of transactional analysis.
   Nursing Process: Implementation
   Cognitive Level: Application

6. **d. Structures of the temporal lobe are critically involved with visual recognition, auditory perception, memory, and emotions.**
   a. This is a frontal lobe function.
   b. This is a parietal lobe function.
   c. This is an occipital lobe function.
   Nursing Process: Assessment
   Cognitive Level: Comprehension

7. **b. Staggering gait, clumsiness, and slurred speech observed in an acute alcoholic state are symptoms of a generalized malfunction of the cerebellum.**
   a. Cerebral cortex is not implicated in psychobiology disorders.
   c. Disorders of the basal ganglia include Parkinson's disease and Huntington's chorea.
   d. Disorders associated with the brain stem involve sleep and motor disturbances.
   Nursing Process: Evaluation
   Cognitive Level: Analysis

8. **a. Current psychobiology indicates that two neurotransmitters, serotonin and norepinephrine, are related to depression.**
   b. Cortisol levels increase in depression.
   c. Dopamine is associated with schizophrenic disorders.
   d. Acetylcholine is not associated with depression.
   Nursing Process: Implementation
   Cognitive Level: Application

9. **d. Freud postulated that all behavior has meaning, even if the person is unaware of why he or she does something.**
   a. The libido is the energy produced by the id.
   b. Thoughts may be illogical because of unconscious or preconscious motivations.
   c. Behavior may be influenced by the unconscious, but it is not considered in control.
   Nursing Process: Planning
   Cognitive Level: Application

10. **a. Resistance may be exhibited as avoiding or rejecting what the therapist suggests.**
    b. Transference occurs when the client responds to the therapist as if the therapist was someone important in the client's past.
    c. Countertransference occurs when the therapist relates to the client as if they were someone else.
    d. Catharsis is the unburdening of oneself.
    Nursing Process: Evaluation
    Cognitive Level: Analysis

11. **b. The anal phase occurs between 18 months and 3 years of age, and the focus is on control of the anal sphincter.**
    a. This stage occurs from 0 to 18 months of age and focuses on oral satisfaction.
    c. This stage occurs between 3 and 5 years of age and focuses on the resolution of the oedipal conflict.
    d. Latency occurs between 5 and 12 years of age and the focus is on same sex relationships.
    Nursing Process: Assessment
    Cognitive Level: Comprehension

12. **b. Phobias respond well to behavioral modification.**
    a. Clients with bipolar disorder require medication primarily.
    c. Schizophrenic clients require medication and social skills training.
    d. Suicidally depressed clients require safety maintenance and individual therapy to encourage verbalization of feelings.
    Nursing Process: Planning
    Cognitive Level: Application

13. **a. Underlying a behavior modification approach is the tenet that all behavior is learned; therefore, newer, more effective behaviors can be learned by the client.**
    b. Behavior is a part of the individual, not separate.
    c. This is a tenet of psychoanalytic therapy.
    d. This is a tenet of Freud's theory.
    Nursing Process: Planning
    Cognitive Level: Application

14. **b. Beck's cognitive triad describes the three common characteristics of depressed persons: negative view of self, ongoing events, and future possibilities.**
    a. This is related to psychobiological theory.
    c. Anger turned inwards is not a component of Beck's theory.
    d. These are related to Ellis's RET.
    Nursing Process: Assessment
    Cognitive Level: Comprehension

15. **c. It is important in strategic therapy to identify previous attempted solutions which may be aggravating the problem.**
    a. Reframing is a powerful verbal tool used to create a second-order change.
    b. In order to know how to intervene, the strategic therapist needs to understand the client's position, or view of the problem.
    d. Second-order change is that which changes the system itself.
    Nursing Process: Evaluation
    Cognitive Level: Analysis

16. **a. Berne proposes that communication is effective and functions if it is complementary. Complementary transactions are between role appropriate ego states.**
    b. This will not necessarily result in healthy and functional interactions.
    c. This will decrease dysfunction but not necessarily result in effective interactions.
    d. The goal of TA is to assist the client to choose the most appropriate ego stance in various situations.
    Nursing Process: Assessment
    Cognitive Level: Comprehension

17. **a. One of the basic tenets of Beck's theory is that automatic thoughts label and interpret situations and result in depression. The problem is the client's automatic thoughts about losing his job.**
    b. This is not directly based on Beck's theory.
    c. This is not directly based on Beck's theory.
    d. This is not related to the diagnosis as described above.
    Nursing Process: Nursing diagnosis
    Cognitive Level: Application

18. **b. The behavioral model focuses on changing behaviors. This diagnosis is related to her relapse behavior.**
    a. Poor self-concept is not a behaviorally oriented problem.
    c. Negative thoughts would be focused on in a cognitive approach.
    d. Introjected feelings are a factor in a psychoanalytic approach.
    Nursing Process: Nursing diagnosis
    Cognitive Level: Application

19. **d. Psychoanalysis works towards uncovering unconscious conflicts and empowering the ego to deal with them.**
    a. This is an outcome of a Rogerian approach.
    b. This is an outcome of RET.
    c. This is a goal of strategic therapy.
    Nursing Process: Outcome identification
    Cognitive Level: Application

20. **a. Strategic therapists use symptom prescriptions, which involves prescribing the actual symptom that the client is seeking relief from.**
    b. Dream analysis is a component of psychoanalysis.
    c. Feeling logs are used in RET.
    d. Relaxation training is part of a behavioral approach.
    Nursing Process: Planning
    Cognitive Level: Application

21. **b. Rogerian is a client-centered therapy, and the therapist allows the client to lead the therapy.**
    a. Reframing the symptoms is a technique used by strategic therapists.
    c. Structural analysis is part of TA.
    d. Homework assignments are used in cognitive therapy.
    Nursing Process: Planning
    Cognitive Level: Application

22. **c. A basic tenet of RET is the use of these irrational ideas, which affect how the person thinks, feels, and behaves.**
    a. Automatic thoughts label without acknowledgment of the thought.
    b. This is not a term used in therapies.
    d. This is part of gestalt therapy and relates to the superego and id.
    Nursing Process: Evaluation
    Cognitive Level: Analysis

23. **a. Friend A uses an adult transaction to an adult, while B responds as a child to a parent.**
    b. Friend A directs her communication to an adult.
    c. Friend A is not communicating from her parent.
    d. Friend A is not communicating from her parent.
    Nursing Process: Evaluation
    Cognitive Level: Analysis

24. **c. Psychoanalytic approach focuses on uncovering the unconscious motivations.**
    a. This is threatening the client.
    b. This would be a client-centered approach.
    d. This is personalizing the client's behavior.
    Nursing Process: Implementation
    Cognitive Level: Application

25. **c. The basic tenet of client-centered therapy is that human beings move toward constructive change and integration.**
    a. The basic tenet of gestalt therapy is that intrapsychic conflicts arise from interactions in society.
    b. This focuses on thoughts.
    d. This focuses on reframing problems.
    Nursing Process: Planning
    Cognitive Level: Application

26. **c. PET scans detect decreased use of glucose in different regions of the brain.**
    a. CT scans are photographs of specific areas of the brain.
    b. EEGs map the brain's electrical activity.
    d. MRIs use the body's magnetic field to create images of the brain.
    Nursing Process: Assessment
    Cognitive Level: Comprehension

27. **b. Neurotransmitters are chemical substances that transmit an impulse from one neuron to another.**
    a. Neurons are nerve cells.
    c. Synapses are areas between neurons.
    d. Gyri are convolutions in the cortex of the brain.
    Nursing Process: Assessment
    Cognitive Level: Comprehension

28. **c. These drugs increase or decrease the synthesis, storage, release, metabolism, or receptor activity of neurotransmitters.**
    a. The cerebellum is responsible for contraction and relaxation of muscle groups.
    b. Dendrites relay impulses toward the nerve soma.
    d. The PNS refers to all of the nervous system except the brain and spinal cord.
    Nursing Process: Evaluation
    Cognitive Level: Comprehension

29. **d. The focus in psychoanalysis is on uncovering unconscious conflicts in the mind—not on biological mechanisms in the brain.**
    a. ECT affects the biology of the brain.
    b. Reserpine is a psychotropic drug that affects neurotransmitters.
    c. Thorazine is a psychotropic drug that affects neurotransmitters.
    Nursing Process: Evaluation
    Cognitive Level: Analysis

30. **a. The sympathetic system increases body alertness.**
    b. This system affects circadian cycles, among other functions.
    c. This system counteracts the responses induced by the sympathetic system.
    d. The EPS regulates reflex movement of muscles and controls body movement.
    Nursing Process: Assessment
    Cognitive Level: Comprehension

Chapter 4

1. **b. Awareness of past family disorders may help pinpoint diagnoses and avoid delays in appropriate treatment modalities.**
   a. Family history is not a definitive predictor of disorder occurrence
   b. This distractor is irrelevant for the question
   c. Discussion may help for many reasons, but will not prevent occurrence of disorders
   Nursing Process: Assessment
   Cognitive Level: Comprehension

2. **c. Psychologic model of mental disorders dates back to time of classical Greece.**
   a, b, and d. Choices are all incorrect based on the content in choice c.
   Nursing Process: Assessment
   Cognitive Level: Comprehension

3. **d. The basis for all aspects of nursing care involving clients with brain based illnesses lies in thorough knowledge of human brain structure and function.**
   a. Client behavior originates in the brain.
   b. Nurses frequently call on knowledge regarding brain bases for illnesses.
   c. Knowledge of brain structure and function are necessary during all levels of care.
   Nursing Process: Assessment
   Cognitive Level: Comprehension

4. **c. Limbic system structures are responsible for many functions, such as sleep, drives (sex, hunger), and emotional response regulation.**
   a. The cerebellum regulates functions such as breathing and heart beat.
   b. The cerebrum is responsible for higher level activity such as speech, thinking, voluntary motor function.
   d. The extrapyramidal motor system regulates involuntary motor function such as walking, posture, maintaining balance between body parts.
   Nursing Process: Assessment
   Cognitive Level: Comprehension

Chapter 5

1. **a. This response is less threatening and allows the client to express her views.**
   b. Ms. S. may be too psychotic to know why, and it is an accusatory statement.
   c. This is a threatening response and may agitate Ms. S.
   d. Ms. S. may not know what a delusion is.
   Nursing Process: Assessment
   Cognitive Level: Comprehension

2. **d. This allows staff to debrief and discuss what happened, whether they followed guidelines, and whether another intervention could have been helpful.**
   a. This is accusatory and will place the staff on the defensive.
   b. This is a defensive posture about an event which may not happen and is not focused on client care.
   c. This is accusatory and does not encourage the staff to discuss what occurred.
   Nursing Process: Implementation
   Cognitive Level: Application

3. **b. The nurse asks to be excused from testifying based on state law.**
   a. This is an exemption used to prevent incriminating oneself.
   c. The nurse has not been authorized by the client to reveal information.
   d. It is preferable to invoke the statute.
   Nursing Process: Implementation
   Cognitive Level: Application

4. **b. Under the Tarasoff decision, health care professionals have a duty to warn an intended identifiable victim.**
   a. Instead of consequences, the therapist should help the client identify coping behaviors to use at home.
   c. Day hospital may be recommended, but attendance is not mandatory.
   d. Client's should not alter their medication dosages without consulting their physician.
   Nursing Process: Planning
   Cognitive Level: Application

5. **a. Paul needs to be taught about the common side effects of lithium (including fine hand tremors) and how to manage these side effects.**
   b. Increasing the medications will increase the side effects.
   c. There is no evidence of drug withdrawal.
   d. There is no evidence of manipulation.
   Nursing Process: Evaluation
   Cognitive Level: Analysis

6. **b. Involuntary clients retain the right to appeal their commitment and the right to legal representation to assist in this.**
   a. The nurse cannot allow her to leave the unit, because she is an involuntary client.
   c. Restricting her to her room would be a violation of her rights.
   d. All clients retain the right to appeal their commitment.
   Nursing Process: Planning
   Cognitive Level: Comprehension

7. **c. The best initial approach is to determine the client's reasons for refusing the medication.**
   a. A client cannot be placed in seclusion for refusing medication. There are specific guidelines for the use of seclusion.
   b. All clients, involuntary as well as voluntary, retain the right to refuse treatment.
   d. The client retains the right not to be medicated against his will, unless he is a danger to himself or others.
   Nursing Process: Implementation
   Cognitive Level: Application

8. **b. A basic explanation of the purposes of seclusion to reduce stress and stimulation is indicated. The nurse should explain that seclusion is not a punishment.**
   a. Although clients need an understanding of their treatment plan and how to work towards discharge, this does not seem indicated by the above data.
   c. This is not useful information for these clients.
   d. This is not useful information for clients.
   Nursing Process: Planning
   Cognitive Level: Comprehension

9. **b. Based on the principle of the right to the least restrictive treatment, this is the most appropriate option.**
   a. There is no evidence that Debby is a danger to herself or others.
   c. Both mother and daughter should be treated.
   d. There is no criteria for emergency admission.
   Nursing Process: Implementation
   Cognitive Level: Application

10. **b. Clients must be a danger to self or others in order to be committed.**
    a. This has no bearing on psychiatric commitment.
    c. This would not preclude psychiatric commitment.
    d. Commitment is involuntary and does not require client consent.
    Nursing Process: Evaluation
    Cognitive Level: Analysis

11. **c. Competency to stand trial is determined by Mr. D.'s ability to understand the charges against him and the consequences of those charges, as well as by his capability to advise his attorney.**
    a. This is not determinative of competency to stand trial.
    b. Child abuse has no impact on current competency to stand trial.
    d. The reason for assaulting the victim is not relevant to competency determination.
    Nursing Process: Assessment
    Cognitive Level: Comprehension

12. **a. Confidentiality of the status of clients mandates this.**
    b. This would acknowledge that Steve is a client.
    c. This is a violation of Steve's right to confidentiality.
    d. This is a violation of Steve's right to confidentiality.
    Nursing Process: Implementation
    Cognitive Level: Application

13. **b. Seclusion/restraint are appropriate when a client is potentially dangerous.**
    a. Although important, this is not first priority.
    c. This is important at a later time when Sue is calmer.
    d. This is important after safety of all is assured.
    Nursing Process: Planning
    Cognitive Level: Application

14. **c. The priority problem is Sue's risk for violence to other clients/staff.**
    a. This is not a priority problem.
    b. Although her management of anger is not effective, it is not the priority problem.
    d. This is not the priority problem.
    Nursing Process: Nursing diagnosis
    Cognitive Level: Comprehension

Chapter 6

1. **c. This is a traditional belief regarding health which includes factors important in varying cultures.**
   a. This does not include spiritual factors, integral to many cultures.
   b. This does not look at internal harmony factors.
   d. This is not inclusive of important cultural factors.
   Nursing Process: Planning
   Cognitive Level: Application

2. **a. This person's irrational reason for not joining the group may indicate a belief in such a superstition.**
   b. This does not indicate such a belief.
   c. There is no indication of this belief.
   d. There is no indication of such a belief.
   Nursing Process: Assessment
   Cognitive Level: Comprehension

3. **a. The best intervention is to assess this belief further with the client to determine whether it is based on cultural beliefs; however, do not interrupt the group to do so.**
   b. This will demean the client and interfere with his becoming a group member.
   c. This is not appropriate to discuss with the group.
   d. It is premature to label this a delusion without further assessment.
   Nursing Process: Implementation
   Cognitive Level: Application

4. **c. Some people believe that wearing amulets will prevent the evil eye. It is important for the nurse to understand these beliefs.**
   a. This does not indicate a belief in the evil eye.
   b. Religiosity can be a symptom of psychotic disorders.
   d. Wearing black signifies mourning in some culture.
   Nursing Process: Assessment
   Cognitive Level: Comprehension

5. **c. Many Hispanic-Americans believe that good results from a balance of "hot and cold" and that illness results from an imbalance.**
   a. This is not a belief among Asian-Americans.
   b. This is not a belief among African-Americans.
   d. This is not a belief among Native Americans.
   Nursing Process: Planning
   Cognitive Level: Comprehension

6. **d. Homeopathic medicine focuses on the person rather than the disease.**
   a. Chiropractic medicine focuses on the disability.
   b. Osteopathic medicine focuses on the musculoskeletal system.
   c. Allopathic medicine does not focus on the person.
   Nursing Process: Planning
   Cognitive Level: Comprehension

7. **d. This would indicate inconsistency with one's heritage.**
   a. This would indicate heritage consistency.
   b. This would indicate heritage consistency.
   c. This would indicate heritage consistency.
   Nursing Process: Assessment
   Cognitive Level: Comprehension

8. **c. A xenophobe would demonstrate a wariness of new ideas, and therefore the nurse would have to implement changes slowly.**
   a. This would not be common in a xenophobe.
   b. This would not be seen in a xenophobe.
   d. This would not be seen in a xenophobe.
   Nursing Process: Planning
   Cognitive Level: Application

9. **b. Many clients can speak English but may have problems with the written material.**
   a. The client has requested this information.
   c. The client's request indicates readiness.
   d. Although important, the nurse who plans to use pamphlets as part of the education process needs to determine client's ability to understand this written material.
   Nursing Process: Evaluation
   Cognitive Level: Analysis

10. **a. African-Americans have a present-over-future orientation.**
    b. This is not the predominant time orientation.
    c. European Americans have a future orientation.
    d. This is not indicated.
    Nursing Process: Planning
    Cognitive Level: Application

11. **d. Native Americans tend to have a future-over-present orientation with no boundaries in terms of space.**
    a. This is not indicative of psychopathology.
    b. This is normal behavior.
    c. This is traditional behavior.
    Nursing Process: Evaluation
    Cognitive Level: Analysis

12. **b. Hispanics are embracing and have tactile relationships.**
    a. Hispanics are present oriented.
    c. Hispanics have tactile relationships.
    d. Hispanics value physical presence.
    Nursing Process: Assessment
    Cognitive Level: Comprehension

13. **a. The preferred approach would be for the nurse to obtain specific information about the client's culture so as to be able to accurately assess and interact with the client.**
    b. This may be inappropriate for the client.
    c. This is not focused on the client's needs.
    d. This may confuse the client and nurse.
    Nursing Process: Implementation
    Cognitive Level: Application

14. **d. This will provide the nurse with more information before any precipitous action is taken.**
    a. This is precipitous and a potential violation of rights.
    b. This is harsh and overbearing.
    c. Although this may be the policy, it is best for the nurse to first determine what the client actually took.
    Nursing Process: Implementation
    Cognitive Level: Application

15. **a. Race has been identified as potentially altering assessment of symptoms and level of functioning.**
    b. Age is not a cultural factor.
    c. Gender is not a cultural factor.
    d. Education is not a cultural factor.
    Nursing Process: Assessment
    Cognitive Level: Comprehension

16. **b. Take care not to assume that clients are angry, aggressive, or hostile if they speak more loudly or emotionally than most European Americans.**
    a. Use titles such as Mr. and Mrs. unless you have established a first name basis for the relationship.
    c. Never attempt to use ethnic dialects; this may be interpreted as poking fun or condescension.
    d. Avoid attempting to impress clients by saying you have friends of same background.
    Nursing Process: Implementation
    Cognitive Level: Application

17. **c. This is the most comprehensive understanding and includes the transmission over time.**
    a. Culture is not related solely to physical characteristics.
    b. Culture involves not only shared heritage but also behaviors and thought processes.
    d. Culture is not a group.
    Nursing Process: Planning
    Cognitive Level: Comprehension

Chapter 7

1. **d. This will elicit the client's judgment in response to a particular situation.**
   a. This is challenging and will not provide information regarding judgment.
   b. This is a direct question to obtain specific information.
   c. This is confrontational and not about the client's judgment.
   Nursing Process: Assessment
   Cognitive Level: Comprehension

2. **d. This is a general question that may help the nurse elicit memory problems.**
   a. This would help to determine the client's orientation to place.
   b. This would help to determine the client's orientation to time.
   c. This would help to determine whether the client knows who the nurse is (not necessarily an indication of memory problems).
   Nursing Process: Planning
   Cognitive Level: Application

3. **c. To test comprehension, the client is given an address or sentence that does not contain familiar associations. The client is asked to remember the content verbatim.**
   a. Recent memory would be assessed by asking the client what they ate for breakfast.
   b. Remote memory can be assessed by asking the client something from their past, such as where they went to school.
   d. The ability to abstract is assessed by asking the client to give meaning to a familiar proverb.
   Nursing Process: Assessment
   Cognitive Level: Comprehension

4. **b. Impaired social interaction is related to the sociocultural life process.**
   a. This is related to biologic life process.
   c. This is related to the sexual life process.
   d. This is related to the psychological life process.
   Nursing Process: Nursing diagnosis
   Cognitive Level: Comprehension

5. **b. This indicates an inability to problem solve.**
   a. This client is expressing his dislike of his doctor.
   c. This is not an example of ineffective problem solving.
   d. This is an example of impaired self-esteem.
   Nursing Process: Assessment
   Cognitive Level: Comprehension

6. **c. This outcome helps the client develop problem-solving skills.**
   a. This is an example of choosing rather than problem solving.
   b. This is not related to problem-solving skills.
   d. This may help in the client's therapy but is not related to client's issue.
   Nursing Process: Outcome identification
   Cognitive Level: Application

7. **b. In this example, the client made a decision regarding the best place for him to reside.**
   a. This is not necessarily improved problem solving.
   c. This would demonstrate working on communication patterns.
   d. This would indicate improved self-esteem.
   Nursing Process: Evaluation
   Cognitive Level: Analysis

8. **a. This describes the criteria for the diagnosis of chronic low self-esteem.**
   b. This goes beyond a sense of powerlessness and includes negative self-opinions.
   c. Hopelessness does not involve feelings of guilt and shame.
   d. Although it is likely this person has ineffective individual coping, this data describes chronic low self-esteem.
   Nursing Process: Nursing diagnosis
   Cognitive Level: Comprehension

9. **d. Outcome criteria for a risk diagnosis are developed from the risk factors, in this case social isolation. This is an appropriate client goal.**
   a. This is not measurable or realistic.
   b. The client may be lonely while sitting in group.
   c. This is a nursing action.
   Nursing Process: Outcome identification
   Cognitive Level: Application

10. **b. This goal is most closely related to the nursing diagnosis.**
    a. This would be appropriate for a diagnosis of hopelessness.
    c. This would also be related to hopelessness.
    d. This would be an outcome criterion for anxiety.
    Nursing Process: Evaluation
    Cognitive Level: Analysis

11. **d. This is involved in the planning step of the nursing process.**
    a. This is an assessment step.
    b. This is an evaluation step.
    c. This is an outcome identification step.
    Nursing Process: Planning
    Cognitive Level: Comprehension

12. **c. Clients need to know symptoms of toxicity and what to do if they occur.**
    a. Clients should not stop this drug on their own.
    b. Clients should not increase their dosage on their own.
    d. Lithium is administered orally.
    Nursing Process: Implementation
    Cognitive Level: Application

13. **b. Descriptive nursing interventions explicitly describe a course of therapeutic activity.**
    a. This is vague.
    c. This is vague.
    d. This is vague.
    Nursing Process: Implementation
    Cognitive Level: Application

14. **c. This is a nursing focused activity, rather than one following the prescribed medical regimen.**
    a, b, and d. These are all examples of activities that follow the medically prescribed regimen.
    Nursing Process: Implementation
    Cognitive Level: Application

15. **a. Attainment of expected client outcomes is the criterion used for evaluation.**
    b. Nursing actions are not evaluated.
    c. The diagnostic statement is not evaluated.
    d. The client's feelings are important but are not the standard for the evaluation step of the nursing process.
    Nursing Process: Evaluation
    Cognitive Level: Analysis

16. **b. It is imperative for the nurse to remain calm when interacting with an anxious client.**
    a. Keep explanations brief and concrete.
    c. Use more direct, closed-ended questions in early hospital phase.
    d. Keep environment calm and decrease stimulation.
    Nursing Process: Planning
    Cognitive Level: Comprehension

17. **b. The nursing diagnosis includes the problem statement and etiology.**
    a. Goal statements are part of outcome identification.
    c. Nursing actions are part of the planning phase.
    d. Assessment tools are part of the assessment stage.
    Nursing Process: Nursing diagnosis
    Cognitive Level: Comprehension

Chapter 8

1. **b. This offers a positive response to a client who is trying out new behavioral decisions.**
   a. This is challenging and threatening.
   c. This is the technique of exploring.
   d. This is the technique of reflecting.
   Nursing Process: Planning
   Cognitive Level: Application

2. **a. Nurses must meet aggression assertively by setting firm limits.**
   b. This will not help modify these behaviors.
   c. Although medication may be helpful to some clients, behavioral strategies are needed to modify behaviors.
   d. This is inappropriate.
   Nursing Process: Implementation
   Cognitive Level: Application

3. **d. This is one of the characteristics of "problem clients."**
   a. "Problem clients" usually claim to be more ill than they are.
   b. They produce feelings of incompetence in staff.
   c. They take up most of nurse's attention and time.
   Nursing Process: Assessment
   Cognitive Level: Comprehension

4. **c. Giving information, as well as restating, reflecting, interpretation, silence and support are responding techniques.**
   a, b, and d. These are nontherapeutic techniques.
   Nursing Process: Planning
   Cognitive Level: Application

5. **b. This is an example of congruency between verbal and nonverbal communication.**
   a. Incongruent would be a contradictory message between verbal and nonverbal.
   c. This message is not contradictory.
   d. The message in the example is very clear.
   Nursing Process: Evaluation
   Cognitive Level: Analysis

6. **d. Paralinguistic behavior includes any audible sound that is not a spoken word.**
   a, b, and c are all examples of body cues.
   Nursing Process: Planning
   Cognitive Level: Comprehension

7. **b. The most therapeutic response is to clearly communicate appropriate boundaries.**
   a. Paul may intrude on other's boundaries with disastrous results.
   c. Touch may be misinterpreted by a psychotic client.
   d. The message in this response is unclear.
   Nursing Process: Implementation
   Cognitive Level: Application

8. **c. Therapeutic communication is intended to assist the client to grow and change.**
   a. This is a purpose of social communication.
   b. This is a purpose of social communication.
   d. These are characteristics of social communication.
   Nursing Process: Evaluation
   Cognitive Level: Analysis

9. **c. This will help the nurse recognize problems as well as positive responses.**
   a. The goal is not to maintain distance from the client's problems, but rather to remain objective about them.
   b. This is not an expected outcome of such a review.
   d. The purpose of such a review is to recognize the nurse's responses, not to maintain a boundary.
   Nursing Process: Outcome identification
   Cognitive Level: Application

10. **c. This response focuses on the client's feelings and encourages further discussion.**
    a. This sounds judgmental and will cut off communication.
    b. Although self-disclosure can be therapeutic, this focuses on the nurse's feelings.
    d. This is nontherapeutic.
    Nursing Process: Implementation
    Cognitive Level: Application

11. **b. The first step in learning to be more assertive is to target behaviors to be changed.**
    a. This would be passive behavior.
    c. This would be acquiescent behavior.
    d. This would be aggressive behavior.
    Nursing Process: Planning
    Cognitive Level: Application

12. **b. The aggressive person stands up for his or her own rights often at the expense of the rights of others.**
    a. This is an assertive person.
    c. This is a passive person.
    d. This is a passive person.
    Nursing Process: Assessment
    Cognitive Level: Comprehension

13. **b. This broad opening will encourage discussion as well as allow the client to decide what to include about his or her family.**
    a. This may result in a one-word answer.
    c. This may result in a yes-or-no answer.
    d. This may not encourage further discussion; the client may respond "yes" or "no".
    Nursing Process: Implementation
    Cognitive Level: Application

14. **a. This encourages the client to consider alternatives without giving advice.**
    b. This is giving advice.
    c. This is also telling the client what to do.
    d. This is another example of giving advice.
    Nursing Process: Planning
    Cognitive Level: Application

15. **b. By validating the client's reality, hopefully the client will continue to ventilate.**
    a. The nurse does not self-disclose to inform the client of how to behave.
    c. The goal is to foster the client's independence.
    d. Therapeutic relationships are to meet the client's needs only.
    Nursing Process: Outcome identification
    Cognitive Level: Comprehension

16. **c. It is important for the student nurse to recognize different uses of touch. An example of procedural touch would be positioning the client's arm for BP measurement.**
    a, b, and d. These are all examples of nonprocedural touch. This does not imply that these are inappropriate.
    Nursing Process: Planning
    Cognitive Level: Comprehension

17. **d. The psychological benefit of humor is the decrease of fears, anxiety, negative emotions, stress and tension.**
    a. It lessens, but will not eliminate, negative emotions.
    b. It will increase alertness.
    c. The goal is to laugh with others, not at someone.
    Nursing Process: Outcome identification
    Cognitive Level: Comprehension

18. **a. The nurse must truly listen and then use the techniques of clarifying and reflecting to begin the problem-solving process.**
    b. The client will not feel understood and valued if such limits are imposed.
    c. This will not assist the client to change and grow.
    d. This is counter-productive.
    Nursing Process: Implementation
    Cognitive Level: Application

19. **d. This communicates to the client that the nurse understands how difficult his problems are for him.**
    a. This is false reassurance.
    b. This indicates that the nurse was not paying attention to what the client said.
    c. This will cut off communication and belittle the client's problems.
    Nursing Process: Evaluation
    Cognitive Level: Analysis

20. **d. This encourages the client to discuss and explore her options so that she can make her own decision.**
    a. This is judgmental and challenging. It will probably cut off communication.
    b. This is also judgmental and reflects the nurse's bias.
    c. This is based on nurse's own value system.
    Nursing Process: Implementation
    Cognitive Level: Application

21. **d. This helps the client to identify feelings and hopefully to continue verbalizing.**
    a. This is challenging and confrontational.
    b. If the nurse tries to dispute the delusion, the client will defend it further. Therefore, the client remains focused on delusional content.
    c. This is changing the topic. It is more therapeutic to assist the client to identify and discuss feelings.
    Nursing Process: Planning
    Cognitive Level: Application

22. **a. The nurse is demonstrating warmth and acknowledging the client's feelings.**
    b. This is an example of the technique of making observations.
    c. This is an example of seeking clarification.
    d. This is an example of reflection.
    Nursing Process: Implementation
    Cognitive Level: Application

Chapter 9

1. **c. The oral character has as its major defenses projection, denial, and introjection.**
   a. The phallic character has as its major defense repression.
   b. The anal character has as its major defenses intellectualization, reaction formation, and isolation.
   d. The genital character has as its major defense sublimation.
   Nursing Process: Evaluation
   Cognitive Level: Analysis

2. **b. This strategy will allow the child to demonstrate interest in helping mom wash dishes without worrying about breakage.**
   a. This is useful in the autonomy versus doubt stage.
   c. This might be detrimental by increasing stress to succeed.
   d. This is not related to the task of initiative.
   Nursing Process: Implementation
   Cognitive Level: Application

3. **a. Coles believed that unique experiences fostering moral and ethical development depend heavily on the models to which the child is exposed.**
   b. This is not related to moral development theory.
   c. This is a part of Kohlberg's theory.
   d. This is a part of Kohlberg's theory.
   Nursing Process: Planning
   Cognitive Level: Application

4. **b. Kohlberg believed that moral development was influenced by the forms of justice the child was exposed to.**
   a. This may impede the introjection of values and mores.
   c. There is no connection with this and moral development per se.
   d. This may impede the child's ability to develop his or her own moral schema.
   Nursing Process: Implementation
   Cognitive Level: Application

Test Bank Answers with Rationales

5. **b. Freud postulated that the genital stage combines the learning of the pregenital stages and develops the ability to love and work.**
   a. This is related to Erikson's adolescent stage.
   c. This is an outcome of Freud's latency stage.
   d. This is an outcome of Erikson's school-age child.
   Nursing Process: Outcome identification
   Cognitive Level: Application

6. **c. A sense of hope is the outcome of Erikson's stage of trust versus mistrust (infant). Inconsistent, unpredictable, and discontinuous care would lead to hopelessness and to a mistrust in self and world.**
   a. There is no evidence for this in above statement.
   b. There is insufficient evidence of this.
   d. There is no evidence of this in above statement.
   Nursing Process: Nursing diagnosis
   Cognitive Level: Application

7. **d. According to Erikson, failure to master academic and social pursuits leads to inferiority and hinders attempts to try new things.**
   a. This is associated with failure to develop will power.
   b. This is associated with failure to develop purpose.
   c. This is associated with failure to develop fidelity.
   Nursing Process: Assessment
   Cognitive Level: Comprehension

8. **a. According to Sullivan, the expected development of the preadolescent leads to the ability to work with peers towards a common goal and to develop a sense of oneness.**
   b. This is related to the juvenile stage (6 to 10 years).
   c. This is seen in late adolescence.
   d. This is related to the childhood stage (2 to 6 years).
   Nursing Process: Outcome identification
   Cognitive Level: Application

9. **b. By targeting self-regulation of emotions, parents may foster more effective self-regulatory strategies that would help their child to develop positive relationships with peers.**
   a. This may be interpreted by the child as a lack of caring.
   c. This does not encourage the child's own development; instead it fosters compliance.
   d. This will not necessarily lead to more effective self-regulatory strategies.
   Nursing Process: Planning
   Cognitive Level: Application

10. **a. The preoperational stage (2 to 7 years) involves here-and-now thinking with intuitive guesses about cause and effect.**
    b. The ability to conserve is observed in the concrete operations stage (7 to 11 years).
    c. The ability to reverse operations is seen in the concrete operations stage (7 to 11 years)
    d. The ability to think in hypothetical terms is seen in formal operations stage (11 to 16 years).
    Nursing Process: Assessment
    Cognitive Level: Comprehension

11. **c. The formal operations level includes the ability for future thinking and for problem solving of complex issues.**
    a. The preoperational level is primarily here-and-now thinking.
    b. The concrete operations level allows the child to think about past and present events but not future ones.
    d. Postconventional is one of Kohlberg's stages of moral development.
    Nursing Process: Evaluation
    Cognitive Level: Analysis

12. **b. The preconventional stage (4 to 10 years) involves a punishment-obedience orientation.**
    a. A good boy/girl orientation is seen in the conventional stage (10 to 13 years).
    c. A law-and-order orientation is also seen in the conventional stage (10 to 13 years).
    d. A hierarchy of principles is seen in the postconventional stage (adolescence).
    Nursing Process: Assessment
    Cognitive Level: Comprehension

13. **c. According to Sullivan, if the child experiences punitive responses to the toilet training accidents, the child may develop a sense of the "not me" self-system.**
    a. This may decrease the child's stress.
    b. Mild parental frustration is seen as helpful in assisting the child to become toilet trained.
    d. As in response "a", this may decrease the child's stress level.
    Nursing Process: Implementation
    Cognitive Level: Application

14. **b. In the concrete operations level, the child can decenter (focus and coordinate) and imagine a series of events.**
    a. In the preoperations stage, the child is unable to relate two classifications at one time, and time is oriented in the present only.
    c. In formal operations, the child can think abstractly and in a future orientation.
    d. Postoperational is not a stage of cognitive development.
    Nursing Process: Evaluation
    Cognitive Level: Analysis

15. **b. A six-year-old can learn to comply with requests when the adults reinforce the compliance with positive reinforcements.**
    a. Varied outcomes is not a step to use in operant conditioning.
    c. Self-efficacy is not a strategy to use in operant conditioning.
    d. A conditioned response is the outcome of the operant conditioning, not a strategy.
    Nursing Process: Planning
    Cognitive Level: Application

16. **a. At the conventional level, there is a good boy/girl orientation.**
    b. At the preconventional level, there is a punishment-obedience orientation.
    c. At the social contract level, moral judgments are motivated by a sense of community respect and disrespect.
    d. At the postconventional level, the person focuses on abstract principles underlying right and wrong.
    Nursing Process: Evaluation
    Cognitive Level: Analysis

17. **b. During the stage of autonomous morality, the child is able to consider intentions and consequences when making moral judgments.**
    a. In the moral realism stage, behavior is seen as all good or bad.
    c. Universal ethical principles is part of Kohlberg's theory.
    d. Social contract is part of Kohlberg's theory.
    Nursing Process: Evaluation
    Cognitive Level: Analysis

18. **a. Information-processing theorists look at a child's specific performance at a given time, what steps are used in development, and under what conditions skills emerge.**
    b. Piaget saw development in terms of competence.
    c. Moral reasoning is assessed for moral development.
    d. This is not used by the information-processing theorists.
    Nursing Process: Assessment
    Cognitive Level: Comprehension

19. **a. The primary concern is Sharon's safety, and signing a "no suicide" pact is important.**
    b. This is not related to the diagnosis.
    c. This is not directly related to the diagnosis.
    d. Although this may be part of the plan, it is not the priority.
    Nursing Process: Outcome identification
    Cognitive Level: Comprehension

20. **c. This specifically addresses the child's development.**
    a. This will elicit prenatal history.
    b. This will identify the presenting problem.
    d. This will identify past attempts to deal with the presenting problem.
    Nursing Process: Assessment
    Cognitive Level: Comprehension

Chapter 10

1. **a. Jung wrote that adults in their twenties and thirties continue to work on separation and personality individuation from their primary families.**
    b. Jung viewed adult development as continuous throughout the life cycle.
    c. Freud considered it important to reevaluate one's life in five-year increments.
    d. Jung viewed adult development as continuous throughout the lifespan.
    Nursing Process: Planning
    Cognitive Level: Application

2. **a. According to Erikson, an individual who regresses to stagnation, boredom, and interpersonal impoverishment is not meeting the tasks in the stage of generativity.**
   b. If the person has problems with the stage of ego integrity, he or she become stagnated in despair.
   c. A person not meeting the tasks of intimacy faces isolation and self-absorption.
   d. The stage of identity is associated with adolescents.
   Nursing Process: Evaluation
   Cognitive Level: Analysis

3. **c. Failure to achieve generativity, the seventh stage, can result in regression to an obsessive need for pseudointimacy.**
   a. This would indicate problems with the first stage.
   b. This is associated with problems of the fourth stage.
   d. This is related to a problem with the sixth stage.
   Nursing Process: Assessment
   Cognitive Level: Comprehension

4. **b. Indications of adapting to the need for integrity include the ability to be satisfied with the accomplishments of one's life as well as the disappointments.**
   a. Intimacy requires the near fusion of one's identity with that of another.
   c. This involves the concern for establishing and guiding the next generation.
   d. This involves the search for one's own beliefs, values, etc.
   Nursing Process: Evaluation
   Cognitive Level: Analysis

5. **b. Defensive personality traits, which originally protected the person from feeling insecure, can be converted into assets as an adult.**
   a. Personality traits are considered to be enduring, ingrained qualities.
   c. Insight is not needed to help the person adapt this trait.
   d. Exploring the client's childhood experiences will not necessarily lead to adaptation.
   Nursing Process: Implementation
   Cognitive Level: Application

6. **a. Social scientists believe that with each life-transitional crisis, unique social rituals help an individual achieve his or her potential.**
   b. Rituals allow individuals to tolerate separateness.
   c. Rituals are effective for all adults.
   d. Rituals make change manageable.
   Nursing Process: Implementation
   Cognitive Level: Application

7. **a. During their thirties, women tend to struggle between the choices of starting a family or focusing on a career first.**
   b. Women who postpone a career fear that this life choice may be sacrificed.
   c. Men are able to work toward both goals with less stress than women.
   d. Men do not experience the same biological clock imperatives as women.
   Nursing Process: Evaluation
   Cognitive Level: Analysis

8. **b. This client is clearly indicating how her inability to conceive has altered her self-esteem.**
   a. Alteration in body image applies to physiologic changes, whereas this client is expressing her loss of self-esteem.
   c. Fear applies to a perception that one is in danger.
   d. Based on the information given, there is not enough evidence of ineffective coping.
   Nursing Process: Nursing diagnosis
   Cognitive Level: Comprehension

9. **c. Women are most affected by losses involving close relationships.**
   a, b, and d. Men tend to become depressed with the loss of an ideal, an achievement-related goal, or a performance issue.
   Nursing Process: Assessment
   Cognitive Level: Comprehension

10. **c. Essential needs according to Maslow begin with basic physiologic processes.**
    a. Safety needs are a second priority on this hierarchy.
    b. The need to be loved is the third level.
    d. Self-esteem needs are the fourth level.
    Nursing Process: Planning
    Cognitive Level: Application

11. a. Self-esteem needs include a desire for adequacy, self-respect, and competence.
    b. This would relate to the third level.
    c. This is associated with the second level.
    d. This relates to the fifth level.
    Nursing Process: Assessment
    Cognitive Level: Comprehension

12. b. The acquisition of wisdom is considered to be the outcome of the ego integrity stage.
    a. Fidelity is related to the identity stage.
    c. Care is associated with generativity.
    d. Love is the result of intimacy.
    Nursing Process: Outcome identification
    Cognitive Level: Application

13. a. A review of the accomplishments, as well as disappointments, in one's life is considered necessary to develop ego integrity.
    b. This is related to the development of intimacy.
    c. This is related to generativity.
    d. This is also connected with generativity.
    Nursing Process: Implementation
    Cognitive Level: Application

14. b. Alterations in strength and endurance typically occur in mid-life.
    a. Reaction time would be decreased.
    c. Muscle tone would be decreased.
    d. Hearing and vision both begin to diminish.
    Nursing Process: Assessment
    Cognitive Level: Comprehension

15. d. Crisis intervention focuses on the client's previous successes and coping mechanisms to help the person manage the crisis.
    a. Group therapy is not treatment of choice for a client in a crisis.
    b. This is used for phobias.
    c. This would increase her dependency.
    Nursing Process: Planning
    Cognitive Level: Application

16. d. Before moving on to the next stage of life, the client needs to accept losses.
    a. Crisis intervention does not focus on insight development.
    b. This would be a behavior-modification approach.
    c. This is not a part of crisis intervention.
    Nursing Process: Implementation
    Cognitive Level: Application

Chapter 11

1. b. Research supports the view that aging involves a combination of internal and external factors.
   a. Environmental factors also affect aging.
   c. Immune function does decline with aging, but it still is able to function at a lower level.
   d. Internal events also impact aging.
   Nursing Process: Planning
   Cognitive Level: Application

2. a. As one ages, the person attempts to maintain continuity of habits, beliefs, norms, and other personality factors.
   b. Activity theory postulates that a high level of activity maintains life satisfaction.
   c. Adaptation theory is more a model to categorize aging changes.
   d. Disengagement theory focuses on withdrawal of the individual and society.
   Nursing Process: Evaluation
   Cognitive Level: Analysis

3. d. It is the additive, or multiple, nature of losses for the elderly that is debilitating.
   a. Elderly clients are able to rely on past coping mechanisms.
   b. On the contrary, many losses are gradual, so the elderly can cope with them.
   c. The meaningfulness of the loss varies for the individual and plays a more significant part than the age of the person in coping.
   Nursing Process: Planning
   Cognitive Level: Application

4. c. Presbycusis is a diminished ability in hearing acuity related to perception of tones.
   a. Presbyopia is the loss of ability of the eye to accommodate to changing distances.
   b. Changes in the sense of touch in the elderly are highly individualized.
   d. The sense of proprioception refers to the individual's sense of balance.
   Nursing Process: Assessment
   Cognitive Level: Comprehension

5. **a. Contrary to belief, many elderly people do enjoy various forms and degrees of intimacy, and caregivers should encourage such feelings.**
   b. This is a myth.
   c. Sperm production seems to be sustained well into old age.
   d. The production of androgens decrease with aging.
   Nursing Process: Implementation
   Cognitive Level: Application

6. **d. Loss of bone mass may lead to osteoporosis and is common in elderly females. It can lead to fractures of the hip and spine.**
   a. This is not a priority; it will decrease with age.
   b. It is expected to decrease with age and is not a priority.
   c. Flexibility decreases with age and is not a priority assessment.
   Nursing Process: Assessment
   Cognitive Level: Comprehension

7. **c. Atrial arrhythmias are common in the elderly because of changes in the structure of the heart muscle fibers.**
   a. Blood pressure normally increases with aging.
   b. Heart rate decreases in normal aging.
   d. Cardiac output decreases with aging.
   Nursing Process: Assessment
   Cognitive Level: Comprehension

8. **c. According to this approach, old age should be a period of individuality and continued self-development through such means as recreational and creative activities.**
   a. This is related to life structure theory.
   b. This is related to Erikson's theory.
   d. This is related to Erikson's theory.
   Nursing Process: Implementation
   Cognitive Level: Application

9. **b. According to Erikson, each stage involves maintaining a balance between the syntonic and dystonic.**
   a. This is related to Jung's theory.
   c. Levinson advocated the need for a mentor.
   d. This would be a medical model.
   Nursing Process: Planning
   Cognitive Level: Comprehension

10. **b. Lowenthal's theory of life structure focuses on the ability of individuals to cope with life transitions.**
    a. This is the goal of Erikson's last stage.
    c. This is related to Maslow's hierarchy.
    d. This is related to Jung's theory.
    Nursing Process: Outcome identification
    Cognitive Level: Application

11. **d. Individual personality traits and past experiences affect how a person reacts to aging, and they need to be considered.**
    a. This is not a factor in social theories.
    b. Family history does not have an impact on social theories.
    c. This is not an important factor.
    Nursing Process: Planning
    Cognitive Level: Application

12. **c. Retirement implies a major role transition for many individuals.**
    a. This is not an expected change in the elderly.
    b. Immobility is not an expected change in the elderly.
    d. This would be a role for the health professional.
    Nursing Process: Assessment
    Cognitive Level: Comprehension

13. **d. Promoting physical appearance will assist in meeting the need for self-esteem (fourth level).**
    a. This is related to need for belonging.
    b. This is related to need for safety and security.
    c. This is related to need for self-actualization.
    Nursing Process: Implementation
    Cognitive Level: Application

14. **b. Individuals with an external locus of control believe they have no control over their destiny and their behaviors have no effect on outcomes.**
    a. This is not associated with external locus of control.
    c. There is no indication of this based on information given.
    d. There is no indication for this based on information given.
    Nursing Process: Nursing diagnosis
    Cognitive Level: Application

15. **d. Feelings of worth, self-confidence, and adequacy are outcomes for a self-esteem disturbance.**
    a. This would be an outcome related to an impairment in safety/security needs.
    b. This outcome is related to self-actualization needs.
    c. This outcome is related to love and belonging needs.
    Nursing Process: Outcome identification
    Cognitive Level: Application

16. **b. This intervention will best assist the client to develop feelings of self-confidence, worth, and adequacy.**
    a. This would assist a client with social isolation.
    c. This is not related to the diagnosis.
    d. This would be helpful for a confused, forgetful client.
    Nursing Process: Implementation
    Cognitive Level: Application

Chapter 12

1. **c. When the level of anxiety has increased to the severe stage, the person manifests the fight-or-flight response with decreased sensory perception and excessively stimulated autonomic nervous system.**
    a. At this level, vital signs are normal, and there is minimal muscle tension.
    b. Vital signs may be slightly elevated with some tension experienced.
    d. The person at the panic level is completely disorganized.
    Nursing Process: Evaluation
    Cognitive Level: Analysis

2. **a. Narrowing of the perceptual field occurs at the severe level of anxiety, and therefore, this diagnosis would be appropriate.**
    b. Closed perception occurs at the panic level of anxiety.
    c. Total loss of control occurs at the panic level.
    d. Combative behavior is indicative of the panic level
    Nursing Process: Nursing diagnosis
    Cognitive Level: Comprehension

3. **a. This is an example of the behavioral model, which attributes the etiology of anxiety disorders to an earlier traumatic experience.**
    b. Steve's symptoms are not related to a physiological cause.
    c. There is no evidence of a deficiency in this scenario.
    d. This is not supported by the above.
    Nursing Process: Evaluation
    Cognitive Level: Analysis

4. **a. Parathesias are indicative of agoraphobia with panic attacks.**
    b. Diarrhea, rather than constipation, is seen.
    c. The client is not feigning or pretending to be afraid.
    d. Hypertension would be expected.
    Nursing Process: Assessment
    Cognitive Level: Comprehension

5. **c. The symptoms of OCD worsen as stress increases.**
    a. These symptoms are involuntary.
    b. This would provide secondary gains and is nontherapeutic.
    d. OCD responds well to medications and therapy.
    Nursing Process: Planning
    Cognitive Level: Application

6. **d. There is involvement of multiple organ systems such as GI, reproductive, and neurological.**
    a. The complaints begin before age 30.
    b. The complaints cannot be explained by general medical disorders.
    c. There is no structural abnormality.
    Nursing Process: Assessment
    Cognitive Level: Comprehension

7. **a. These symptoms meet the DSM-IV criteria for somatization disorder.**
    b. This is not indicative of pain syndrome, in that there is no association with a medical condition.
    c. Generalized anxiety disorder does not include multiple organ complaints.
    d. There is no mention of obsessions or ritualized behaviors.
    Nursing Process: Evaluation
    Cognitive Level: Analysis

8. **d. Psychological factors are identified as being related to the onset or exacerbation of the symptom.**
   a. This is also true of somatization disorder.
   b. The symptom is not limited to pain or sexual function.
   c. The symptom is not intentionally feigned.
   Nursing Process: Evaluation
   Cognitive Level: Analysis

9. **c. This will lead to the client developing strategies to manage anxiety.**
   a. This is not realistic.
   b. Suppressing his symptoms will not lead to anxiety management.
   d. The client may need medication to assist in learning to manage anxiety, but it is usually short-term.
   Nursing Process: Outcome identification
   Cognitive Level: Application

10. **a. Difficulty in concentrating is indicative of anxiety.**
    b. This describes depressive symptoms.
    c. This is a misnomer and would not necessarily provide accurate data.
    d. This describes aggressive/anger disorder symptoms.
    Nursing Process: Planning
    Cognitive Level: Comprehension

11. **d. This is a realistic goal that would then allow Sue to interact with others.**
    a. This is inappropriate.
    b. This focuses on her symptoms.
    c. This is a very short-term measure that does not focus on the problem.
    Nursing Process: Outcome identification
    Cognitive Level: Application

12. **b. Participation in a support group is recommended for clients with PTSD.**
    a. There is no evidence that Jill has poor coping skills.
    c. There is no evidence of anger towards her boyfriend.
    d. This implies that Jill somehow is responsible for the rape.
    Nursing Process: Outcome identification
    Cognitive Level: Application

13. **a. This would indicate growth in learning the precipitants of her anxiety.**
    b. This is not realistic.
    c. Although beneficial, this is not related to above goal.
    d. This will reduce the client's egocentricity but is not related to above goal.
    Nursing Process: Evaluation
    Cognitive Level: Analysis

14. **c. Caffeine, nicotine, and other stimulants increase anxiety symptoms.**
    a. This is nontherapeutic.
    b. This is not a strategy to improve anxiety management.
    d. This is nontherapeutic.
    Nursing Process: Planning
    Cognitive Level: Application

15. **c. The priority is to determine whether the symptoms are related to anxiety or a medical problem.**
    a. This may be a strategy after further assessment is done.
    b. This may be done after determination of the problem.
    d. This may also be done after determining the problem.
    Nursing Process: Implementation
    Cognitive Level: Application

16. **a. The initial step is to define the phobic stimulus.**
    b, c, and d are all follow-up steps.
    Nursing Process: Planning
    Cognitive Level: Application

17. **a. This will help Mike to identify his feelings, and then he can manage them more effectively.**
    b. This is nontherapeutic.
    c. The symptoms reflect unresolved feelings, not only fear.
    d. This will not help the disorder.
    Nursing Process: Outcome identification
    Cognitive Level: Comprehension

18. **d. Cognitive behavioral therapy works toward identifying the target symptoms and then changing the cognitions associated with these.**
    a. This would be a psychodynamic approach.
    b. Anxiety disorders are not considered delusional.
    c. This would not be a helpful approach.
    Nursing Process: Evaluation
    Cognitive Level: Analysis

19. **b. Visual imagery is an anxiety-reduction technique.**
    a. This would increase anxiety.
    c. The client should focus on a single object rather than the whole room.
    d. The client with increased anxiety may not be able to interact in a group, and this will not reduce the anxiety.
    Nursing Process: Implementation
    Cognitive Level: Application

20. **d. This is an appropriate goal in helping Dwayne manage this problem.**
    a. Dwayne needs to inform others of dissatisfaction in a nonthreatening manner.
    b. Dwayne should refer to himself with the first person pronoun: "I think . . . ."
    c. Dwayne should use assertive behavior to meet his needs.
    Nursing Process: Outcome identification
    Cognitive Level: Application

Chapter 13

1. **c. It is imperative to assess whether the client has suicidal ideation, plan, and means in order to plan for safety maintenance.**
   a. This is an important area to assess since most depressed clients have weight loss, but it is not the priority.
   b. This is an important area to assess but not the priority.
   d. This is a component of the assessment but not the priority.
   Nursing Process: Assessment
   Cognitive Level: Comprehension

2. **b. The client with mania has an exaggerated view of his abilities.**
   a. This would be typical of a client with depression.
   c. This sounds like a realistic adult statement.
   d. This also sounds like a realistic adult statement.
   Nursing Process: Assessment
   Cognitive Level: Comprehension

3. **d. Clients with depression frequently have a dependent personality and are prone to depression when they feel overwhelmed.**
   a. Egocentric personality types would be focused on themselves at expense of others.
   b. This is seen more in clients with schizoid and paranoid disorders.
   c. Narcissistic personality is seen in persons with histrionic and narcissistic disorders.
   Nursing Process: Assessment
   Cognitive Level: Comprehension

4. **c. Dysthymia is a chronic low-level depression frequently lasting for several years.**
   a. Dysthymia has a slow, insidious onset.
   b. Delusional thinking is not a common manifestation in dysthymia.
   d. Suicidal thoughts are common in clients with dysthymia.
   Nursing Process: Evaluation
   Cognitive Level: Analysis

5. **a. The highest priority at this point is her risk for injury related to dehydration and agitated behavior.**
   b. This would be an area to work on in the long term since mania is viewed as depression turned inwards.
   c. Sally has been noncompliant with her medications, but this will not be the priority at this time.
   d. Sally has a sleep pattern disturbance, but the first priority will be risk for injury.
   Nursing Process: Nursing diagnosis
   Cognitive Level: Comprehension

6. **b. Behavioral characteristics of atypical depression include leaden paralysis, hypersomnia, and weight gain.**
   a. Seasonal affective disorder is characterized by symptoms between Oct/Nov until March/April.
   c. Psychomotor agitation can be observed in melancholic depression.
   d. Increased depression in the morning is seen in melancholic depression.
   Nursing Process: Assessment
   Cognitive Level: Comprehension

7. **a. The priority is stabilization of the client, and therefore, vital signs are monitored for several hours post ECT.**
   b. Oral fluids are contraindicated until the gag reflex returns.
   c. The client typically is sleepy and confused and would be unable to participate in group this soon post ECT.
   d. ECT effectiveness is measured after several treatments.
   Nursing Process: Implementation
   Cognitive Level: Application

8. **a. Clients with mania frequently ignore their basic needs.**
   b. Setting limits, although important, is not the priority.
   c. Her manic state precludes a thorough assessment at this time.
   d. Suicide is not a priority at this time.
   Nursing Process: Planning
   Cognitive Level: Application

9. **b. It is important for the client taking lithium to maintain a normal sodium intake.**
   a. The client should ingest at least 2-3 liters per day.
   c. Taking lithium with food minimizes gastrointestinal effects.
   d. Regular monitoring of serum lithium levels is important to prevent toxicity.
   Nursing Process: Evaluation
   Cognitive Level: Analysis

10. **b. Most clients with bipolar disorder require medication treatment for their lifetime.**
    a. Clients should never stop their medication without consulting their physician.
    c. Once a therapeutic serum level is achieved, the client will continue on maintenance lithium medication.
    d. Diuretics are contraindicated for the client on lithium.
    Nursing Process: Evaluation
    Cognitive Level: Analysis

11. **a. Diuretics alter fluid and electrolyte balance, increasing risk of lithium toxicity.**
    a. Antipsychotic medications are frequently prescribed with lithium to manage the acute manic client.
    c. Antianxiety drugs are not contraindicated with the use of lithium.
    d. Antibiotics do not alter fluid and electrolyte balance.
    Nursing Process: Evaluation
    Cognitive Level: Analysis

12. **c. This client is exhibiting signs of possible depression, and the nurse should explore this.**
    a. The nurse should do a basic assessment before referral.
    b. These are not typical signs of aging; they indicate depression.
    d. The nurse should perform a basic mental status exam before referral.
    Nursing Process: Implementation
    Cognitive Level: Application

13. **d. Ability to manage basic ADL demonstrates improvement in major depression.**
    a. Understanding of the disorder often occurs once the client has improved and is able to cognitively process the information.
    b. Initiation of community social activity occurs when the client has increased energy.
    c. Assertive communication is learned and practiced after the client's depression is decreased.
    Nursing Process: Outcome identification
    Cognitive Level: Comprehension

14. **b. The client needs to understand the food and medication interactions, which can cause hypertensive crisis with Nardil.**
    a. Mood does not have an impact on the side effects of Nardil.
    c. The support network does not influence medication therapy.
    d. Activity level is not directly associated with side effects of Nardil.
    Nursing Process: Planning
    Cognitive Level: Application

15. **d. Cognition may be impaired in major depression; thus the client is encouraged to participate in the care planning as capable.**
    a. Clients should have input in their plan of care as much as possible.
    b. There is no evidence that mania is a concern.
    c. ECT is a collaborative intervention to be determined with the physician.
    Nursing Process: Planning
    Cognitive Level: Comprehension

16. **c. M.B. is physically impaired and exhibits symptoms of depression.**
    a. There is no evidence of altered thought processes.
    b. There is no evidence of knowledge deficit.
    d. There is no data to support a diagnosis of altered self-esteem.
    Nursing Process: Nursing diagnosis
    Cognitive Level: Comprehension

17. **c. This direct approach invites the client to participate in a firm but gentle manner.**
    a. This is false reassurance.
    b. Social interaction needs to be promoted with withdrawn depressed clients.
    d. Avoid focusing intensely on negative thoughts and feelings.
    Nursing Process: Implementation
    Cognitive Level: Application

18. **b. Clients with depression are at increased risk for suicide when they have been on antidepressant medications for 2 weeks until the full therapeutic effect is achieved in 4-6 weeks.**
    a. Self-esteem is important, but not the priority at this time.
    c. There is no evidence of noncompliance.
    d. There is no indication of anxiety in data presented.
    Nursing Process: Nursing diagnosis
    Cognitive Level: Comprehension

19. **b. Antidepressant medication works on the balance of neurotransmitters, particularly serotonin and norepinephrine.**
    a. These medications do not cure this disorder, rather assist in managing it.
    c. This is an appropriate dose for elavil.
    d. Medications can help regardless of his effect.
    Nursing Process: Outcome identification
    Cognitive Level: Comprehension

20. **d. A behavioral intervention establishes a reward for accomplishing a specific behavior.**
    a. This represents a psychoanalytic approach.
    b. Administering medication is a biological approach.
    c. This represents an interpersonal intervention.
    Nursing Process: Implementation
    Cognitive Level: Application

21. **b. The more specific the plan, the greater the risk the person will attempt suicide.**
    a. Many clients who attempted suicide try again until successful.
    c. Many suicidal persons verbally give clues about their feelings.
    d. Many factors have an impact on whether an attempt is successful, and if not, it does not indicate intent.
    Nursing Process: Planning
    Cognitive Level: Comprehension

22. **a. Verbalization helps to relieve pent-up feelings and allows them to be validated.**
    b. This is nontherapeutic for a client who is suicidal.
    c. This might increase guilt feelings and, therefore, suicidal thoughts.
    d. It is therapeutic to encourage the client to verbalize feelings, not to avoid them.
    Nursing Process: Implementation
    Cognitive Level: Application

23. **b. The most important principle is to decrease stimulation; this will assist in decreasing manic symptoms.**
    a. Manic clients respond poorly to criticism from others.
    c. Increasing stimulation is contraindicated.
    d. Manic clients have a very short attention span.
    Nursing Process: Planning
    Cognitive Level: Application

24. **c. Because of her mania, Pat cannot respond to verbal commands, and she needs to be escorted to a less stimulating area.**
    a. This does not address Pat's mania.
    b. Pat cannot respond to verbal commands.
    d. Some intervention is needed for her mania at this point.
    Nursing Process: Implementation
    Cognitive Level: Application

Chapter 14

1. **a. Echopraxia and other psychomotor symptoms are typically seen in catatonic schizophrenia.**
    b. Paranoia is seen in paranoid schizophrenia.
    c. Regression is found more frequently in disorganized schizophrenia.
    d. Clanging is manifested in disorganized schizophrenia.
    Nursing Process: Assessment
    Cognitive Level: Comprehension

2. **c. Improvement would be noted when the client can validate with the nurse, or others, what is real.**
    a. Telling the nurse what the voices say does not indicate improvement.
    b. This is not an indicator of improvement.
    d. This may be dangerous if the voices give commands to harm self or others.
    Nursing Process: Evaluation
    Cognitive Level: Analysis

3. **d. This is a manageable and appropriate goal for the ambivalent client.**
   a. This would be unrealistic.
   b. Negativity is one way ambivalence is displayed, and so this may not even indicate improvement.
   c. This is not an expected behavior of clients.
   Nursing Process: Outcome identification
   Cognitive Level: Comprehension

4. **a. The highest priority is the maintenance of basic physiological needs while the client is in a catatonic stupor.**
   b. Although important, this is not the highest priority.
   c. Although his verbal communication is impaired, it is not the priority.
   d. This would not be the initial priority.
   Nursing Process: Nursing diagnosis
   Cognitive Level: Comprehension

5. **c. These symptoms are suggestive of an alteration in thought processes: delusions, loosened associations.**
   a. There is no evidence presented that this client may act violently.
   b. Although her symptoms may help her defend against stress, this diagnosis is not appropriate.
   d. Her verbal communication is intact; it is her thoughts that are disordered.
   Nursing Process: Nursing diagnosis
   Cognitive Level: Comprehension

6. **c. This is an appropriate outcome for this diagnosis.**
   a. A delusion is a fixed false belief, and so it is not expected that the client will allow anyone to dispute it.
   b. There is no indication of boundary disturbance.
   d. It is nontherapeutic to focus on the delusional content.
   Nursing Process: Outcome identification
   Cognitive Level: Comprehension

7. **d. Therapeutic approaches with a delusional client include presenting reality and not focusing on delusional content.**
   a. Confronting the delusion will lead to Susan's need to defend this.
   b. This would be focusing on the delusion.
   c. This would also be focusing on the delusion.
   Nursing Process: Implementation
   Cognitive Level: Application

8. **c. Sally's recognition of her self and staff for who they are is an indicator that she is functioning in reality.**
   a. Although this is an important client behavior, it is not related to identified symptom.
   b. This would indicate a lack of improvement.
   d. This would not necessarily indicate improvement.
   Nursing Process: Evaluation
   Cognitive Level: Analysis

9. **a. Poor impulse control is exhibited by these behaviors.**
   b. There is no indication of anger in the above data.
   c. Derealization involves a loss of ego boundaries.
   d. Inappropriate affect would be manifested by the client laughing at a sad event or crying at a happy time.
   Nursing Process: Evaluation
   Cognitive Level: Analysis

10. **c. Although these are all useful interventions for a client with schizophrenia, engaging the client in activities designed to promote success is specifically geared toward improvement of self-esteem.**
    a. This will work towards improving communication.
    b. This will improve communication.
    d. This will help the client learn effective ways to manage stress.
    Nursing Process: Implementation
    Cognitive Level: Application

11. **c. Antipsychotic medications work by blocking dopamine receptors at the dendrite ends, keeping dopamine out of the extrapyramidal system.**
    a. The opposite is true, as explained above.
    b. The symptoms are not related to the dosage of the medications.
    d. These effects are not commonly seen with the use of antidepressant medications.
    Nursing Process: Evaluation
    Cognitive Level: Analysis

12. **b. The clue to making a diagnosis of disordered thinking is Donna's statement on nonreality-based thoughts.**
    a. There is no indication of altered mood states.
    c. Withdrawal is symptomatic of many conditions and may not be pathological.
    d. Decreased impulse control is anticipated in such a client.
    Nursing Process: Nursing diagnosis
    Cognitive Level: Comprehension

13. **b. This will help to clarify and focus the client in reality.**
    a. This might cut off the interaction.
    c. This may confuse a client whose thinking is autistic.
    d. The acceptance of the neologism plays into the client's delusional system, and 'why' questions are considered threatening.
    Nursing Process: Implementation
    Cognitive Level: Application

14. **c. Goals planned with the client need specific criteria to facilitate their evaluation and possible readjustment.**
    a. Signs and symptoms belong in the assessment section.
    b. Each care plan is based on a specific nursing diagnosis.
    d. Evaluation is performed after implementing the plan.
    Nursing Process: Planning
    Cognitive Level: Comprehension

15. **d. Emotional blunting, as well as social withdrawal, eccentric behavior, and illogical thinking are the common symptoms of residual schizophrenia.**
    a. Delusions are found in acute exacerbations, not residual form of schizophrenia.
    b. Disorganized speech pattern is seen in acute exacerbations of schizophrenia.
    c. Catatonic posturing is observed in catatonic schizophrenia.
    Nursing Process: Assessment
    Cognitive Level: Comprehension

16. **c. An appropriate outcome which would indicate readiness for Sam to be discharged is his ability to recognize when he becomes anxious and connect this with hearing the voices.**
    a. This would be focusing on the hallucinations.
    b. This would increase his inappropriate appearance to others.
    d. This is inappropriate.
    Nursing Process: Outcome identification
    Cognitive Level: Application

17. **a. Ask questions that are open-ended and nonthreatening. Use 'how,' 'what,' and 'when'.**
    b. This response threatens the client.
    c. 'Why' questions are demanding and threatening to clients.
    d. This avoids the problem and does not encourage verbalization.
    Nursing Process: Implementation
    Cognitive Level: Application

18. **b. Since Laura is mute and catatonic, she may not be able to communicate needs or problems. It is imperative to assess if she is in pain or is thristy, cold, etc.**
    a. Although an appropriate intervention, it is not the priority.
    c. This is an important intervention, but it will take time, especially with a mute, catatonic client.
    d. This is an appropriate intervention, but not the priority.
    Nursing Process: Implementation
    Cognitive Level: Application

19. **c. Always allow the client his body space, keep hands at side, and assume an open posture.**
    a. Keep voice calm and modulated.
    b. Allow the client his space; do not stand closer than eight feet.
    d. Give clear instructions and be brief.
    Nursing Process: Planning
    Cognitive Level: Comprehension

Chapter 15

1. **d. The client with antisocial personality disorder is impulsive, manipulative, and dishonest. Clients with this disorder are frequently involved in illegal behaviors.**
    a. This is appropriate for a client with borderline personality disorder.
    b. This is appropriate for borderline personality disorder.
    c. This would apply to schizoid and paranoid personality disorders.
    Nursing Process: Nursing diagnosis
    Cognitive Level: Comprehension

2. **a. Clients with narcissistic personality disorder are grandiose, with a constant need for admiration from others.**
    b. Clients with narcissistic personality disorder are nonempathetic towards others.
    c. The client with schizoid personality disorder lacks trust in others.
    d. The client with borderline personality disorder has a labile affect.
    Nursing Process: Assessment
    Cognitive Level: Comprehension

3. **c. Sarah's symptoms indicate an avoidant personality disorder: fears rejection, avoids relationships, censors expression of thoughts and feelings because of fear of negative reactions.**
   a. This client would present with unstable interpersonal relationships, labile affect, and complaints of emptiness.
   b. This type is overly dramatic, manipulative, and attention-seeking.
   d. This type is indifferent to, and lacks a concern for, any interpersonal contacts.
   Nursing Process: Assessment
   Cognitive Level: Comprehension

4. **b. This person depends on others to make decisions and assume responsibility for major areas of his or her life.**
   a. This is indicative of the avoidant personality.
   c. This is indicative of the avoidant personality.
   d. This is indicative of the narcissistic personality.
   Nursing Process: Planning
   Cognitive Level: Application

5. **d. Clients with antisocial personality disorder are described as charming because of their ability to 'size up' and manipulate others.**
   a. Narcissistic clients demand constant attention.
   b. Clients with antisocial personality disorder do not tolerate delay of gratification or frustration.
   c. Clients with antisocial personality disorder have a poorly developed super ego.
   Nursing Process: Planning
   Cognitive Level: Application

6. **c. The goal is for Josh to comply with expected behaviors.**
   a. The goal is to learn more appropriate ways of behaving.
   b. Behavior modification does not focus on development of insight.
   d. Clients with antisocial personality disorder do not lack interaction skills.
   Nursing Process: Outcome identification
   Cognitive Level: Application

7. **b. Clients with borderline personality disorder frequently engage in self-mutilation in an attempt to manage their chaotic feelings.**
   a. There is no data to support this.
   c. The risk is higher for self-directed violence.
   d. There is insufficient data to support this.
   Nursing Process: Nursing diagnosis
   Cognitive Level: Comprehension

8. **c. Incorrect interpretation of external events and a belief that all events refer to the self are typical of clients with schizotypal personality disorder.**
   a. This is indicative of schizoid personality disorder.
   b. This is indicative of borderline personality disorder.
   d. This is seen in paranoid personality disorder.
   Nursing Process: Assessment
   Cognitive Level: Comprehension

9. **a. The priority is the prevention of self-harm via a contract with the client.**
   b. This would be done with this client over time.
   c. This is an intervention to work on, but not the priority.
   d. This is not related to the above data.
   Nursing Process: Implementation
   Cognitive Level: Application

10. **a. Hopefully the client will develop the ability to express her feelings appropriately.**
    b. This is not a hoped-for outcome.
    c. This does not indicate management of these feelings.
    d. Suppressing of feelings is not therapeutic.
    Nursing Process: Evaluation
    Cognitive Level: Analysis

11. **c. This person is nonremorseful, defensive when confronted, and liable to justify illegal acts.**
    a. This person will have difficulties with interactions.
    b. This person is typically bizarre in presentation with few interpersonal interactions.
    d. This person has intense, angry relationships, is impulsive, and may self-mutilate.
    Nursing Process: Assessment
    Cognitive Level: Comprehension

12. **b. This is directly related to her symptoms and underlying pathology.**
    a. There is no data to support this diagnosis.
    c. The data presented does not support this diagnosis.
    d. There is no evidence of a thought disorder.
    Nursing Process: Nursing diagnosis
    Cognitive Level: Comprehension

13. **c. Suicidal gestures and attempts to injure or mutilate self are indicative of borderline personality disorder.**
    a. Clients with narcissistic personality disorder are attention-seeking and demanding but not at risk of injury to selves.
    b. Clients with histrionic personality disorder are overly dramatic but not self-injuring.
    d. Clients with antisocial personality disorder act violently against others, not selves.
    Nursing Process: Evaluation
    Cognitive Level: Analysis

14. **a. This helps the client to understand his own behavior and its effect on others and to work on changes.**
    b. This will increase the client's isolation and problems interacting with others.
    c. Avoiding problems is nontherapeutic; instead, help the person learn more effective strategies.
    d. Alleviating problem behaviors is important, but first the person must recognize these and their purpose before changing the pattern.
    Nursing Process: Implementation
    Cognitive Level: Application

15. **c. This would be an important topic for the group to explore and it may help to defuse Jim's anger in a constructive manner.**
    a. Seclusion is not indicated by this data. Jim did not lose control.
    b. Restraints are inappropriate; Jim did not lose control.
    d. This will not help in learning how to manage these feelings more appropriately.
    Nursing Process: Implementation
    Cognitive Level: Application

16. **a. OT can help Janet recognize and explore healthy ways to reduce stress.**
    b. PT can help reduce her back pain, but her primary problem is suicide gestures and self-mutilation.
    c. Acupuncture can help reduce pain, but this is not the primary problem.
    d. Janet's sexual addiction is one of the unhealthy ways she manages stress, so stress reduction would be a preferred intervention.
    Nursing Process: Planning
    Cognitive Level: Application

17. **c. Identifying his feelings of sadness and loss will help him understand the meaning of the relationship and resolve his depression.**
    a. Ralph is able to express needs prior to the depression.
    b. Before moving on to another relationship, Ralph must understand the feelings generated in this one.
    d. Although important, Ralph must first identify feelings of loss.
    Nursing Process: Evaluation
    Cognitive Level: Analysis

Chapter 16

1. **b. The number of drug-free days is the most reliable indicator of success for a substance abuser.**
   a. Although important, it does not indicate success.
   c. This is not a measure of success for a substance abuser.
   d. This does not indicate success of a rehabilitation program.
   Nursing Process: Evaluation
   Cognitive Level: Analysis

2. **c. This will help the client to recognize the degree to which their drinking is a problem.**
   a. This may help with knowledge deficit, but not with denial.
   b. The nurse should not consider the situation hopeless.
   d. This will not necessarily help the client recognize that he or she has a drinking problem.
   Nursing Process: Implementation
   Cognitive Level: Application

3. **c. Based on data presented, this is the most appropriate nursing diagnosis. This client's method of 'coping' has been with alcohol.**
   a. Although denial is a common symptom of substance abusers, this client stated he is dependent on alcohol.
   b. His separation from his wife may cause loneliness, but it is not priority diagnosis.
   d. There is no evidence to support this diagnosis.
   Nursing Process: Nursing diagnosis
   Cognitive Level: Comprehension

4. **b. In order for Mr. Jones to remain sober, he will need to admit that he is an alcoholic.**
   a. There is no evidence that he is noncompliant while in the hospital.
   c. Mr. Jones has had problems remaining abstinent in the past, and he minimizes his dependence on alcohol. He must first acknowledge the problem.
   d. It is hoped that once Mr. Jones acknowledges his alcoholism, he can begin to work on better coping skills.
   Nursing Process: Outcome identification
   Cognitive Level: Application

5. **d. Close monitoring of his vital signs will determine if he is physiologically stable.**
   a. Applying ice to his tongue will not ensure his physical stability.
   b. Oral fluids may be contraindicated while he is in DT's.
   c. It is preferable to keep the room well lit to decrease his illusions.
   Nursing Process: Planning
   Cognitive Level: Application

6. **a. Sharon is enmeshed with her husband's disease, and both need treatment.**
   b. This is not an example of healthy concern.
   c. Sharon may consider herself a martyr, but the CNS would consider her enmeshed.
   d. This is not an example of introversion, or going within oneself.
   Nursing Process: Evaluation
   Cognitive Level: Analysis

7. **b. Psychological theories related to substance abuse describe this client as having a depressive personality organization.**
   a. This would be considered a healthy personality.
   c. This person would be more likely to have a disorder involving violence or abuse.
   d. The codependent is the person who remains in a relationship with the substance abuser and who 'rescues' them again and again.
   Nursing Process: Assessment
   Cognitive Level: Comprehension

8. **a. Sweating, especially at night, may possibly signal adolescent drug use.**
   b. There may be a change in nutritional intake, but not increased thirst necessarily.
   c. There may be drowsiness following ingestion, whether it is day, evening, or night.
   d. Headaches are not a sign of adolescent drug use.
   Nursing Process: Planning
   Cognitive Level: Comprehension

9. **b. These are signs of alcohol withdrawal, called delirium tremens.**
   a. Werniecke's encephalopathy is a neurological disease characterized by ataxia, opthalmoplegia, confusion, and nystagmus.
   c. Alcoholic hallucinosis involves disorientation, confusion and hallucinations.
   d. Korsakoff's syndrome is an amnesiac syndrome caused by a deficiency of the B vitamins.
   Nursing Process: Evaluation
   Cognitive Level: Analysis

10. **b. Ataxia is associated with this organic brain syndrome.**
    a. Confabulation is associated with Korsakoff's syndrome.
    c. Peripheral neuropathy is associated with Korsakoff's syndrome.
    d. Hallucinations are associated with alcoholic hallucinosis.
    Nursing Process: Assessment
    Cognitive Level: Comprehension

11. **d. A quiet nonstimulating environment is recommended for the client in DTs.**
    a. A client in DTs is not able to participate in group discussions.
    b. Until the client is stable, the nurse cannot work on denial.
    c. Oral fluids may be contraindicated for the client in DTs.
    Nursing Process: Planning
    Cognitive Level: Comprehension

12. **a. During the detox stage, the priority is on stable vital signs and prevention of complications.**
    b, c, and d. These are all outcomes which would follow the detox stage.
    Nursing Process: Outcome identification
    Cognitive Level: Comprehension

13. a. **Pete needs to recognize that he will always be a recovering addict, and he can't put it all behind him.**
    b. Although this may be part of his recovery work, it is not the expected outcome.
    c. This will not be of benefit in terms of remaining abstinent.
    d. This is judgmental and may not be appropriate.
    Nursing Process: Outcome identification
    Cognitive Level: Comprehension

14. a. **Following stopping of cocaine ingestion, clients frequently experience a suicidal depression.**
    b. This would not be the priority diagnosis at this point.
    c. This would occur when the client is 'high' on cocaine, not during withdrawal.
    d. The client is hypoactive in cocaine withdrawal.
    Nursing Process: Nursing diagnosis
    Cognitive Level: Comprehension

15. a. **Heroin is an opiate, and the most immediate problem is respiratory depression.**
    b. This will be dealt with after stable respirations are established.
    c. This is not a priority for this client.
    d. This is not a problem at this point.
    Nursing Process: Nursing diagnosis
    Cognitive Level: Comprehension

16. d. **This is most significant of chronic alcoholism**
    a. This signifies increased blood volume.
    b. SGPT is a liver enzyme test which may be altered with chronic alcoholism as well as other causes of liver disease.
    c. LDH signifies muscle damage and is not specific to alcoholism.
    Nursing Process: Assessment
    Cognitive Level: Comprehension

17. a. **Medication should be administered based on the individual's needs and presence of withdrawal symptoms.**
    b. Medication is usually tapered over a two-week period.
    c. Medication is usually tapered over a two-week period.
    d. It would be inappropriate to awaken the client for detox medication.
    Nursing Process: Planning
    Cognitive Level: Application

18. c. **Tolerance means a person needs to take increasing amounts of the substance to achieve the desired high.**
    a. This is not a substance abuse problem.
    b. This may indicate dependence.
    d. If a person is dependent on a substance, they would experience withdrawal symptoms when they stop ingesting the substance.
    Nursing Process: Evaluation
    Cognitive Level: Analysis

19. c. **This is least likely to upset the client and more likely to obtain desired information.**
    a. This will probably upset the client and hinder information flow.
    b. It is important to obtain all relevant history from client and family.
    d. The client may never bring up his or her drug use, and this may put client at risk if there is a chance of withdrawal.
    Nursing Process: Assessment
    Cognitive Level: Comprehension

20. b. **This data will provide best estimate of likelihood of withdrawal.**
    a. This would indicate state of intoxication, not withdrawal.
    c. Although useful data, this is not the most significant in terms of likelihood of withdrawal.
    d. This would not be useful.
    Nursing Process: Assessment
    Cognitive Level: Comprehension

21. a. **Methadone is a synthetic opiate developed as a substitute for other illegal opiates.**
    b. Amphetamines are central nervous system stimulants, not depressants such as opiates.
    c. Methadone is not a replacement for barbiturates.
    d. There is no substitute for hallucinogenic currently.
    Nursing Process: Evaluation
    Cognitive Level: Application

22. d. **This is an accurate description of addiction, whereas abuse refers to misuse of a substance.**
    a. These terms are incorrectly used interchangeably at times.
    b. This is an inaccurate definition.
    c. This is inaccurate.
    Nursing Process: Planning
    Cognitive Level: Application

23. a. There is an increased risk in families with a history of alcohol abuse.
    b. This is not true.
    c. The opposite is true.
    d. Heredity seems to have more influence in development of this disease.
    Nursing Process: Implementation
    Cognitive Level: Application

24. b. These symptoms are found in delirium tremens.
    a. This does not refer to any substance withdrawal.
    c. Tachycardia and elevated blood pressure are seen in DT's.
    d. These symptoms signify opiate withdrawal.
    Nursing Process: Assessment
    Cognitive Level: Comprehension

Chapter 17

1. c. The best strategy is to present reality in a gentle manner.
    a. This is an example of confabulation, but it is important to reorient the client.
    b. This is not a delusion, and it is never therapeutic to confront delusions.
    d. This will not help to maintain orientation.
    Nursing Process: Planning
    Cognitive Level: Application

2. b. This will best achieve the objective of accurate testing.
    a. His input in the assessment is important, and insisting he leave may increase his wife's anxiety.
    c. The use of this exam is an integral component of the overall assessment, which will also include observations.
    d. Testing in familiar, comfortable surroundings will yield more reliable results.
    Nursing Process: Assessment
    Cognitive Level: Comprehension

3. c. There is a report of inability to manage ADLs, inability to learn new computer system, and reliance on sister to communicate for her.
    a. There is insufficient evidence of low self-esteem.
    b. There is no evidence of anxiety.
    d. There is no evidence to support body image disturbance.
    Nursing Process: Nursing diagnosis
    Cognitive Level: Comprehension

4. b. This is an accurate description of Alzheimer's disease.
    a. Alzheimer's is not a secondary dementia.
    c. Alzheimer's is not a secondary dementia.
    d. This describes multi-infarct dementia.
    Nursing Process: Evaluation
    Cognitive Level: Analysis

5. b. This outcome addresses the individual's functional level.
    a. Long-term placement may be an option but not necessarily the first choice.
    c. This does not allow for any consideration of the progression of the client's illness and current functional level.
    d. Many client's with Alzheimer's disease have a loss of physical functioning, which this does not address.
    Nursing Process: Outcome identification
    Cognitive Level: Comprehension

6. d. This addresses his needs for nutrition and safety, and his dementia.
    a. It is unlikely he will regain speech.
    b. English classes are not indicated, nor is it necessary to transfer to a different facility.
    c. Assistance with meal prep may be needed, not necessarily taking away his ability to manage some food prep.
    Nursing Process: Outcome identification
    Cognitive Level: Comprehension

7. b. This will restore her safety and self-esteem.
    a. Isolating will decrease her self-esteem and may increase her confusion.
    c. Discontinuing the program is detrimental to the other clients.
    d. Behavioral interactions should be attempted prior to medication administration.
    Nursing Process: Planning
    Cognitive Level: Application

8. b. All of these would indicate success in a therapeutic activity program.
    a. Accurate recent memory is not an expected outcome.
    c. Improved abstract reasoning is not expected.
    d. Ability to remember multiple steps is not realistic.
    Nursing Process: Evaluation
    Cognitive Level: Analysis

9. **c. These actions will encourage a positive emotional environment and preserve the client's self-esteem.**
   a. Directions must be given and understood one at a time to help a client with impaired memory.
   b. Activities should be "no fail"; a loud voice is contraindicated.
   d. Added time is usually needed by the client with Alzheimer's disease.
   Nursing Process: Implementation
   Cognitive Level: Application

10. **a. Fluctuating levels of consciousness are indicative of an acute onset delirium.**
    b. This is seen in dementia.
    c. This is seen in depression.
    d. This is seen in depression.
    Nursing Process: Assessment
    Cognitive Level: Comprehension

11. **b. Alcoholism is one potential toxic cause of secondary dementia.**
    a. Vitamin B12 deficiency is an electrolyte disturbance producing dementia.
    c. Hepatic disease is an electrolyte disturbance producing dementia.
    d. Tuberculosis is an infective cause of dementia.
    Nursing Process: Assessment
    Cognitive Level: Comprehension

12. **c. Increased forgetfulness, particularly of former usual activities is symptomatic.**
    a. This is healthy behavior.
    b. This indicates her wish to remain independent and is healthy.
    d. Although this may be unsafe, depending on how slow she drives, it is not an indication of Alzheimer's disease.
    Nursing Process: Assessment
    Cognitive Level: Comprehension

13. **a. Susan is delusional with paranoia, which is common in clients with Alzheimer's disease.**
    b. There is no evidence of powerlessness.
    c. Susan is unable to cope because of Alzheimer's, but the data presented does not support this diagnosis.
    d. There is no evidence of defensive coping.
    Nursing Process: Nursing diagnosis
    Cognitive Level: Comprehension

14. **b. Delirium is a reversible condition in which the cause, if identified, can be eliminated.**
    a. Managing symptoms is appropriate for chronic dementias.
    c. This is an outcome for dementia.
    d. Regression is not a symptom of delirium.
    Nursing Process: Outcome identification
    Cognitive Level: Comprehension

15. **a. In this first stage the symptoms can include recent memory loss.**
    b. This is indicative of the middle stage II.
    c. This is indicative of the terminal stage III.
    d. This is indicative of the middle stage II.
    Nursing Process: Evaluation
    Cognitive Level: Analysis

16. **b. Bathing three times a week is a realistic goal for this client.**
    a. Bathing daily may be overzealous for someone who has not bathed for a month.
    c. This is inappropriate for a client in the home and is a nursing action rather than an outcome.
    d. Although hopefully Gail will remain free of skin diseases, this goal is not related to the nursing diagnosis.
    Nursing Process: Outcome identification
    Cognitive Level: Comprehension

17. **c. The prime intervention should reduce all stimulation so that the client can calm down.**
    a. Employ positive, not neutral, interactions.
    b. Touch may be misinterpreted.
    d. Be careful of invading the client's boundaries.
    Nursing Process: Implementation
    Cognitive Level: Application

18. **d. This would indicate some success.**
    a. Hopefully, the client will become more involved.
    b. This would not indicate success of the program.
    c. Hopefully, incidents of sundowning would decrease.
    Nursing Process: Evaluation
    Cognitive Level: Analysis

19. **a. Use of a daily activity schedule helps to remind the client of activities and what they should be doing.**
    b. Large motor activities aid in retention of perceptual skills.
    c and d. Simple word games and discussion groups promote stimulation of language.
    Nursing Process: Planning
    Cognitive Level: Application

Chapter 18

1. **a. Many childhood illnesses continue into adulthood.**
   b. Often a child masks his illness by the manner in which he behaves, which makes diagnosing difficult.
   c. Medications have proved to be effective in treating specific mental disorders.
   d. Outcomes of treatment depends on multiple variables and age of the client is not considered a factor.
   Nursing Process: Assessment
   Cognitive Level: Comprehension

2. **c. A person with moderate retardation has developed some social and communication skills but seldom advances beyond the second grade level.**
   a. Joe is severely retarded.
   b. Steve is mildly retarded.
   d. Beth is mildly retarded.
   Nursing Process: Assessment
   Cognitive Level: Comprehension

3. **a. Repetitive and stereotypical use of language is considered in the diagnostic criteria for this disorder.**
   b. The developmental skill for creative, imaginative play is lacking.
   c. There is usually an indifference or aversion for affection and peer interaction present.
   d. The need to maintain sameness is demonstrated in their behavior.
   Nursing Process: Assessment
   Cognitive Level: Analysis

4. **d. Being unable to concentrate for a period of time is a hallmark for ADHD.**
   a. This is characteristic of separation anxiety and not related to this disorder.
   b. This is an example of oppositional behavior and more data is needed prior to making a diagnostic statement.
   c. Fascination with spinning, moving objects is characteristic of pervasive developmental disorder.
   Nursing Process: Assessment
   Cognitive Level: Application

5. **a. While Brad is unable to control himself, external controls should be used to assist him.**
   b. The team already is in the position of authority.
   c. Limit setting will not provide Brad extra attention.
   d. Brad will continue to be responsible for his own behavior.
   Nursing Process: Implementation
   Cognitive Level: Application

6. **c. Reactive theory supports this belief.**
   a. Structural theory supports predetermined ability for developing behavior.
   b. This is not characteristic of family therapy.
   d. This is not applicable to this statement.
   Nursing Process: Assessment
   Cognitive Level: Comprehension

7. **b. Unhealed fractures indicate that medical intervention was not sought at the time of injury.**
   a. A bloody nose and black eyes indicate a more recent injury.
   c. Clinging to a parent in a strange environment is normal behavior.
   d. Fear of the unknown and of pain could contribute to the struggling behavior.
   Nursing Process: Assessment
   Cognitive Level: Application

8. **b. Providing him information as to expectations and the consequences of breaking the rules provides much needed structure and guidance.**
   a. Isolating him will not facilitate learning appropriate behavior and can decrease self-esteem.
   c. There was no data indicating that he was in danger of hurting himself or others that would require this intervention.
   d. No specific behavior was described that would warrant medication.
   Nursing Process: Implementation
   Cognitive Level: Application

9. **d. Roy may still be a danger to himself and requires a safe environment.**
   a. Food should be provided but is not the priority need at this time.
   b. Providing comfort by pain relief and efforts to reduce his psychological pain is important but not the highest priority.
   c. A sense of belonging and knowing that he is cared about will support his recovery but are not the highest priorities at this time.
   Nursing Process: Implementation
   Cognitive Level: Comprehension

10. **b. There are no clinically significant delays in language or cognitive development with Asperger's.**
    a, c, and d. Both autistic and Asperger's disorders display these behaviors.
    Nursing Process: Assessment
    Cognitive Level: Comprehension

11. a. **Blaming others is characteristic of oppositional-defiant disorder.**
    b. Being mildly retarded is not associated with this disorder.
    c. Judy is not displaying symptoms of this disorder but may need further evaluation to determine what may be contributing to her problem.
    d. Having to be reminded and then following through with the work is not characteristic of this disorder.
    Nursing Process: Assessment
    Cognitive Level: Comprehension

12. **b. Beginning to separate from one's parents is an expected task of adolescence.**
    a. Developing a trusting relationship with peers has been an ongoing activity and not related to the period of adolescence.
    c. Participating in sports is important to some adolescents, but mastering the sport is not significant to adolescent development.
    d. Adolescence is the time to develop special interest in future goals, but goal completion is not a developmental task.
    Nursing Process: Planning
    Cognitive Level: Comprehension

13. **b. Play therapy is effective in helping the child communicate and release feelings about problems.**
    a. A five-year-old will likely have difficulty expressing feelings verbally.
    c. Family therapy may be useful but not as a means to assist Torrie to release her feelings.
    d. It is unlikely that role play would assist Torrie in releasing her feelings about what had happened to her. This intervention is more effective with older clients.
    Nursing Process: Implementation
    Cognitive Level: Application

14. **c. This statement displays empathy and caring for the client's feelings.**
    a. This is offering false hope and not dealing directly with the client's feelings.
    b. There is no guarantee that time will heal his wounds, and this statement offers false hope.
    d. The nurse has changed the focus from the client to herself and her own needs.
    Nursing Process: Implementation
    Cognitive Level: Analysis

15. **b. Acting out is a typical behavior which prevents the client from having to express his true feelings.**
    a. Brad would likely participate with other clients rather than choose to be alone.
    c. The situation did not provide information supporting family difficulty, which would result in this behavior.
    d. Although Brad may not complete his homework, this would not likely be to mask his feelings.
    Nursing Process: Planning
    Cognitive Level: Application

16. **a. Volunteering with persons who were abused indicated resolution of her own issues, which permits her to help others.**
    b. This statement indicates denial of the situation that existed.
    c. Avoiding programs that involve abuse indicates that her pain is still very real to her and she has not completed her work.
    d. Choosing not to date may indicate that she is fearful that she may be hurt again.
    Nursing Process: Evaluation
    Cognitive Level: Analysis

17. **b. This statement states the expectation that Patty will change this behavior.**
    a. Isolating Patty in her room will not promote a change in behavior and may increase her level of frustration.
    c. An age-appropriate time-out is an effective intervention, but one hour is too long for a 10-year-old client.
    d. This statement is not specific as to what constitutes a decrease in acting-out behaviors.
    Nursing Process: Outcome identification
    Cognitive Level: Analysis

18. **c. This activity involves planning and preparation of the food, as well as sharing with other persons.**
    a. This is a more passive activity and involves little effort from the clients.
    b. Although this would be a good activity, it would not meet the criteria stated for the selected activity.
    d. Playing basketball would not necessarily interest all of the clients on the unit.
    Nursing Process: Planning
    Cognitive Level: Analysis

19. **c. Voicing judgment serves to block the expression of feelings; therefore, remaining nonjudgmental encourages self-expression.**
    a. The nurse is a role model for clients and adopting their terminology may result in less respect from them.
    b. The client is responsible to make his own decision and offering personal opinions will hinder that process.
    d. Empathy is a desirable quality in the nurse and enables the nurse to feel the pain being expressed.
    Nursing Process: Implementation
    Cognitive Level: Analysis

20. **a. It is common for parents to share feelings of guilt when the child requires placement even though they may have done whatever they could to help the child.**
    b. His statement did not reflect anger.
    c. Denial was not expressed by the father.
    d. Rather than relief, there was an expression of frustration.
    Nursing Process: Assessment
    Cognitive Level: Analysis

21. **c. Children have difficulty understanding termination of relationships.**
    a. It is unlikely her change in behavior was to achieve attention.
    b. This is not a valid way to evaluate progress.
    d. It is unlikely that she wants to stay in the hospital.
    Nursing Process: Assessment
    Cognitive Level: Analysis

22. **d. Anhedonia, absence of pleasure, is a common manifestation in depression.**
    a. Having problems with breaking the law is characteristic of conduct disorder.
    b. Crying is more commonly observed in the depressed adult, and it is unlikely that this client would choose to remain in bed.
    c. Blaming others is common in oppositional and conduct disorders.
    Nursing Process: Assessment
    Cognitive Level: Analysis

23. **b. The use of firearms is the most commonly used method of committing suicide in the adolescent.**
    a, c, and d. These are used less often for committing suicide.
    Nursing Process: Implementation
    Cognitive Level: Comprehension

24. **d. Pounding in a safe, structured environment would enable the child to release anger outside himself onto a neutral object.**
    a. The activity of kicking the ball may release anger, but the setting is unsafe and off limits for this activity.
    b. A paint by number picture limits self-expression, which is needed to assist in the relief of anger.
    c. Working on an intricate project may result in increased anxiety, leading to further anger.
    Nursing Process: Planning
    Cognitive Level: Application

25. **b. The nurse may wonder from this remark whether Elizabeth still may try to gain attention from her friends and harm herself again.**
    a. This statement reflects an understanding of Elizabeth's behavior and the consequences.
    c. This is a positive statement indicating Elizabeth is aware of available resources.
    d. This is a positive statement indicative that Elizabeth is feeling less depressed.
    Nursing Process: Assessment
    Cognitive Level: Analysis

Chapter 19

1. **b. The fashion industry and media equate thinness with beauty and success.**
   a. People with eating disorders do not generally choose nutritious foods and are malnourished.
   c. There is no evidence to support this statement.
   d. There is no evidence showing that people from divorced and blended families have increased eating disorders.
   Nursing Process: Assessment
   Cognitive Level: Comprehension

2. **d. People with eating disorders are unable to identify and respond to bodily sensations.**
   a. Inability to use effective coping skills is common in people with eating disorders.
   b. People with eating disorders typically have insecure relationships.
   c. A person with an eating disorder is generally compliant.
   Nursing Process: Assessment
   Cognitive Level: Analysis

3. **a. Thinking a situation is all good or all bad is an example of dichotomous thinking.**
   b. This is an example of erroneous control issues.
   c. This is an example of personalization.
   d. This is an example of personalization.
   Nursing Process: Assessment
   Cognitive Level: Analysis

4. **d. Dental enamel erosion occurs because of acid gastric contents in the emesis.**
   a, b, and c. These are not considered results of purging.
   Nursing Process: Assessment
   Cognitive Level: Analysis

5. **a. Clients with anorexia nervosa are fearful of gaining weight and do not want to know it.**
   b. Adding extra layers of clothing can cause an increase in weight.
   c. It is the custom to hide the scale numbers from view to prevent the client from reacting to the weight reading.
   d. The client is not anxious to be weighed and usually needs to be asked by the nurse.
   Nursing Process: Implementation
   Cognitive Level: Analysis

6. **a. Doris is overgeneralizing and needs to focus on areas of concern.**
   b. It is unlikely that Doris expects to gain anything other than being thin.
   c. Although Doris should be aware of the possibility of becoming ill, this will be more effective after her problems are identified.
   d. This will not assist Doris with dealing with her problem at this time.
   Nursing Process: Implementation
   Cognitive Level: Analysis

7. **b. Dance and movement therapy assist the client in getting in touch with feelings and body space.**
   a. These tests provide information about personality traits but are not used to encourage self-disclosure.
   c. Journalizing and poetry writing allow self-disclosure; however, letter writing is generally too restrictive for therapeutic self-disclosure.
   d. Cooking and meal planning classes do not support self-disclosure.
   Nursing Process: Implementation
   Cognitive Level: Analysis

8. **c. A client who expresses willingness to engage in treatment will become involved and benefit more from the therapeutic interventions.**
   a. Although the question denotes concern, it will not alter the client's level of anxiety.
   b. The nursing assessment is not intended to encourage communication but to collect data to use in planning care.
   d. The nurse has no data indicative of the client's shame and guilt.
   Nursing Process: Assessment
   Cognitive Level: Application

9. **b. Amenorrhea is common in eating disorders possibly related to altered hypothalamic function.**
   a, c, and d. These are not usually related to changes in the body resulting from eating disorders.
   Nursing Process: Assessment
   Cognitive Level: Comprehension

10. **d. The client was attempting to ignore the problem by refusing to acknowledge her eating disorder.**
    a. Repression is a mechanism that prevents unwanted thoughts from conscious awareness.
    b. Rationalization is an attempt to make unacceptable feelings and behaviors tolerable.
    c. Sublimation involves displacing unacceptable drives into acceptable activities.
    Nursing Process: Assessment
    Cognitive Level: Analysis

11. **c. Mary is not using food as a control issue or power struggle.**
    a. John's behavior has the potential to create a control issue.
    b. Sam is using food as a reward, which could result in the continuation of same behavior throughout life.
    d. Ruth may have more difficulty relating to people who abuse the use of food.
    Nursing Process: Planning
    Cognitive Level: Analysis

12. **c. Clinical trials indicate high incidence of seizure disorders from this medication when given to the bulimic client.**
    a. There is no evidence of increased appetite and food intake as related to Butroprion.
    b. There is no evidence of interaction with other meds the bulimic would be prescribed.
    d. There is no report of this drug causing a rise in blood pressure.
    Nursing Process: Implementation
    Cognitive Level: Comprehension

13. **b. The client with an eating disorder frequently also has a depressive disorder.**
    a, c, and d. These are not usually associated with eating disorders.
    Nursing Process: Assessment
    Cognitive Level: Comprehension

14. **a. Zoloft is an SSRI and has proved effective in treating this condition.**
    b and c. These are used for anxiety reduction and are habit forming.
    d. Lithium is given for manic behavior.
    Nursing Process: Intervention
    Cognitive Level: Comprehension

15. **a. Electrolyte imbalances are common with eating disorders, and determining the levels is necessary prior to replacement therapy.**
    b. There is no data provided indicating the client is a suicide risk.
    c. It is unlikely that the client will eat at this time even if food is provided.
    d. Placing her on bed rest may be necessary; however, access to the bathroom must be monitored to prevent continuation of previous behaviors.
    Nursing Process: Implementation
    Cognitive Level: Comprehension

16. **d. Helping Jane to identify thoughts will enable her to learn effective coping mechanisms to deal with them.**
    a. Calling her parents would prevent Jane from having to deal with her own discomfort.
    b. The nurse has taken control of the situation without allowing Jane the opportunity to explore her own issues.
    c. The nurse should encourage Jane to do the work rather than try to rescue her from her pain.
    Nursing Process: Implementation
    Cognitive Level: Analysis

17. **b. Demonstrating the ability to deal with stress more effectively is essential for discharge.**
    a. Discharge criteria is generally based on maintaining the desired weight without additional loss.
    c. Having the knowledge of nutrition does not insure that the client will apply it to her situation.
    d. Exercising three times a day is considered excessive.
    Nursing Process: Evaluation
    Cognitive Level: Comprehension

18. **c. The nurse is responding to the mother's sense of failure and encouraging elaboration.**
    a. This is true, but it serves as a block to further interaction with the mother.
    b. Giving advice does not allow for clarification of the mother feeling responsible for her daughter's illness.
    d. This is not a realistic approach and does not address the mother's concerns.
    Nursing Process: Implementation
    Cognitive Level: Analysis

19. **b. There is an obvious lack of boundaries in an enmeshed family.**
    a. Individuality is discouraged in enmeshed families.
    c. There is little healthy conflict resolution in enmeshed families.
    d. An enmeshed family places considerable importance on appearances and public acceptance.
    Nursing Process: Implementation
    Cognitive Level: Application

20. **c. The client with anorexia nervosa has an unrealistic perception of her body image.**
    a and b. The anorexic client does not visualize herself as attractive or malnourished.
    d. The anorexic client does not view herself as like a role model.
    Nursing Process: Evaluation
    Cognitive Level: Application

21. **a. Hypokalemia is a result of potassium deficiency, possibly related to purching.**
    b. Calcium deficiency was not addressed in the situation.
    c. Metoclopramide is used for gastroparesis.
    d. Ferrous sulfate is given for an iron deficiency.
    Nursing Process: Implementation
    Cognitive Level: Comprehension

22. **b. Helping Clemmie recall previous times when she could enjoy food without purging will offer hope that she can have this experience again.**
    a. This may occur; however, it is not the goal of this intervention.
    c. Providing special foods for Clemmie is ineffective in helping her to learn improved eating habits, and it provides secondary gains.
    d. This intervention will not promote compliance.
    Nursing Process: Implementation
    Cognitive Level: Application

23. **b. The realization that one is more alike than different decreases secondary gains.**
    a. This is not the goal of group therapy and would not necessarily prevent clients from focusing on food.
    c. Clients need to focus on their own issues.
    d. There is no evidence to support this statement.
    Nursing Process: Planning
    Cognitive Level: Comprehension

24. **b. Having an understanding of an illness and what to expect decreases fear and anxiety and empowers clients to cope more effectively.**
    a. Eating disorders are not caused by family dysfunction.
    c. This is not the responsibility of the family.
    d. This is no guarantee of illness prevention.
    Nursing Process: Planning
    Cognitive Level: Analysis

25. **c. Stating satisfaction with a picture of how she actually looks indicates an improved body image.**
    a. Selecting clothes too large indicates that Tracy still views her body as extremely large.
    b. Tracy is stating her boyfriend's opinion rather than how she views herself.
    d. Tracy is not stating her view of herself but expressing what her mother had said.
    Nursing Process: Evaluation
    Cognitive Level: Analysis

Chapter 20

1. **c. Aversion disorder is characterized by avoidance of genital sexual contact with a partner.**
    a. Orgasmic disorder, male or female, is characterized by delayed orgasm following sexual excitement.
    b. Hypoactive sexual desire disorder is characterized by absence of drive for sexual activity.
    d. Dyspareunia refers to genital pain associated with intercourse.
    Nursing Process: Assessment
    Cognitive Level: Comprehension

2. **d. Since the 1960s, there has been an increase in research concerning the subject of sexuality and sexual dysfunctions.**
    a. Kaplan identified the need for using behavioral techniques in treating sexual disorders.
    b. Freud did not base his work on scientific data.
    c. Freud, Newton, and Ellis preceded Masters and Johnson in studying sexual dysfunction.
    Nursing Process: Assessment
    Cognitive Level: Comprehension

3. **b. The nurse must be aware of her personal feelings and views about sexual issues to best assist a client on the sexual disorders unit.**
   a. Previous experience may prove to be helpful; however, it is not required.
   c. Thinking that all types of sexual dysfunction can be corrected is unrealistic.
   d. The nurse is not expected to discuss personal issues in the interview or with the clients.
   Nursing Process: Planning
   Cognitive Level: Comprehension

4. **d. The nurse should begin with the least sensitive area and allow time for the client to become somewhat comfortable before focusing on sexual concerns.**
   a, b, and c. All address sexual issues, which are sensitive topics.
   Nursing Process: Assessment
   Cognitive Level: Application

5. **b. Antidepressants are known to decrease sexual desire.**
   a, c, and d. These do not provide enough data to indicate their contribution to a sexual disorder.
   Nursing Process: Planning
   Cognitive Level: Analysis

6. **d. Fetishism refers to using various objects for sexual arousal.**
   a. Exhibitionism refers to exposing genitals to others.
   b. Frotteurism refers to achieving sexual pleasure from rubbing against a stranger in a public place.
   c. Pedophilia refers to sexual attraction to a young child.
   Nursing Process: Nursing diagnosis
   Cognitive Level: Comprehension

7. **d. Stating there is nothing wrong with the way he behaves indicates his denial that a problem exists.**
   a. Childhood abuse should be considered in assisting him with his problem but places blame on others.
   b. Stating that he acted inappropriately only when stressed is rationalizing his behavior.
   c. This shows recognition of wrong behavior and presence of remorse.
   Nursing Process: Evaluation
   Cognitive Level: Analysis

8. **d. Mr. Luther has not accepted the fact that he has a problem and therefore refuses to comply with the plan of care.**
   a. If anger at being hospitalized does exist, it also indicates his denial that he has a problem.
   b. There is no evidence to support embarrassment.
   c. There is no indication to support this assumption.
   Nursing Process: Nursing diagnosis
   Cognitive Level: Analysis

9. **c. The client must acknowledge that he has a sexual disorder before he will be helped with the problem.**
   a. Withdrawing from the program indicates that he does not want to continue treatment.
   b. Wanting his wife involved in treatment is an indication that he has acknowledged his problem.
   d. He may need medication at times during the treatment, but this does not relate to effectiveness of treatment.
   Nursing Process: Evaluation
   Cognitive Level: Analysis

10. **b. The NET test is used to determine erectile responses during the sleep cycle.**
    a. This is incorrect.
    c. Incorporating visual erotic stimuli is a different assessment tool.
    d. This is incorrect.
    Nursing Process: Planning
    Cognitive Level: Comprehension

11. **c. Genital pain is a manifestation of dyspareunia.**
    a. The inability to maintain adequate lubrication during intercourse is a female sexual arousal disorder.
    b. Lack of desire and avoidance of sexual activity is hypoactive sexual disorder.
    d. Involuntary contraction of perineal muscles refers to vaginismus.
    Nursing Process: Assessment
    Cognitive Level: Application

12. **c. Because of side effects, the client must give written consent before taking Depo-Provera.**
    a. Depo-Provera dosage is not determined specifically by body weight and height.
    b. Alcohol consumption is not related to this med; however, history of abuse must be considered in the treatment.
    d. Providing information about the drug is part of informed consent; however, it does not have to be done only in printed form.
    Nursing Process: Implementation
    Cognitive Level: Application

13. **a. Identification of triggers that may increase continuation of dysfunctional behavior will decrease his risk to society.**
    b. Interaction with others is a part of any group but not the purpose of this particular group.
    c. Legal implications will not likely be addressed in this group.
    d. Assisting with time structuring is done in occupational therapy or similar adjunct therapy group.
    Nursing Process: Implementation
    Cognitive Level: Comprehension

14. **b. Refusal to take prescribed meds indicates the client is denying the problem exists.**
    a. Wanting to see family members is a positive sign.
    c. Sitting alone writing poetry is a way of reflecting and expressing feelings constructively.
    d. This is inappropriate but does not indicate a potential relapse.
    Nursing Process: Assessment
    Cognitive Level: Application

15. **a. An ego syntonic pedophile is cognitively aware that the behavior is inappropriate but is not troubled by it.**
    b. Being uncomfortable with the behavior describes an ego dystonic pedophile.
    c. This is using projection to place blame on the parents.
    d. This describes an ego dystonic pedophile.
    Nursing Process: Assessment
    Cognitive Level: Analysis

16. **a. Fred must learn to recognize what occurs prior to his making the obscene calls in order to stop this behavior.**
    b. There is no data to support this statement.
    c. There is no data to support this; however, many receivers of obscene calls do consider this to be a problem.
    d. There is no data to support this.
    Nursing Process: Implementation
    Cognitive Level: Analysis

17. **d. Stating that his babysitter did the same to him is his attempt to justify his behavior by rationalization.**
    a. This reflects use of projection by attributing his thoughts and impulses to the children.
    b. Choosing to avoid accepting the fact he has a problem is denial.
    c. This reflects projection.
    Nursing Process: Nursing diagnosis
    Cognitive Level: Analysis

18. **d. Having enlarged breasts at time of puberty is a characteristic finding in Klinefelter's Syndrome.**
    a. Aspermatogenesis is an expected finding.
    b. The level of FSH is decreased in this disorder.
    c. The newborn displays male characteristics rather than female.
    Nursing Process: Assessment
    Cognitive Level: Comprehension

19. **b. The therapist needs to know the way both Mr. and Mrs. Moses view the problem in order to be effective in helping them.**
    a. Focusing on body feeling during intimacy is involved in sensate focusing, which is a premature outcome at this time.
    c. Identifying specific stressors is necessary at a later session.
    d. There is no data to support her feelings, and this is too sensitive for initial outcome.
    Nursing Process: Outcome identification
    Cognitive Level: Analysis

20. **b. The blood pressure should be monitored for possible elevation.**
    a. Testosterone levels decrease.
    c. Clients frequently report weight gain.
    d. Motor activity and energy level usually decrease.
    Nursing Process: Implementation
    Cognitive Level: Application

Chapter 21

1. **d. Adjustment disorders are short term disturbances in mood or behavior resulting from identifiable stressors.**
   a. Psychotic manifestations are not present.
   b. Adjustment disorders can occur in any age group.
   c. Anxiety and depression symptoms may be present, but emphasis is on dealing with identifying and resolving specific stressful issue.
   Nursing Process: Planning
   Cognitive Level: Comprehension

2. **c. Diagnostic criteria states at least six months for chronic.**
   a and b. These lengths are considered acute.
   d. This is also chronic.
   Nursing Process: Planning
   Cognitive Level: Comprehension

3. **c. This statement affords the opportunity to compare self-perceptions with perceptions of others.**
   a. This could be damaging to the client.
   b. This is not the intention of the intervention.
   d. Ruth needs to express her feelings.
   Nursing Process: Implementation
   Cognitive Level: Analysis

4. **c. In order to assist the client, the stressful event and interpretation of the existing problem must be identified.**
   a. If the family is a support system, including them may be beneficial, but first identification of the stressor and problem must be done.
   b. This is important, but until the stressor and problem are identified, anxiety level continues to rise.
   d. This is a necessary intervention but not directly related to the question.
   Nursing Process: Implementation
   Cognitive Level: Application

5. **a. When preexisting coping skills are not adequate to deal with a stressor, symptoms may appear.**
   b. This is not applicable to situation.
   c. Usually, client recognizes there is a problem.
   d. This is not related to onset of the disorder.
   Nursing Process: Nursing diagnosis
   Cognitive Level: Application

6. **b. The stress of the argument was likely the stimulus for the headache.**
   a. There is no indication of her feeling unloved.
   c. Client did not lose control.
   d. There is no information supporting a problem given.
   Nursing Process: Nursing diagnosis
   Cognitive Level: Analysis

7. **a. His identity and purpose were associated with his job, so when he no longer is working, he may experience adjustment difficulties.**
   b. No information about finances was provided and he likely would have had a plan.
   c. No data was given supporting lack of interests given.
   d. No data was given indicating he would be alone.
   Nursing Process: Nursing diagnosis
   Cognitive Level: Analysis

8. **c. Cultural practices dealing with grief and loss differ, and failure to incorporate their significance in the treatment plan may lessen resolution of the client's problem.**
   a. Talking about the loss helps the client deal with it.
   b. It may be a normal response to feel sadness for one who is hurting.
   d. Getting help from qualified persons to assist with problem resolution is valuable if the client approves.
   Nursing Process: Implementation
   Cognitive Level: Analysis

9. **d. Erikson supports age-appropriate resolution of developmental tasks.**
   a, b, and c. These are not related to Erikson's theory.
   Nursing Process: Planning
   Cognitive Level: Comprehension

10. **c. Amber is exhibiting a problem with lack of social interaction since she has assumed the role of being responsible for her siblings.**
    a. There is no data to support her being a danger to herself.
    b. There is no information suggesting this diagnosis.
    d. Although her mother died, no information suggesting this problem was indicated.
    Nursing Process: Nursing diagnosis
    Cognitive Level: Analysis

11. **c. This question will determine whether the client is able to identify a particular stressor occurring recently.**
    a. This would assist in gaining information about important persons in client's life.
    b. This will provide only factual information about status of client's therapy.
    d. This determines ability to cope.
    Nursing Process: Assessment
    Cognitive Level: Application

12. **d. Recognizing socially and culturally appropriate expression of grief when planning care indicates respect and enables the staff to incorporate her customs into her plan of care.**
    a. This is not an indicator of magnitude of grief experience.
    b. Including a support system may become a part of the plan; however, the goal is for the client to do the grief work herself.
    c. The goal is for the client to do the work herself.
    Nursing Process: Assessment
    Cognitive Level: Analysis

13. **c. Accepting the fact that grief is a normal process and will be resolved shows an understanding by the client.**
    a. This indicates denial since there likely will be times when these feelings will exist.
    b. This indicates inability to deal with feelings unless doing a special activity with others.
    d. Anger stage should have been resolved earlier in the grief process.
    Nursing Process: Evaluation
    Cognitive Level: Analysis

14. **c. She could be in danger of harming herself since she is in a strange environment and has expressed no desire to live.**
    a. This should be considered in her treatment plan with goal of improving behavior.
    b. This will likely be considered to determine her feelings about the divorce.
    d. This also should be addressed as a problem in need of change.
    Nursing Process: Nursing diagnosis
    Cognitive Level: Application

15. **b. This question may help client identify what likely triggered this episode of ineffective coping.**
    a. This provides information about who may be available for support.
    c. This solicits factual data.
    d. This may determine whether client has adequate coping skills.
    Nursing Process: Assessment
    Cognitive Level: Analysis

16. **c. The nurse is seeking clarification in order to identify the client's problem.**
    a. It's unlikely the nurse understands; this serves to block communication.
    b. Reassuring may block communication. This is not responding to client's feelings and verbal expression.
    d. Premature assumption and does not respond to client cues.
    Nursing Process: Implementation
    Cognitive Level: Analysis

17. **a. Listing past experiences of loneliness will enable Jane to recognize a pattern of having similar feelings and help her recall previous coping methods.**
    b. Keeping a journal is more effective when done regularly and not only when upset, which would not assist in identification of patterns of feelings.
    c. This will not meet goal of identifying pattern of feelings.
    d. This does not support meeting goal.
    Nursing Process: Planning
    Cognitive Level: Analysis

18. **a. Absence of symptoms is indication of resolution of the problem.**
    b. Medications are not usually indicated for adjustment disorders, and if so, a decrease does not signify problem resolution.
    c. Decreased socialization may not have been a presenting problem.
    d. Base weight data is indicated since a gain may indicate eating to deal with stress.
    Nursing Process: Evaluation
    Cognitive Level: Analysis

19. **a. In the majority of cases, identification of the stressor and using effective coping mechanisms results in resolution.**
    b. Potential for self-harm is not a criteria for this diagnosis.
    c. If used, medications are for the purpose of assisting in dealing with the issues, not masking them.
    d. This is not applicable to this situation.
    Nursing Process: Implementation
    Cognitive Level: Application

20. **d. Physical exercise may assist in releasing stress and promoting feelings of well-being.**
    a. Knitting is tedious and requires steadiness, which the client does not have.
    b. Client is probably too jittery for this activity.
    c. This is incorrect for the same reasons as a and b.
    Nursing Process: Planning
    Cognitive Level: Analysis

21. **a. The desire to actively participate with others in meal preparation demonstrates that she is less depressed and can involve herself in a group activity.**
    b. Most mental health facilities require clients to get their meds at the med room. Her continued need for p.r.n.s shows she still displays symptomatology.
    c. Most likely she would permit the minister to visit even when depressed.
    d. Group therapy is part of the treatment program.
    Nursing Process: Evaluation
    Cognitive Level: Analysis

22. **b. Statement indicates Mark has no leisure or exercise activity nor does he have interactions with friends, which he needs during this stressful period.**
    a. This is not a problematic statement.
    c. This indicates his understanding of the importance of exercise.
    d. This shows he is thinking of ways to change present isolative behavior.
    Nursing Process: Assessment
    Cognitive Level: Analysis

23. **b. This provides opportunity to observe interactions with others in a setting similar to the real world.**
    a. This would be expensive and frustrating for the client. Less significant than observing behaviors.
    c. There are no lab studies specific to this symptomatology.
    d. This is less effective than observation.
    Nursing Process: Implementation
    Cognitive Level: Application

24. **d. Not harming self in the hospital is the expected client behavior.**
    a. Client should be encouraged to openly express feelings of self-harm.
    b. Client is encouraged to verbalize feelings to staff, who can provide necessary intervention.
    c. This is a useful intervention for expression of feelings but may prevent client from verbalizing his destructive feelings.
    Nursing Process: Outcome identification
    Cognitive Level: Analysis

25. **b. Listening to relaxation tapes indicates Mr. Todd has learned some effective methods to cope with the problem.**
    a. This indicates a belief that the drug is necessary to solve problem.
    c. This is incorrect for the same reasons as a.
    d. This reflects relying on someone else to solve his problem.
    Nursing Process: Evaluation
    Cognitive Level: Analysis

Chapter 22

1. **d. Understanding oneself is imperative for the nurse in order to assist someone else to heal emotionally.**
   a. Administering medications accurately is necessary but does not directly enhance the development of a therapeutic relationship.
   b. The nurse should interact with the team in planning care but this does not directly relate to the client-nurse relationship.
   c. Same rationale applies as for b.
   Nursing Process: Implementation
   Cognitive Level: Comprehension

2. **d. A specific goal is established with the client, which gives meaning for the relationship.**
   a. The focus is shared in a social relationship.
   b. Establishment and maintenance of boundaries is essential in a therapeutic relationship.
   c. Definite beginning and ending times are stated, as well as the duration of individual sessions.
   Nursing Process: Evaluation
   Cognitive Level: Comprehension

3. **a. In the role of counselor, the nurse listens to the client's experiences and assists in clarifying feelings.**
   b. The client may cast the nurse into roles of past experiences in an effort to clarify feelings, which is the surrogate role.
   c. The role of the resource person gives specific information to the client.
   d. The role of the technical expert is to navigate the complexities of the health care system.
   Nursing Process: Implementation
   Cognitive Level: Application

4. **c. Assisting the client to become a more responsible healthy person is the goal of a therapeutic relationship.**
   a. Support is necessary but not the goal.
   b. This is not the intended goal, although having a time limit is recommended.
   d. Planning care is a nursing and/or treatment team function and should include client input, but it is not the goal of the relationship.
   Nursing Process: Planning
   Cognitive Level: Comprehension

5. **d. This shows nonjudgmental acceptance of the client and recognition of feelings experienced by the client. It indicates caring and concern and does not block communication.**
   a. This indicates agreement and does not allow client to express feelings.
   b. Assigning another nurse would reinforce maladaptive behavior and feed into symptoms without confronting the issue.
   c. This focuses on nurse behavior rather than dealing with client feelings.
   Nursing Process: Implementation
   Cognitive Level: Analysis

6. **b. Examining oneself and becoming self-aware are essential for the nurse.**
   a. All nurses do not require individual therapy.
   c. This is not involved in examining self.
   d. This refers to learning from other professionals about one's performance.
   Nursing Process: Planning
   Cognitive Level: Comprehension

7. **c. Leaning forward conveys the message of interest and caring.**
   a. It is best to alternate periods of eye contact since constant maintenance may increase anxiety.
   b. The desk serves as a barrier and separates the nurse from the client.
   d. The client is the focus of the interaction.
   Nursing Process: Implementation
   Cognitive Level: Comprehension

8. **d. Empathy is an objective understanding of how one feels or views a situation and is conveyed by active listening to one's feelings.**
   a. Respect demonstrates unconditional positive regard conveyed through consistency and active listening.
   b. Genuineness refers to verbal and behavioral congruence and authenticity.
   c. Sympathy denotes agreement, compassion, and understanding.
   Nursing Process: Implementation
   Cognitive Level: Application

9. **a. Boundaries are the social, physical, and emotional limits of the interaction.**
   b. This is established during orientation stage.
   c. This is established during orientation stage.
   d. Emergence of undesired material may prove to be a significant issue for the client.
   Nursing Process: Planning
   Cognitive Level: Comprehension

10. **a. This is orientation, which is the first phase and begins when the client enters the system.**
    b. This is the middle phase, characterized by maintenance and analysis of the contract.
    c. This is the final stage and should reflect on accomplishments made.
    d. This is not a phase of the relationship.
    Nursing Process: Implementation
    Cognitive Level: Application

11. **b. The nurse listens for recurring patterns of interactions the client experiences in his stories.**
    a. This describes echolalia, a type of speech found in specific psychiatric illnesses.
    c. Unhealthy human responses are the basis for formulating a nursing diagnosis.
    d. Problem solving may occur after themes are identified, but themes as such are not a method of problem solving.
    Nursing Process: Assessment
    Cognitive Level: Application

12. **b. Being consistent in keeping one's word implies that the nurse is trustworthy and does what she promises.**
    a. The client may need to be confronted about her demanding behavior and learn new techniques for meeting her needs, rather than receiving a positive response.
    c. This is important in order to know what the client is saying, but it is not the best method of establishing trust.
    d. The client needs an opportunity to interact with other staff and peers. Also, a therapeutic relationship is time-limited.
    Nursing Process: Outcome Identification
    Cognitive Level: Analysis

13. **b. This demonstrates warmth, caring, and the desire to help the client.**
    a. True, but the nurse will also perform independent nursing actions to assist the client.
    c. This implies the meds will take care of his problems, overlooking contribution of staff and therapeutic milieu.
    d. Giving information is important but does not necessarily convey attitude of helper and ally.
    Nursing Process: Evaluation
    Cognitive Level: Analysis

14. **c. Task groups focus on defining the tasks and the work needed to accomplish the tasks.**
    a. This is not a defining characteristic of task groups.
    b. This is not significant to describing task groups.
    d. This refers to dealing with issues that are taking place at the present time.
    Nursing Process: Planning
    Cognitive Level: Application

15. **a. The goal of group therapy is to help persons develop more functional and satisfying relationships, based on the fact that psychopathology often comes from disordered relationships.**
    b. This may be true; however, people need to focus on individual issues on a one-to-one basis.
    c. True, but this is not the reason to offer group therapy.
    d. True, but the goal is on assisting the client to get well, and cost is not the assumption on which group therapy works.
    Nursing Process: Planning
    Cognitive Level: Application

16. **a. Tom is realizing he is not alone in his discomfort.**
    b. This reflects corrective recapitulation of the family group.
    c. This is an example of cohesiveness.
    d. This is an example of catharsis.
    Nursing Process: Evaluation
    Cognitive Level: Application

17. **b. Maxwell Jones developed this concept in the 1950s.**
    a. Freud explained human behavior in psychologic terms and demonstrated that behavior can be changed.
    c. She was the first to recognize nursing's responsibility for creating and controlling client's environment.
    d. He described "therapeutic factors" that help clients, regardless of type group.
    Nursing Process: Implementation
    Cognitive Level: Comprehension

18. **d. The aggressor acts negatively with hostility and criticism toward others.**
    a. This describes the compromiser.
    b. This describes the harmonizer.
    c. This describes the dominator.
    Nursing Process: Assessment
    Cognitive Level: Application

19. **c. The ideal number of clients for an inpatient group is six to ten, according to Yalom.**
    a. The clients who suffered abuse in childhood would benefit from this type of group.
    b. This would meet the criteria and would support the decision for such a group.
    d. This client would benefit from women's group.
    Nursing Process: Planning
    Cognitive Level: Analysis

20. **b. This statement shows the family has made an effort to deal with the lack of communication and problem of alienation without any one member bearing complete responsibility.**
    a. Playing football was important to the son's self-esteem and psychological development. Withdrawing from the team indicated he was feeling solely responsible for the family problem.
    c. The mother is bearing entire burden; however, her not working does not insure a smoothly run home.
    d. This indicates that the father had withdrawn from family participation and is bearing entire burden.
    Nursing Process: Outcome identification
    Cognitive Level: Analysis

21. **d. Statement indicates respect, acknowledges the situation, and refocuses on the therapeutic relationship.**
    a. This infers that the family is a problem for the client.
    b. This offers false reassurance and implies that the feelings are negative.
    c. This represents avoidance of dealing with the client's feelings and fulfilling role of the nurse.
    Nursing Process: Implementation
    Cognitive Level: Analysis

22. **c. Ms. Dean is expressing normal feelings associated with loss, which is therapeutic for her.**
    a. This does not indicate returning to former state or unreadiness to leave.
    b. This does not imply a hidden meaning but an open expression of her feelings.
    d. Further evaluation is not needed for expression of normal feelings of loss.
    Nursing Process: Evaluation
    Cognitive Level: Analysis

23. **a. Involving the group members in decision making is characteristic of the democratic leadership style.**
    b. This is autocratic style of leadership.
    c. This is laissez-faire style of leadership.
    d. This is autocratic style of leadership.
    Nursing Process: Evaluation
    Cognitive Level: Analysis

24. **a. Assisting Mrs. Lee afforded her a safe, non-threatening opportunity to assume responsibility for meeting her own needs.**
    b. This removes the responsibility from Mrs. Lee in getting her needs met.
    c. Ignoring the behavior permits the client to continue in the same manner without learning its effect on others.
    d. There is no reason to triangle in another person; also, this continues to prevent Mrs. Lee from learning self-responsibility.
    Nursing Process: Implementation
    Cognitive Level: Analysis

Chapter 23

1. **c. Atypical antipsychotics cause fewer EPS and are characterized by improved response of negative symptoms.**
   a. No evidence supports this.
   b. No evidence supports this.
   d. They are not available in depot form.
   Nursing Process: Implementation
   Cognitive Level: Comprehension

2. **c. An increased temperature is the cardinal sign of NMS.**
   a. Decrease in blood pressure may be associated with Haldol and should be rechecked, but this is not significant to NMS.
   b and d. These are not significant findings.
   Nursing Process: Evaluation
   Cognitive Level: Comprehension

3. **c. Dry mouth and blurred vision are anticholinergic effects.**
   a. Decreased dopamine causes extrapyramidal side effects.
   b. Blockade of histamine causes sedation.
   d. This results in hypotension, especially orthostatic hypotension.
   Nursing Process: Assessment
   Cognitive Level: Application

4. **a. Behaviors characterize tardive dyskinesia, resulting from treatment with phenothiazines, usually after prolonged use.**
   b. Sleepiness could result from CNS effects of various medications.
   c and d. These are extrapyramidal side effects resulting from imbalance between dopamine and acetylcholine in extrapyramidal tracts.
   Nursing Process: Assessment
   Cognitive Level: Application

5. **b. Haldol Decanoate is a long-acting injection providing slow release over a two-to-four-week period.**
   a. There is no mention of support system given; this also places responsibility on someone else.
   c. It is doubtful that this would help, and it probably was previously done.
   d. This would not increase likelihood of compliance.
   Nursing Process: Implementation
   Cognitive Level: Application

6. **b. Tricyclic antidepressants block reuptake mechanism, making larger amounts of norepinephrine and serotonin available and for a longer time.**
   a. Decreased dopamine available is result of antipsychotic meds.
   c. MAOIs inhibit monoamine oxidase in cell mitochondria.
   d. Benzodiazepines increase effects of gammaaminobutyric acid.
   Nursing Process: Implementation
   Cognitive Level: Comprehension

7. **b. Orthostatic hypotension can result from Alpha blockade, and constipation is common.**
   a. Urinary retention and mild tremors may occur.
   c. This is a side effect of antipsychotics.
   d. This is a side effect of antipsychotics.
   Nursing Process: Evaluation
   Cognitive Level: Application

8. **d. Liver contains tyramine, which can cause a hypertensive crisis when combined with MAOIs.**
   a. Photosensitivity is not a problem with these meds.
   b. There is no interaction between sodium and MAOIs.
   c. Many cold preparations contain sympathomimetics that interact with MAOIs.
   Nursing Process: Evaluation
   Cognitive Level: Analysis

9. **c. A headache is a warning sign of a hypertensive crisis. The nurse should assess his blood pressure and inquire about other symptoms.**
   a. Stiffness is not related to his taking this med.
   b. Elevated temperature is not an initial sign of impending hypertensive crisis.
   d. Constipation can be a side effect and should be monitored, but it is not the priority concern.
   Nursing Process: Assessment
   Cognitive Level: Analysis

10. **a. Compared to other antidepressants, there are fewer side effects.**
    b. SSRIs are more costly at this time.
    c. There is no research to support client compliance as a factor.
    d. They are absorbed slowly, and peak serum concentrations are obtained in 4-10 hours.
    Nursing Process: Implementation
    Cognitive Level: Comprehension

11. **b. Changing the dietary salt intake will affect lithium levels. Adding salt can cause lower levels, and reducing salt can increase levels.**
    a. Serum levels are done 12 hours after the last dose of lithium to be accurate.
    c. Water restriction can result in adverse side effects.
    d. Weight gain is a concern for some clients.
    Nursing Process: Outcome identification
    Cognitive Level: Analysis

12. **a. The presence of a benzodiazepine enhances the activity of GABA.**
    b. There is no effect on availability.
    c. This is not a function of GABA.
    d. This is the opposite effect of GABA.
    Nursing Process: Implementation
    Cognitive Level: Comprehension

13. **b. Xanax and Valium are the two fastest absorbed benzodiazepines, which accounts for the "buzz" effect.**
    a. This is not the reason for this experience.
    c. This describes mechanism of barbiturates.
    d. This is not related to this symptom.
    Nursing Process: Evaluation
    Cognitive Level: Analysis

14. **c. Combining a benzodiazepine with alcohol or other CNS depressant is potentially fatal.**
    a. There are no food interactions documented with this drug.
    b. Client should not increase dosage without physicians order.
    d. Client can likely return to work unless experiencing sedation, which may interfere with certain types of work.
    Nursing Process: Outcome identification
    Cognitive Level: Application

15. **c. Valproate is contraindicated during pregnancy because of teratogenic effects and the drug's association with neural tube defects.**
    a, b, and d. These present no problem contraindicating this medication.
    Nursing Process: Assessment
    Cognitive Level: Analysis

16. **a. The drug's short half-life results in the return of symptoms. Giving the med late in day leads to insomnia.**
    b. There is no effect on sleepiness.
    c. This is not the rationale for this question.
    d. This does not affect toxicity.
    Nursing Process: Implementation
    Cognitive Level: Analysis

17. **d. The light must strike the eye directly to be effective.**
    a. Direct sunlight on the skin is not effective.
    b. Time of administration does not effect treatment.
    c. Recommended distance is 3 feet.
    Nursing Process: Implementation
    Cognitive Level: Comprehension

18. **c. The client must be NPO prior to having ECT.**
    a. Client is expressing normal feelings.
    b. Client exhibits anxiety, which is an expected reaction.
    d. Client implies her hopefulness that this will help.
    Nursing Process: Assessment
    Cognitive Level: Analysis

19. **a. She is recognizing therapeutic effects of the med in assisting her to work with the therapist on her issues.**
    b. This indicates lack of knowledge about the medication and the need for additional teaching.
    c. This displays lack of acceptance of having a problem.
    d. This is an attempt to avoid scheduled activities and escape by sleeping.
    Nursing Process: Evaluation
    Cognitive Level: Analysis

20. **d. These are symptoms of pseudoparkinsonism.**
    a. This might occur as a result of prolonged use.
    b and c. These are not manifest by these symptoms.
    Nursing Process: Assessment
    Cognitive Level: Analysis

Chapter 24

1. **b. Meditation can produce beneficial effects in all systems.**
   a. Meditation is relatively easy to learn and can be done alone.
   c. People may benefit from meditation regardless of type of anxiety.
   d. Anxiety is invariably decreased during and after meditation.
   Nursing Process: Implementation
   Cognitive Level: Comprehension

2. **a. The client learns to gain conscious control over situations thought to be beyond voluntary command.**
   b. Client can learn to do biofeedback without machine.
   c. Success of technique depends on client's use of mental processes to control body action.
   d. Biofeedback is not dependent on mood of client.
   Nursing Process: Planning
   Cognitive Level: Analysis

3. **b. Humor may positively affect heart and respiratory rates, muscle tension, and several other body systems according to research.**
   a. Several hospitals and other health care settings are prescribing humor as part of treatment.
   c. Humor may increase defenses that prolong acceptance of reality.
   d. Age is not a specific factor affecting the benefits of humor, but humor can be made age specific.
   Nursing Process: Assessment
   Cognitive Level: Application

4. **d. After given all current information, clients have the right to make their own decisions about their care.**
   a. The nurse had full knowledge of reported traditional health options.
   b. Nurses in this position remain objective and empathic but do not interfere with client's choices.
   c. Confrontation was not necessary in this situation.
   Nursing Process: Implementation
   Cognitive Level: Analysis

Chapter 25

1. **b. Clergy and community caretakers can offer support needed to help the bereaved through the grief process.**
   a. All persons do not require individual counseling after experiencing a crisis.
   c. This is not a finding from this report.
   d. Crisis is not a natural phenomena.
   Nursing Process: Assessment
   Cognitive Level: Comprehension

2. **b. A situational crisis occurs when a specific, external event, such as losing a job, disturbs one's psychological equilibrium.**
   a. Adventitious crises are incurred by acts of God, providence, or fate.
   c. This is a maturational crisis.
   d. This is a maturational crisis.
   Nursing Process: Nursing Diagnosis
   Cognitive Level: Comprehension

3. **c. The nurse needs information as to why Peter sought help at this time.**
   a. This places blame on Peter for his wife's leaving.
   b. This is a good question that will be asked later in the interview.
   d. This is the same as b.
   Nursing Process: Intervention
   Cognitive Level: Analysis

4. **d. She is using displacement by screaming at her sister, which is not an effective way for her to cope.**
   a. Talking to a friend is acceptable and therapeutic.
   b. Crying will relieve stress and help Tammy deal with her feelings.
   c. Journaling is acceptable and therapeutic.
   Nursing Process: Evaluation
   Cognitive Level: Analysis

5. **c. Social isolation denies the availability of social interactions and opportunities to develop meaningful relationships.**
   a. This does not address issue of loneliness.
   b. This is a potential problem but does not address issue of loneliness.
   d. She is reacting to a sudden loss and is not experiencing delayed grief.
   Nursing Process: Nursing diagnosis
   Cognitive Level: Analysis

6. **c. The length of time for crisis intervention is usually 4 to 6 weeks.**
   a, b, and d. These are all incorrect.
   Nursing Process: Assessment
   Cognitive Level: Comprehension

7. **b. Stage 4 is when tension increases and major disorganization occurs.**
   a. This is stage 1.
   c. This is stage 3.
   d. This is not one of Caplan's crisis developmental phases.
   Nursing Process: Planning
   Cognitive Level: Comprehension

8. **d. The crisis team can provide on-the-spot emotional support for the friends and families.**
   a. This is not a function of a crisis team.
   b. Determining the level of coping may occur as part of the process.
   c. The crisis team will be with the families while offering emotional support.
   Nursing Process: Implementation
   Cognitive Level: Application

9. **a. The nurse needs to determine the precipitating event.**
   b. This may provide additional information but not always available.
   c. It is unlikely that this would be of value at this time.
   d. This is not an initial intervention.
   Nursing Process: Assessment
   Cognitive Level: Application

10. **a. Jake needs to be able to express his feelings and deal with the pain.**
    b. Leaving would postpone resolution of his feelings.
    c. There is no evidence of his need for a mental health admission.
    d. There is no data to support that he has a minister. Jake needs to talk rather than be talked to.
    Nursing Process: Planning
    Cognitive Level: Analysis

Chapter 26

1. **a. The therapist qualified to lead the particular group is responsible for interpreting the parents, activity and involvement.**
   b. Being familiar with the goals of a specific group will promote an understanding and lend support to the group leaders.
   c. The nurse may make suggestions, but the physician is required to order the particular therapy for the client.
   d. Dealing with the financial ability of the client and the group charges is not in the realm of nursing intervention.
   Nursing Process: Planning
   Cognitive Level: Comprehension

2. **c. The movements involved in dance therapy enables the client to become more aware of the body by self-expression.**
   a, b, and d. Psychodrama, music, and recreation are excellent therapies but will not promote body awareness.
   Nursing Process: Planning
   Cognitive Level: Comprehension

3. **a. The client is able to express feelings on the emotional, physical, and symbolic level, whereas verbal therapies are limited by linear communication.**
   b. The primary facilitator of the selected adjunct therapy is required to have formal education and supervised experience.
   c. The opportunity to use defense mechanisms is generally limited in adjunct therapies.
   d. Availability is dependent of resources provided (not necessarily available in each treatment setting).
   Nursing Process: Planning
   Cognitive Level: Analysis

4. **c. Learning to identify maladaptive behaviors and develop skills to change is a goal of an independent living skills group.**
   a. This would be learned in self-care maintenance group.
   b. This is not a function of independence living group.
   d. This is learned in relaxation therapy.
   Nursing Process: Evaluation
   Cognitive Level: Analysis

5. **b. Recognizing and pointing out to him any positive changes in his behavior provides encouragement.**
   a. Limit setting offers security and should be instigated when necessary.
   c. Interacting with more seriously ill clients will not deter his reaching his goal, and isolation may convey the message of inferiority.
   d. Intervention may be necessary to prevent the client from losing control.
   Nursing Process: Implementation
   Cognitive Level: Analysis

6. **a. Offering to dance with the client indicates that he is worthy and may also serve as a safe starting point for the client.**
   b. Determining whether or not this was his first dance would not encourage participation and may cause embarrassment.
   c. Sitting with the client may offer comfort, but isolating him from others will not encourage participation.
   d. Another client should not be giving the responsibility for Mr. Smith's involvement but should focus on their own need.
   Nursing Process: Implementation
   Cognitive Level: Analysis

7. **d. These art supplies tend to promote regression to a more immature period of development.**
   a and b. These supplies tend to promote defenses against regression.
   c. Large unlined paper encourages free expression.
   Nursing Process: Planning
   Cognitive Level: Analysis

8. **b. Moreno, in the early 1900s, viewed people as "natural role players" and believed that health was promoted from the spontaneous expression of diverse roles.**
   a. Marian Chase did not develop psychodrama.
   c. Freud was the father of psychoanalysis.
   d. Ulman was an art therapist who worked with psychotic clients.
   Nursing Process: Assessment
   Cognitive Level: Comprehension

9. **b. The role of the alter ego is to play significant others in the clients life.**
   a. Doubles operate as the inner voice.
   c. Group therapy provides the opportunity for catharsis, which is considered a therapeutic factor, according to Yalom.
   d. The director or psychodramatist directs the group.
   Nursing Process: Assessment
   Cognitive Level: Comprehension

10. **a. Jim needs more structure, which a defined space affords.**
    b. There are no defined limits on the paper, which would lead to frustration to Jim.
    c. Jim requires a more structured activity.
    d. Finger paints tend to promote regressive behavior.
    Nursing Process: Planning
    Cognitive Level: Analysis

11. **d. This response treats the art project with respect and value, and the nurse refrained from commenting on the artistic value of the work.**
    a. This indicates that the art project did not meet the nurse's standards for completion.
    b. This gives nurse's opinion that not painting meant John disliked to paint.
    c. This indicates that John did something wrong, which could decrease his self-esteem.
    Nursing Process: Evaluation
    Cognitive Level: Analysis

12. **b. The "warm up" phase may include relaxation techniques, stretching, and talking, which heighten awareness and decrease anxiety.**
    a. This is not the objective of dance/movement therapy.
    c. Although the purpose is not to improve cardiovascular functioning, the intake of oxygen would increase rather than decrease.
    d. This will not guarantee no injuries but may lessen the chances.
    Nursing Process: Implementation
    Cognitive Level: Comprehension

13. **b. Florence Nightingale observed that clients involved in the care and feeding of pets experienced increased feelings of self-worth and self-esteem.**
    a. There is no research to support work with nursing students.
    c. Using recreation therapy with mentally ill is not attributed to Nightingale.
    d. There is no record of Nightingale's use of recreation therapy with physically handicapped.
    Nursing Process: Assessment
    Cognitive Level: Comprehension

14. **c. The group is a safe environment in which to encourage the clients to process their reactions.**
    a. The nurse should be qualified to assist clients at this time.
    b. Leaving the group will prevent the clients from adequately processing their feelings and dealing with their grief.
    d. Being upset and anxious are possible reactions to lack of grief resolution and do not indicate activity failure.
    Nursing Process: Implementation
    Cognitive Level: Analysis

15. **a. Music therapy is a structured activity that promotes self-organization and social connectedness.**
    b. This may happen but is not the purpose of music therapy.
    c. There are a number of other activities that reduce anxiety and stress; music therapy may also, but it is not the purpose.
    d. Psychodrama and other therapies are effective in meeting this objective.
    Nursing Process: Assessment
    Cognitive Level: Comprehension

Chapter 27

1. **b. Interpersonal violence is usually committed by someone the victim knows.**
   a. Alcohol and drugs are not necessarily involved in interpersonal violence.
   c. Victim usually knows the perpetrator.
   d. The perpetrator is aware of what he/she is doing.
   Nursing Process: Assessment
   Cognitive Level: Comprehension

2. **c. Providing a safe environment is the first step in assisting a client who is a victim of domestic violence to talk.**
   a. An additional person may increase the client's anxiety and feelings of insecurity.
   b. Separating her from the abuser is assumed in providing a safe environment.
   d. The client may not disclose without prompting from the nurse.
   Nursing Process: Implementation
   Cognitive Level: Application

3. **d. Developing an emergency plan is critical for a battered woman.**
   a. Supporting her hopefulness is deceitful in that the battering likely will not end without the batterer seeking help.
   b. This will not stop the violence although it may offer her some protection.
   c. Violence frequently increases over time.
   Nursing Process: Implementation
   Cognitive Level: Application

4. **c. The best approach is one that is open, honest, and conveys concern for the welfare of the child.**
   a. Direct questions must be asked in order to obtain a history.
   b. Concerns about the possibility of abuse must be addressed in a sensitive manner.
   d. The family will be able to provide essential information required in the history.
   Nursing Process: Assessment
   Cognitive Level: Application

5. **b. Fear of being removed from home and the possibility of being institutionalized is a powerful motive for keeping abuse a secret.**
   a, c, and d. These are possibly true but not the most common reasons.
   Nursing Process: Assessment
   Cognitive Level: Analysis

6. **a. The batterer uses violence as a means of controlling his partner in order to meet his own needs.**
   b. Alcohol may be related, but it is not the cause of abuse.
   c. There is no evidence to support mental illness as a factor in abuse.
   d. Assertive behavior may result in increased abuse.
   Nursing Process: Planning
   Cognitive Level: Comprehension

7. **b. The most powerful reason for failing to disclose is fear of being blamed or disbelieved and the belief that he will not be supported.**
   a. This is not the most common reason for not reporting, although it can be traumatic.
   c. This is possibly true but not the most common reason for not reporting.
   d. This is possibly true but can be considered as part of b.
   Nursing Process: Assessment
   Cognitive Level: Analysis

8. **d. Only suspicions are required by the state's mandatory child abuse and neglect reporting laws.**
   a. The nurse is legally responsible for reporting abuse; therefore, the supervisor's permission is unnecessary.
   b. Strong evidence is not required for reporting.
   c. Parents do not have to be notified prior to reporting.
   Nursing Process: Planning
   Cognitive Level: Application

9. **b. Securing the client's safety is the priority for care.**
   a, c, and d. These are good interventions but not highest priority.
   Nursing Process: Implementation
   Cognitive Level: Analysis

10. **d. The nurse must first examine personal feelings and assumptions about child abuse in order to be objective and therapeutic in providing care.**
    a. This is not the first step in providing care to abused families.
    b. Removal from the family is not always recommended. Other interventions, such as stress reducing techniques may decrease possibility of future abuse.
    c. This may or may not be required, depending on the situation.
    Nursing Process: Implementation
    Cognitive Level: Analysis

11. **a. Timmy fits the highest risk group, which are children under 3 years of age because they are more fragile at that period.**
    b, c, and d. These children are older than the group with highest fatality rate.
    Nursing Process: Assessment
    Cognitive Level: Application

12. **b. Primary prevention focuses on identification of families at risk and avoidance of initial abusive episodes.**
    a. This is tertiary prevention.
    c. This is secondary prevention.
    d. This does not specify type services or how they would apply to interventions.
    Nursing Process: Evaluation
    Cognitive Level: Analysis

13. **b. Altered parenting is the appropriate diagnosis. The expectation that an 18 month old should not soil his diapers is unrealistic.**
    a. This is incorrectly stated.
    c. Abuse has already occurred, and the etiology is incorrect.
    d. There is no data indicating child will be removed from the home.
    Nursing Process: Nursing diagnosis
    Cognitive Level: Analysis

14. **b. Usually the victim moves slowly when making the decision to leave the batterer.**
    a. This has no relationship to decision to leave in most cases.
    c. This may be a factor, but there is no evidence to support.
    d. It is unlikely the batterer will give permission for victim to leave.
    Nursing Process: Implementation
    Cognitive Level: Application

15. **b. Since the abuse has occurred in the past and is increasing in intensity, Mrs. Cone needs to state her awareness of the danger in the situation.**
    a. It is a false assumption that the victim is responsible for the abuse.
    c. This is not practical since she has not begun to pursue litigation against her husband at this time, which would be a first step toward divorce.
    d. Retaliating is not an effective method of problem solving.
    Nursing Process: Outcome identification
    Cognitive Level: Analysis

16. **a. At least two photographs are taken of each trauma area.**
    b. Assessment for sexually transmitted diseases is part of the rape protocol.
    c. Rape protocol is used if there is evidence of sexual acts against client's will.
    d. Protective services must be notified in cases of child abuse.
    Nursing Process: Assessment
    Cognitive Level: Comprehension

17. **c. The desensitization to violence results in people being apathetic with the impact of violence on others.**
    a. This is a false statement.
    b and d. There is no evidence to support these statements.
    Nursing Process: Assessment
    Cognitive Level: Comprehension

18. **c. Physical discipline gives the message that aggressive punishment is necessary to gain compliance.**
    a. Time-out (appropriate for age) provides the opportunity for the child to process information related to the incident.
    b and d. Losing privileges teaches the relationship between behavior and consequences.
    Nursing Process: Assessment
    Cognitive Level: Application

19. **a. Flashbacks and recurrent dreams of the event are listed as PTSD criteria.**
    b. This is agorophobia reaction.
    c. This characterizes a dependent personality.
    d. Having no difficulty talking about a situation is not characteristic of this disorder.
    Nursing Process: Assessment
    Cognitive Level: Application

20. **b. Often the abused child cannot put into words his or her feelings or describe the event that took place. Play therapy affords tools through which the child can work.**
    a. Other adjunct therapies are more effective in helping the child act out behaviors.
    c. This is not the purpose of play therapy.
    d. Acting will likely be done in a psychodrama group.
    Nursing Process: Planning
    Cognitive Level: Comprehension

Chapter 28

1. **b. This is the correct answer.**
    a. This is egoistic suicide.
    c. This is altruistic suicide.
    d. This is fatalistic suicide.
    Nursing Process: Assessment
    Cognitive Level: Comprehension

2. **b. Freud viewed suicide as hostility directed inward toward the internalized love object.**
   a. This is Sullivan's view.
   c. This is Menninger's view.
   d. This is Jung's view.
   Nursing Process: Assessment
   Cognitive Level: Comprehension

3. **a. Irregularities in dopamine, serotonin, and norepinephrine have been discovered.**
   b, c, and d. There is no evidence to support these.
   Nursing Process: Assessment
   Cognitive Level: Comprehension

4. **c. Although there are no drugs specifically for suicide behavior, antidepressants for mood disorders may be indicated.**
   a. There are meds that affect the mood disorders associated with suicidal behaviors.
   b. Antipsychotics are used for thought disorders primarily.
   d. This is a myth about suicide.
   Nursing Process: Implementation
   Cognitive Level: Analysis

5. **c. Frontal lobe dysfunction is associated with cognitive content dimension of depression.**
   a. This is a major relay station for messages from all parts of the body.
   b. This discriminates sounds, verbal and speech behavior.
   d. This regulates voluntary movement.
   Nursing Process: Assessment
   Cognitive Level: Comprehension

6. **c. Decreasing unpleasant events and increasing pleasant events such as relaxation and stress-management techniques is based on learning theory.**
   a, b, and d. These are not related to the learning theory.
   Nursing Process: Implementation
   Cognitive Level: Application

7. **d. Statistical data in 1993 provided this information.**
   a. The rate of suicides is increasing.
   b. Children seldom commit suicide.
   c. The highest rates of suicide are found in the elderly and youth population.
   Nursing Process: Planning
   Cognitive Level: Comprehension

8. **a. Hanging contributes to more in-hospital suicides than any other method. The fact that the tie is in his possession should be taken seriously.**
   b and c. These do not indicate a concrete plan has been made to harm themselves.
   d. The client should be carefully monitored, but he is not talking of a current plan.
   Nursing Process: Assessment
   Cognitive Level: Analysis

9. **b. The single best predictor of suicidal thinking is the presence of a mood disorder.**
   a, c, and d. These are incorrect.
   Nursing Process: Assessment
   Cognitive Level: Comprehension

10. **c. The client who has previously attempted suicide is likely to do so again, especially if severely depressed.**
    a. This is a false statement.
    b. He likely will admit to the seriousness of the attempt.
    d. It is unlikely that this would be reported during the assessment. Writing a will can be a factor if one has a suicide plan.
    Nursing Process: Planning
    Cognitive Level: Application

11. **c. He would be placed on suicide watch, which entails continuous or more frequent observation of him.**
    a. There is no evidence to support his hiding information.
    b. The physician must be notified, however, the need to provide a safe environment is the priority.
    d. It is not required that he will be placed in a locked area if a less restrictive area provides the level of safety he requires.
    Nursing Process: Planning
    Cognitive Level: Analysis

12. **b. A loaded gun is the most lethal, and he could use it quicker than the other items.**
    a. Prozac used alone will not likely be lethal.
    c. A garden hose can be used for hanging, but preparation would take more time.
    d. Alcohol, if used alone, would not likely be fatal.
    Nursing Process: Implementation
    Cognitive Level: Analysis

13. **d. The nurse should monitor his behavior more closely because of the anniversary and allow him the opportunity to express his feelings about the relationship with his wife. Special days cause reflection on past times, and suicide is more likely to occur.**
    a. This indicates he is making plans for discharge.
    b. Statement implies this is not enjoyable as in past times, but client did not state he avoids it completely.
    c. He is trying to understand himself and his behavior.
    Nursing Process: Assessment
    Cognitive Level: Analysis

14. **b. Adolescents who commit suicides had more often lost their mothers to suicide. The nurse should consider potential for self-harm a possibility.**
    a. Running away implies she is struggling with some issues in her life.
    c and d. These indicate dysfunctional family relationships, which are contributing to her behavior.
    Nursing Process: Nursing diagnosis
    Cognitive Level: Analysis

15. **a. Avoiding self-harm is the outcome of highest priority.**
    b. He needs to report feelings to the mental health staff on the unit rather than wait for the doctor, who is not on the unit at all times.
    c. This may be indicated, but it is not highest priority.
    d. His fast driving reflects an unconscious intent of self-harm, and recognizing this is a desired outcome but not of highest priority.
    Nursing Process: Outcome identification
    Cognitive Level: Analysis

16. **c. The most vulnerable periods for suicide attempts are within the first 24 hours after admission and as discharge approaches when the client feels better and has more energy.**
    a, b, and d. These are incorrect answers.
    Nursing Process: Evaluation
    Cognitive Level: Analysis

17. **d. Denying the desire to harm himself indicates that he is not imminently suicidal.**
    a. Meaning is unclear but likely means he will not tell anyone who will try to help him. This needs clarification.
    b. Isolation from others indicates lack of available support.
    c. Having a support person to contact is a part of the discharge planning criteria.
    Nursing Process: Evaluation
    Cognitive Level: Analysis

18. **b. The nurse must take James' behavior seriously and evaluate the situation. There are interventions such as personalized no-harm contracts that can be used.**
    a. This is illegal and unethical.
    c. He needs the support, but answer does not deal with nurses' responsibility.
    d. This action would be detrimental to James.
    Nursing Process: Implementation
    Cognitive Level: Analysis

19. **a. Listing reasons to live is a positive intervention.**
    b. There is no data that anger toward others was a problem.
    c. There is no data indicating unresolved anger.
    d. This is a negative intervention.
    Nursing Process: Planning
    Cognitive Level: Analysis

Chapter 29

1. **b. Tightness in the chest is a physical manifestation of acute grief.**
    a. Loss of appetite is a common complaint during the grief process.
    c. Cardiovascular problems predominate in chronic grief.
    d. Insomnia is a common problem.
    Nursing Process: Assessment
    Cognitive Level: Comprehension

2. **c. Bereavement symptoms are of shorter duration than those experienced with depression.**
   a, b, and d. These are manifestations of depression and are not common in bereavement.
   Nursing Process: Nursing diagnosis
   Cognitive Level: Comprehension

3. **c. Statement implies member is feeling guilty about having not gotten to him before he died so that she could have saved him.**
   a, b, and d. These are normal expressions of grief and are therapeutic for the members.
   Nursing Process: Assessment
   Cognitive Level: Analysis

4. **b. Anger is common and often expressed toward the person who died.**
   a. This does not indicate a plea for help.
   c. This is not an explosive episode.
   d. This is not indicated in the situation, which does imply she was involved with others to make plans.
   Nursing Process: Nursing diagnosis
   Cognitive Level: Analysis

5. **a. In order to work through the grief process, Mrs. Jamison needs to feel the pain. Taking medications may prolong the grief process. The situation did not imply how long she would be taking them.**
   b. Offering to be with her at this time displays care and support.
   c. This is a much needed service at a hectic time.
   d. It is likely advice may be needed to deal with financial concerns.
   Nursing Process: Assessment
   Cognitive Level: Analysis

6. **d. Shock and disbelief are the most common initial responses.**
   a. Despair and protest follow shock and disbelief.
   b. Disorganization and confusion follow protest and despair.
   c. This is not usually initial response.
   Nursing Process: Nursing diagnosis
   Cognitive Level: Comprehension

7. **c. "Grief work" is the means by which one moves through grief process.**
   a. Assistance may be necessary to assist one to deal with loss.
   b. Often, previous coping methods continue to be effective; however, new methods may be useful also.
   d. This may be a part of the process but does not define "grief work."
   Nursing Process: Implementation
   Cognitive Level: Application

8. **a. Jamie fears that if she expresses her pain, she may lose control over her feelings.**
   b. There is no data to support.
   c. This is not likely a concern for Jamie.
   d. Support is implied in the situation.
   Nursing Process: Assessment
   Cognitive Level: Analysis

9. **c. The phase of resolution or recovery is a gradual process in which "the good days begin to outnumber the bad."**
   a. This does not indicate completion of "grief work" but that progress has been made.
   b. Criteria for termination is not indicated in situation.
   d. It is important to reflect on old memories and not try to forget.
   Nursing Process: Evaluation
   Cognitive Level: Analysis

10. **b. Failure to express grief following significant loss describes inhibited grief.**
    a. Preoccupation with the deceased may be exaggerated to the extent that the survivor exhibits symptoms or characteristics of the deceased.
    c. This is exaggeration of one or more components of grief, such as guilt or anger.
    d. Everyone needs to feel the pain of loss, regardless of gender.
    Nursing Process: Nursing diagnosis
    Cognitive Level: Application

11. **b. The father of a son who is schizophrenic is likely experiencing chronic sorrow, which is a response to ongoing loss.**
    a. The mother is not likely experiencing any type of grief but perhaps anxiety.
    c. There is no cause for any type of grief.
    d. Wife may experience grief, but does not meet criteria for chronic sorrow.
    Nursing Process: Assessment
    Cognitive Level: Analysis

12. **a. The possibility that Mrs. Dean may be experiencing pathologic grief should be investigated first.**
    b. This is important to know, but how the client is doing on her own in the grief process is most valuable.
    c. Psychological factors are a part of complete assessment which contributes to correct diagnosis.
    d. Displaying sympathy and concern is not the goal of this statement.
    Nursing Process: Assessment
    Cognitive Level: Analysis

13. **a. Anticipatory loss is associated with an expected loss.**
    b. There is no data to support, but resolution may take less time.
    c. Guilt over the implication that one has given up hope is common.
    d. There is a high incidence of depression associated with anticipatory grief.
    Nursing Process: Assessment
    Cognitive Level: Comprehension

14. **b. Realistic appraisal of the loss gives a clearer perspective of the situation and encourages acceptance of current life circumstances.**
    a. Keeping a journal of only pleasant memories does not help Ruth process the negative feelings.
    c. This may help but might have been more applicable when she was dealing directly with the problem.
    d. Family and friends are important, but Ruth must work through the grief process herself and deal realistically with her feelings.
    Nursing Process: Outcome identification
    Cognitive Level: Analysis

15. **b. The member was expressing ambivalence and low self-esteem related to dysfunctional grieving.**
    a. Member did not imply she had a plan to harm herself.
    c. This comment would not elicit attention.
    d. This is not an expression of anger.
    Nursing Process: Nursing diagnosis
    Cognitive Level: Analysis

16. **d. The nurse must first learn if there is danger of harming himself or others to determine the level of safety.**
    a, b, and c. These are important to include in the plan after safety is established.
    Nursing Process: Assessment
    Cognitive Level: Analysis

17. **a. Failure to express feelings may result in their being internalized, resulting in illnesses such as depression or physical problems.**
    b. This is an opinion statement which will block communication.
    c. This places responsibility on daughter to fix the problem.
    d. This is possible, but not the best answer for this situation.
    Nursing Process: Assessment
    Cognitive Level: Analysis

18. **b. Physical exercise provides a safe, effective method for expending anxious energy, anger, and tension.**
    a. Participation in group exercise may offer a chance to interact with others, but it is not the primary reason to exercise.
    c. Some types of exercise promote a time for thinking, but this is not primary reason.
    d. Feeling of well-being may result from physical exercise and is assumed in answer a.
    Nursing Process: Outcome identification
    Cognitive Level: Analysis

19. **b. Maturational is correct.**
    a, c, and d. These do not apply to the situation experienced.
    Nursing Process: Assessment
    Cognitive Level: Application

20. **c. Experiencing cognitive and physical disturbances is a normal reaction in acute grief, and Donald needs to feel the pain and process the loss.**
    a. His behavior indicates he is dealing with the pain.
    b. There is no data to support this feeling.
    d. There is no data to support that he is suicidal.
    Nursing Process: Nursing diagnosis
    Cognitive Level: Analysis

Chapter 30

1. **b. It is common for a person learning of an HIV seropositive diagnosis to experience symptoms of anxiety and even panic.**
   a. Signs and symptoms do not suggest suicide ideations.
   c. Disappointment is common and may be part of his anxiety reaction.
   d. If present, guilt may be contributing to his anxiety.
   Nursing Process: Assessment
   Cognitive Level: Comprehension

2. **b. He is most likely fearful that friends and family will reject him since he has AIDS.**
   a. If he were afraid of dying, he probably would not want to be alone.
   c. There is no data to support lack of knowledge.
   d. He is not at the stage of anger at this time.
   Nursing Process: Nursing diagnosis
   Cognitive Level: Analysis

3. **c. Consideration of the characteristics of distress is most important and determines the type and dosage of medication that will be prescribed.**
   a. Length of time since illness was diagnosed is not a factor.
   b. This does not relate to this question.
   d. Medications are available in forms other than oral.
   Nursing Process: Assessment
   Cognitive Level: Comprehension

4. **d. Suicide thoughts are common in the AIDS client. The nurse accepted his behavior and demonstrated her desire to help him.**
   a. This statement implied that James was trying to do something wrong and was caught.
   b. This implies that he had no choice in choosing what he could read.
   c. To ask his opinion was positive, but the reason for asking focused on the nurse's needs.
   Nursing Process: Implementation
   Cognitive Level: Analysis

5. **c. Hallucinations and other psychotic behaviors are common in acute psychotic dementia.**
   a, b, and d. Psychomotor retardation is found in primary type dementia, which is characterized by signs of depression.
   Nursing Process: Nursing diagnosis
   Cognitive Level: Application

6. **a. It is likely that a contributing factor to the higher rate of deaths in women is delay in seeking treatment.**
   b, c, and d. These are not contributing factors.
   Nursing Process: Assessment
   Cognitive Level: Comprehension

7. **a. Common early symptoms include fever, night sweats, and nausea.**
   b. These are symptoms of AIDS dementia complex.
   c. These are not expected findings.
   d. These are not expected findings.
   Nursing Process: Assessment
   Cognitive Level: Comprehension

8. **c. Dinah's primary concern was that she might test seropositive.**
   a. This is not a likely reason.
   b. Without her consent her parents would not know.
   d. This is not as likely a reason as c.
   Nursing Process: Assessment
   Cognitive Level: Analysis

9. **b. Realignment of goals is necessary since carrying out previous roles is not possible.**
   a. He will need longer to accept this and needs a more positive approach.
   c. This may be necessary, but he needs to feel needed also.
   d. The family is not the focus of the question.
   Nursing Process: Outcome identification
   Cognitive Level: Analysis

10. **a. Frequently associating with others experiencing a similar problem is most helpful in providing information as well as support.**
    b. He does not meet criteria for adult home admission because of his need for skilled care.
    c. Continuing to be involved with others socially is not as high a priority at this time.
    d. The family must develop a plan for his care because his condition will continue to deteriorate.
    Nursing Process: Planning
    Cognitive Level: Application

11. **a. This response reflects on the client's feelings and encourages communication.**
    b. True, but this reinforces the possibility of becoming infected, which reduces client's self-worth.
    c. This is not responding to the client's feelings.
    d. This tends to play down client's concerns.
    Nursing Process: Implementation
    Cognitive Level: Analysis

12. **d. Nurse D states the belief that everyone is worthy of the nurse's best effort.**
    a. Universal precautions are practiced in every area dealing with direct client care and not only with AIDS clients.
    b. Nurse B avoided directly answering the question.
    c. Nurse C's response does not indicate her ability to work with the clients and their families.
    Nursing Process: Evaluation
    Cognitive Level: Analysis

Chapter 31

1. **b. Socrates is correct.**
   a. Thales believed the cause of events might exist within situation itself.
   c. Aristotle used principles of logic and the senses to gather data.
   d. Hippocrates, father of medicine, treated body, mind, and spirit.
   Nursing Process: Planning
   Cognitive Level: Comprehension

2. **c. Nirvana means the state of perfect peace in the Buddhist culture.**
   a. This is a belief of the Zen philosophy practiced now primarily in Japan.
   b. This is the purpose of Yoga.
   d. This is a Taoism belief.
   Nursing Process: Implementation
   Cognitive Level: Comprehension

3. **d. The Zen philosophy supports this belief.**
   a. This reflects social conformity.
   b. This is a part of Hinduism.
   c. This supports belief in Christ.
   Nursing Process: Planning
   Cognitive Level: Comprehension

4. **a. Holistic health views individuals as total beings and more than a sum of their parts.**
   b. Holistic health supports integration, not separation.
   c. Holistic health believes in individual differences.
   d. Genetic factors are considered important influences.
   Nursing Process: Implementation
   Cognitive Level: Comprehension

5. **b. Trying to find some meaning in one's suffering indicates possible spiritual distress.**
   a. This is not an unusual behavior for those who regularly attend church.
   c. This indicates desire to continue learning.
   d. Daily devotionals are usual for some persons.
   Nursing Process: Assessment
   Cognitive Level: Application

6. **d. Irrelevant demands often require minimal attention.**
   a. These are stressful demands.
   b. These are benign-positive demands.
   c. This is unrelated to situation.
   Nursing Process: Evaluation
   Cognitive Level: Comprehension

7. **c. Therapeutic touch, a term coined by a nurse, Delores Krieger, is derived from "laying on of hands" associated with Eastern, European, and religious philosophies.**
   a. This is an inaccurate statement with no data to support.
   b. This is possibly true but not related to basis of therapeutic touch.
   d. This is an inaccurate statement.
   Nursing Process: Assessment
   Cognitive Level: Comprehension

8. **b. Losing a job meets criteria for a psychologic stressor.**
   a. This is a physiologic stressor.
   c. This is not a current problem.
   d. This is a physiologic stressor.
   Nursing Process: Nursing diagnosis
   Cognitive Level: Application

9. **d. Losing control over one's life as a result of sudden injury or illness is initially the most difficult.**
   a. This is not likely his biggest concern and also a fixable problem.
   b. There is no mention of distance in the situation given.
   c. The information provided is not suggestive of self-esteem problems.
   Nursing Process: Outcome identification
   Cognitive Level: Analysis

10. **a. Mr. Lee is using his illness to gain control over his son's life, requiring that he stay with him.**
    b. This is a positive statement indicating his efforts to help.
    c. He is expressing concern that her life will not be completely disrupted because of his problem.
    d. This indicates hope for the future.
    Nursing Process: Assessment
    Cognitive Level: Analysis

11. **d. It is based on self-protective mechanism due to arousal of the parasympathetic system.**
    a. This is atributed to Hans Selye.
    b. This is not a stress theory.
    c. This refers to Lazarus's transactional theory.
    Nursing Process: Planning
    Cognitive Level: Comprehension

12. **c. Pain relief results from release of endorphins.**
    a. There was no effect on serotonin.
    b. Situation does not involve dopamine.
    d. There was no effect noted.
    Nursing Process: Implementation
    Cognitive Level: Application

13. **b. Asking a client to state in her own words what she is experiencing is the most valuable in learning what is occurring.**
    a. This is important in providing additional information and can be used in planning care.
    c and d. These would provide excellent information to use in conjunction with client's perception of the pain.
    Nursing Process: Assessment
    Cognitive Level: Application

14. **a. Homeopathic medicine is based on the belief that a drug causing disease symptoms in a healthy person can cure those symptoms in an ill person.**
    b. Situation not applicable to witchcraft.
    c. Ayurvedic views body as natural pharmacy that can make natural drugs for self-healing.
    d. Herbal medicine incorporates supplements and other therapies for healing.
    Nursing Process: Implementation
    Cognitive Level: Application

15. **b. Mental imagery is correct.**
    a. Yoga involves controlled breathing and sequence of body positions to strengthen and stretch entire body.
    c. Biofeedback is used to give conscious control over involuntary body functions.
    d. Thought stopping involves concentrating on unwanted thoughts and suddenly interrupting the thought and emptying the mind.
    Nursing Process: Implementation
    Cognitive Level: Application

16. **a. Disorders such as hypertension can reflect psychological problems, and Mrs. Miers's behavior warranted further investigation.**
    b. This is possible, but no data was given to support it.
    c. More data is needed to determine effect of losses, if any.
    d. Her nonverbal behavior did not suggest this, but it should be investigated.
    Nursing Process: Evaluation
    Cognitive Level: Analysis

17. **c. Epidemiologic studies portray general events preceding morbidity and mortality of individuals.**
    a, b, and d. These are research findings unrelated to epidemiologic studies.
    Nursing Process: Assessment
    Cognitive Level: Application

18. **c. A desirable outcome for Mr. Ross would be to express feelings rather than deny the existence of his problem.**
    a. This promotes continuation of denial.
    b. No data is provided in situation to support isolation being a problem.
    d. Failure to acknowledge feelings about lifestyle changes does not promote wellness.
    Nursing Process: Outcome identification
    Cognitive Level: Analysis

19. **d. Mr. Brown may find life to be less meaningful after having been forced to give up his more independent lifestyle.**
    a. This indicates acceptance of his health state and desire to seek activities.
    b. Reflection on past times is normal.
    c. It is expected that an elderly person would express interest in life after death.
    Nursing Process: Evaluation
    Cognitive Level: Analysis

20. **c. The priority at this time is to manage the pain and make him comfortable.**
    a. This is an expected problem and should be considered.
    b. He obviously can communicate in English since he attends a local university.
    d. This may be a problem later, but not the priority at this time.
    Nursing Process: Nursing diagnosis
    Cognitive Level: Analysis

21. **a. Total expenditure of energy occurs at stage of exhaustion.**
    b. "Flight or fight" mechanism is response at alarm stage.
    c. Energy is available at stage of resistance.
    d. This is not a stage of Selye's theory.
    Nursing Process: Implementation
    Cognitive Level: Comprehension

22. **b. The person who perceives stress as a challenge has a greater ability to master the event, which characterizes the concept of hardiness.**
    a, c, and d. These are not a component of hardiness.
    Nursing Process: Implementation
    Cognitive Level: Comprehension

23. **a. Asking about the pain identifies a specific area of concern and indicates her feeling more secure with the nurse.**
    b. This is not an indicator, because the ability to sleep may result from the meds.
    c. This is not an indicator.
    d. Meds for anxiety are prescribed every four hours generally.
    Nursing Process: Outcome identification
    Cognitive Level: Analysis

24. **c. It is important to learn from the client what she views as the reason for admission in order to establish client goals.**
    a. This is not applicable to the situation.
    b. The physician most likely recommended her admission and is aware.
    d. Although this information will be documented this is not the reason for the question.
    Nursing Process: Nursing diagnosis
    Cognitive Level: Analysis

25. **a. Biofeedback gives continuous feedback about results of attempts at control, using monitoring equipment.**
    b. This is not the purpose of biofeedback.
    c. This describes chiropractic medicine.
    d. Biofeedback does not involve medications.
    Nursing Process: Planning
    Cognitive Level: Application

Chapter 32

1. **b. Chronic mental illness refers to persistent emotional disorders that interfere with ADLs, self-direction, IPR, social learning, and economic self-sufficiency.**
   a. Some manifestations of the disease will likely be present throughout the entire life.
   c. Chronic illness is not curable, but psychotrophics can decrease symptoms.
   d. Family stress can result for a variety of reasons, not only mental disorders.
   Nursing Process: Planning
   Cognitive Level: Comprehension

2. **a. Bert is most likely afraid of failing if he makes a change.**
   b. There is no data to support disinterest.
   c. Bert may enjoy his job but likely would prefer a more permanent employment.
   d. Bert is old enough that family support is not essential.
   Nursing Process: Planning
   Cognitive Level: Analysis

3. **a. An adult who developed CMI later in life, having known success, may experience severe depression, which places him at risk for suicide.**
   b. Generally a schizophrenic with no evidence of depression will not commit suicide.
   c. No data is provided to place child at high suicide risk.
   d. Chances are less if diagnosed early in life.
   Nursing Process: Assessment
   Cognitive Level: Analysis

4. **c. Failure to take psychotrophic meds as prescribed leads to return of problematic behaviors.**
   a. Lack of supervision may be a factor in noncompliance.
   b. Involvement in a dysfunctional family may affect noncompliance.
   d. Impaired judgment is also a result of noncompliance.
   Nursing Process: Nursing diagnosis
   Cognitive Level: Application

5. **d. The majority of chronic mentally ill live with their families.**
   a, b, and c. Some of this population do live in these places, but not the majority.
   Nursing Process: Assessment
   Cognitive Level: Comprehension

6. **d. The nurse is supporting the parents decision to have some time for themselves.**
   a. This reflects on their burden rather than their question.
   b. This places the son's needs ahead of the parents.
   c. Providing care for the son was not an issue.
   Nursing Process: Implementation
   Cognitive Level: Application

7. **b. The most likely reason for the alcohol is to relieve unpleasant symptoms.**
   a. This is unlikely. There is no data to indicate depression.
   c. Alcohol decreases inhibitions, but it is doubtful that this is his reason for drinking.
   d. No data given to support
   Nursing Process: Assessment
   Cognitive Level: Application

8. **a. She is blaming herself for Timmy's illness.**
   b. She is displaying anger at the doctor for Timmy's problem.
   c. She is denying that Timmy is mentally ill.
   d. She is indicating acceptance of the situation and looking at the positive aspects.
   Nursing Process: Assessment
   Cognitive Level: Analysis

9. **b. The parents need time together without other family member and the responsibility of Jason's care.**
   a. A picnic requires work and will not provide time alone for the parents.
   c. This defeats the goal of time for parents to be together.
   d. Finding child care for a mentally ill child is difficult.
   Nursing Process: Planning
   Cognitive Level: Application

10. **a. The expected outcome that he will not verbalize intentions to harm others is directly related to his problematic behaviors.**
    b. Ralph was demonstrating psychotic behaviors at the time he threatened the neighbors.
    c and d. These are important but not directly related to his admission behaviors.
    Nursing Process: Outcome identification
    Cognitive Level: Application

11. **b. Transferring clients from one institution to another is common in an effort to ensure that the client will receive the level of care needed at the time.**
    a, c, and d. These are incorrect.
    Nursing Process: Assessment
    Cognitive Level: Comprehension

12. **b. Generally, intoxicated individuals are not served.**
    a, c, and d. Services are provided to homeless persons regardless of retardation, depression, or marital status.
    Nursing Process: Planning
    Cognitive Level: Comprehension

13. **b. Developing a sense of trust is essential to the establishment of a therapeutic relationship.**
    a and c. Determining family support and client's perception of the illness is information the client should provide after he is comfortable with the nurse.
    d. Providing privacy is a factor promoting establishment of trust.
    Nursing Process: Assessment
    Cognitive Level: Comprehension

14. **b. The client's response would be an indicator of hopelessness and depression.**
    a. Question is not specific to the topic of violence.
    c. Question would not provide information as to presence of hallucinations.
    d. Question is not specific to living arrangements.
    Nursing Process: Assessment
    Cognitive Level: Comprehension

Chapter 33

1. **a. The focus of home health nursing is on care of the individual in the home setting.**
   b. Community health nursing employs a transindividual perspective in providing care.
   c. Various home health agencies provide services to persons who need them, not just those discharged from community hospitals.
   d. Many insurances and services reimburse the agency at least partial payment.
   Nursing Process: Implementation
   Cognitive Level: Comprehension

2. **c.** *Concentrated* refers to care delivered on a short-term basis designed to meet a specific acute need.
   a. Intermediate services are short-term and assist the client and family to achieve a planned, higher level of functioning.
   b. Maintenance services are provided when the client has reached a stable, higher-level of functioning.
   d. Primary prevention is a level of prevention and not a level of care.
   Nursing Process: Implementation
   Cognitive Level: Analysis

3. **d.** The nurse must be aware that she is a guest in the client's home, unlike in the hospital where the client is the guest.
   a. In some situations the home setting is not relaxed, and the nurse must be alert to potential problems.
   b. There are not always a large number of family members. Some persons have no one.
   c. The home health nurse will have the supplies needed for the specified client and will know how to obtain additional supplies.
   Nursing Process: Implementation
   Cognitive Level: Comprehension

4. **b.** The nurse's accepting the coffee and opportunity to interact with the client and guest provided support and the opportunity to assess the client in a different way.
   a. This encourages distance between the nurse and client and focuses on the nurse's need to do everything "right."
   c and d. These place the nurse's need first and fail to acknowledge the client's feelings.
   Nursing Process: Intervention
   Cognitive Level: Analysis

5. **b.** Talking with a fellow nurse about working with the Hispanic culture is the fastest way to get information that Mr. Cone needs since his visit is the next day.
   a, c, and d. These are useful in furthering Mr. Cone's cultural understanding, however, they are not for immediate assistance.
   Nursing Process: Planning
   Cognitive Level: Analysis

6. **b.** Initially the nurse must explain her role and what the nurse can expect from her.
   a, c, and d. Although important, none of these is the highest priority.
   Nursing Process: Planning
   Cognitive Level: Comprehension

7. **d.** Scheduling the visit during the daylight hours is safer, and also the nurse will avoid heavy traffic from persons returning from school and work.
   a. The client may not be able to provide the information you need.
   b. The time to notify the supervisor is prior to leaving to visit the client.
   c. Carrying a concealed weapon should not remove the necessity of taking other precautions.
   Nursing Process: Implementation
   Cognitive Level: Comprehension

8. **c.** The Millers seem to be trying in that she did accomplish 50% of the expected goal. Praise may encourage her to do better the next week. Setting a lower goal may increase compliance.
   a. Telling her that she has no choice is disrespectful and not supportive of their efforts.
   b. No data was given to imply that Mr. Miller was not objective.
   d. No data was given to support that skin breakdown is a factor.
   Nursing Process: Evaluation
   Cognitive Level: Analysis

9. **b.** The case manager assumes a coordinating role in the home setting and is responsible for overseeing the treatment plan.
   a. The physician does not assume this role.
   c. No data was given to indicate need for an aide. Besides, the aide is not responsible for coordinating the plan of care.
   d. No data was given to support client's need of an appointed guardian.
   Nursing Process: Planning
   Cognitive Level: Comprehension

10. **a.** The mentally ill client should receive care in the least restrictive environment possible.
    b. No data is given to support placing clients with like disturbances together.
    c. Some clients are unable to use this service and others may abuse it.
    d. Family members are not always available nor qualified for this responsibility.
    Nursing Process: Planning
    Cognitive Level: Comprehension

11. **b.** Case finding is a part of secondary prevention.
    a and c. Primary and tertiary levels do not include case finding.
    d. This is not a level of prevention.
    Nursing Process: Implementation
    Cognitive Level: Application

12. **c. Screening for hypertension is a means of preventing problems and promoting health.**
    a. This is a secondary prevention.
    b. This is a secondary prevention.
    d. This a tertiary prevention.
    Nursing Process: Assessment
    Cognitive Level: Application

13. **c. The nurse is required to write a descriptive note indicating need for home health services.**
    a. Nurses aides are unlicensed and provide care to home health clients.
    b. Family support is not related to question.
    d. There is no improvement shown in some cases, which indicates need for continued services.
    Nursing Process: Evaluation
    Cognitive Level: Analysis

Chapter 34

1. **c. The role of the chaplain is multidenominational; not focused on formal religions. Chaplains don't focus on specific religions; they are multidenominational, which allows them to address the spiritual needs of all those who request or require their guidance. Chaplains do not suggest there is a divine power or God. It is up to the client to decide his or her own views about this.**
   Nursing Process: Evaluation
   Cognitive Level: Analysis

2. **b. Addressing the client's immediate needs and feelings in an open-ended manner is the most therapeutic response.**
   The client needs someone to speak to now and cannot wait for the chaplain; although the client may be referred to the chaplain for more interventions.
   The nurse should not negate the client's concerns or dismiss them as trivial. The nurse's view of God is not appropriate; nor is the suggestion to confess.
   Nursing Process: Implementation
   Cognitive Level: Application

3. **a. Bargaining with the client and structuring time is most therapeutic. Client needs to have some time for both personal needs and therapeutic programming.**
   Telling the client he can only talk to the chaplain about his religious views; and cannot express them at any other time is too constricting and punitive.
   Telling the client he is inappropriate and disruptive is too harsh. The nurse may say the behavior is troubling, medications may be warranted, but not the first response.
   Nursing Process: Implementation
   Cognitive Level: Application

4. **b. Nurse addresses the client's troubled feelings and voices concerns. She assures client of safety and treatment that may help.**
   Dismissing the client's views, even if inappropriate is not therapeutic. Also, the nurse then asks the client to tell her what "he" (the devil) is saying. There are more appropriate ways to ask the client about the content of hallucinations.
   Telling the client to wait until the chaplain comes, to express his views, may be too late. It's best to deal with the problem now. Then the chaplain can continue pursuing the problem with the client.
   Nursing Process: Implementation
   Cognitive Level: Application